—THE JOY OF—
BEAUTY

THE JOY OF
BEAUTY

A Complete Guide to
Lasting Health and Beauty
for Today's Woman

LESLIE KENTON

CENTURY PUBLISHING
LONDON

First published in Great Britain in 1983 by
Century Publishing Co. Ltd,
76 Old Compton Street, London W1V 5PA

ISBN 0 7126 0088 4

Grateful acknowledgment is made for permission
to reprint the following copyrighted material:
Meditation, pages 23–24
From F. C. Happold, *Prayer and Meditation*

Printed in Great Britain by
Butler & Tanner Ltd
Frome and London

Foreword

This is a book about beauty—beauty of the body and of the spirit. It is about health too. For without health, physical beauty fades fast and beauty of the spirit is stifled.

It is divided into two parts. *Book One: The Foundations* deals with the four dimensions of health and beauty—The Self, Fuel, Movement, and Stillness. Together they make up a lifestyle designed not only to preserve youth and promote good looks but also to keep you vibrantly well and help you make the most of your potential—physically, emotionally, and perhaps, to some extent, spiritually too. *Book Two: Maintenance* contains information about promoting and caring for good looks: skin care, hair care, body care, makeup, and reducing.

The two parts go together. Without the foundations, no amount of external care will guard a face from premature aging or restore sleekness to cellulite-troubled legs. But without the things covered in the second part, the ageless delight of self-care—which to some extent is a part of every woman's femaleness no matter what her age, economic circumstances, or political bent—would be lacking.

The book is called *The Joy of Beauty* because to me beauty is a joy. It is a joy because true beauty is nothing less than the expression of the individual nature of a particular woman. There is nothing superficial about it. It has nothing to do with imitation no matter how much glossy magazines would have us believe otherwise. Neither is it something one can get from buying a jar of face cream or sweeping on the latest shimmery eye shadow. These things have their place too, but they are not central to a woman's beauty. They are more the icing on the cake.

What is central is *authenticity*. To be beautiful you need to be what you are. For most of us this means discovering just what this is beneath the complex collection of ideas, moral imperatives, and cultural habit patterns that surround us as we grow up. It also means learning to make the most of your own potential for health, creativity, and self-expression in how you move and speak, look, and adorn yourself. And every woman has far more potential for beauty than she ever realizes. I hope this book will provide some of the tools to help in fulfilling it.

Acknowledgments

In writing this book I have made use of knowledge and techniques gathered over a period of ten years from a variety of sources, many of them overlapping, so that in the end I find it hard sometimes to remember just where and from whom I learned what. I would particularly like to thank Dr. Phillip Kilsby who first made me aware of the power of diet for healing, Dr. Gordon Latto and his wife Dr. Barbara Latto whose unfailing encouragement and help have always kept me fascinated with the field, and Dr. Andrew Strigner whose extraordinary capacity to seek the best in human beings has instilled that quality in me.

I am grateful to Dr. Ralph Bircher for the depth of his research and for sharing it with me, Dr. Dagmar Leichti for her help and encouragement, Celia Wright for her guidance in the use of megavitamins, John Stirk and David Stebbing for their work in exercise, Max Cade for helping me to understand stress and Swami Prakashanand Saraswati, Lama Thuben Yeshe, and Lama Zopa Rimpoche for helping me learn to deal with it, Geoffrey Treissman for introducing me to the powers of yoga, Danielle Ryman for introducing me to the potency of aromatherapy, and British perfumer Nancy McConkey at the Fragrance Studio for helping make the delights of perfume a little less of a mystery to me.

I have drawn on the research and findings of so many scientists and the practical experience of so many helpers in the fields of health and psychology in putting together my information and making use of it that it would be impossible to list them all. I am, however, very grateful and want to make clear that any errors or misrepresentations of their good work I may have made are entirely my own.

Finally I would like to thank Debra Isaac for her endless patience in typing this lengthy manuscript, Graham Jones for his encouragement and support while I was burrowed into my study writing for days on end, and my children Jesse, Susannah, and Branton who throughout the years have put up with every experiment in diet, exercise, and meditation, and every new idea with an open-mindedness and acceptance worthy of saints.

Contents

Book One: The Foundations

"Beauty is truth, truth beauty,"—that is all
Ye know on earth, and all ye need to know.

John Keats
Ode on a Grecian Urn

Book One
The Foundations

The First Dimension

The Self

❧

Introduction

Each woman is in reality two women. The first, the *outer* woman, is a collection of physical characteristics, habits of speech and movement, and ways of thinking and of expressing herself. This outer part is the result of past experience, conditioning, and values—either your own or, more often, those given you by your family, educational background, and society, plus a great many preconceived ideas you have about who you are and what you can and can't do. The outer woman can come in many different forms. She may be conventionally attractive, plain, sexy, dynamic, withdrawn, aggressive, apparently assured, or terribly uncertain about herself.

For each outer woman there is also an inner counterpart—an individual self that is utterly unique. A stable center of strength and growth, this inner self sees the world in her own way, has her own needs, desires, and her own brand of creativity, and is a law unto herself. The self holds the power to create, change, build, and nurture. The outer woman is the vehicle for what the self creates.

When her self is allowed free expression, a woman can be truly beautiful without the need for artificiality or imitation, concealment, or excessive adornment. Her body will be strong and well, her skin clear and healthy, and her movements, speech, and actions will radiate a kind of vitality that is unmistakably charismatic, because it is *real*—an outward expression of who she truly is.

Often, though, the inner and the outer woman have diverged so that there is conflict. The inner truth of a woman can be particularly clear and direct while her outer expression is a mass of confusion in how she dresses, speaks, acts, and looks. Usually this is because she is being stifled by ideas of how she is *supposed* to be, think, act, dress, and look. Where there is no free channel for expression of the inner self, there is much disharmony. Eventually both her health and beauty will suffer. Perhaps even more important, she will probably feel she lacks identity—has no firm idea of who she is or what she wants.

The first dimension of beauty, the *self*, is the most fundamental of all. It is all about discovering who you are and helping to bring the inner self and the outer together so that the way you look and speak, move, and act is *authentic*, not something imitated or artificially imposed.

Discovering the power of the self and expressing it involves transformation. This process can be tremendously exciting. Sometimes it can also be very hard, for it means peeling away the superfluous mechanical façades we all collect—the ways of appearing and acting that have little to do with who we really are but that have come to seem safe and secure. But this process is thrilling, too, and growing itself is beautiful—you needn't look for a specific end result to justify it. Being truly beautiful is being authentic. It is all about becoming who you really are.

So don't be tempted to skip over this section in haste to get on to the "real stuff" of exercises and diet. In truth, this is the most important section of all when it comes to fulfilling your beauty potential, and it is from this section that the whole of the rest of the book stems. Bear with me, if you will: ask yourself the questions it poses and see what answers they bring. When you have finished the book and absorbed all its specific information, you will be glad you have.

1

On Becoming Who You Are

To be beautiful, you must be who you are. Who you are is far more interesting, vital, and attractive than anything or anyone you might pretend to be—a fact that, sadly, is often forgotten. For we live in a world which teaches us, however unwittingly, that whatever we are is not as good as what we should, could, or might be. It also tells us that we need someone or something else outside ourselves to give our lives meaning.

The media are full of programs, articles, advertisements, and imperatives that urge you to "be a better lover," "wear this fashion," "build a better kitchen," or that purport to tell you how to look more sexy, be more assertive, make your life work, and so forth.

It is all an amazing game. And it works very well. It keeps selling dresses, books, and automobiles—and it keeps people *wanting*. The only problem is that in the process it also creates an enormous amount of misery and dissatisfaction as women continue to look outside themselves for yardsticks to measure themselves by. This is because, no matter how well it works, the "want-need-get" game obscures one really important truth: that what you need to be complete, beautiful, healthy, happy, and fulfilled is not "out there," "one day," or "if I only had . . . ," it is already *here*—inside you—right now. It does not need to be bought, sought, seduced, or copied. It simply needs to be discovered within you and then used. That is where the awareness of the self—the particular individual you are physically, mentally, and emotionally—comes in.

THE NEW PSYCHOLOGY

Once concerned primarily with programming the behavior of rats and humans and with examining and describing the aberrations of the psyche, psychology has broadened its scope. Since World War II, several schools of thought have emerged that are remarkably different from the behaviorist, Freudian, and post-Freudian ones. These new approaches to the study of man's psyche are not as concerned with the classifications of mental illnesses as their predecessors have been, nor with developing techniques of changing the mentally ill into normal people. Instead, psychologists such as Abraham Maslow, Roberto Assagioli, and Carl Rogers have tried to discover how human potential, much of which is usually dormant, can be tapped so that people are able to live more productive, happy, and fulfilling lives.

The new psychologies, although they vary from one branch to another in language and practice, are all based on the same important premise: that people have the inherent ability to create their own lives from the inside out once they are aware of the self and the potential power it has. This is an enormously important notion when it comes to beauty and health, for it is the key to becoming whatever you potentially are and to removing any self-imposed limitations—conscious or unconscious—that get in the way of your vitality, beauty, and natural grace.

It all began in the late thirties when Maslow came to New York City (then the center of the philosophical and psychological world) to study with the charismatic anthropologist Ruth Benedict and the psychologist Max Wertheimer. He found them both exceptional people, different from anyone else he'd known. "My training in psychology equipped me not at all for understanding them," he later wrote. "It was as if they were not quite people but something more than people." They were more vital, more intelligent, more committed, happier, and healthier. What, Maslow asked himself, made them so special? Were they simply "super people," especially endowed—something the rest of us could never hope to be?

With his particular bent for methodical study, Maslow watched them, taking notes on their behavior and personality characteristics until one day, he says, "I realized in one wonderful moment that their two patterns could be generalized," that he was "talking about a *kind* of person." Then he looked around him to see whether the same personality characteristics and behavior occurred in others. And, he reported, "I did find it —in one person after another." This discovery set him on a lifelong study of what he called *self-actualizing* men and women and made him ask some important questions such as: What makes them special? What gives them their physical strength and creativity? Is it possible for the so-called normal or ordinary person to develop the same qualities as the self-actualizers? And, finally, just how much are all human beings capable of when they are free to use their potential?

SELF-ACTUALIZATION

Maslow used the term "self-actualizing" to describe what he saw as the tendency a human organism has to fulfill its higher potentialities such as creativity, courage, love, charity, happiness, as soon as its more basic needs for food, affection, shelter, and self-respect are met. He found that people in whom the self-actualizing tendency is highly developed have several things in common. They are the healthiest people in society, mentally and physically. They also tend more frequently to have what Maslow describes as "peak experiences"—that is, moments of great happiness, rapture, ecstasy—in which life's conflicts are at least temporarily transcended or resolved.

Peak experiences give one the feeling that life is worthwhile, that it has meaning. During a peak experience, just as when you fall in love, give birth, or create a work of art, you perceive the world as being unified; the usual dichotomies between selfish and unselfish, self and other, seem to disappear.

Self-actualizing people have another thing in common too: their values tend to be very much the same—simplicity, wholeness, effortlessness, truth, honesty, uniqueness, completion, perfection—in fact, the same values one might expect the "universal" man aimed at by the mystics to possess.

THE FULLY FUNCTIONING PERSON

Other psychologists, anthropologists, and philosophers have described Maslow's self-actualizing person too. Carl Rogers, perhaps most appropriately of all, refers to it as the "fully functioning person." Out of their work and the work of others like Assagioli, a new picture of human nature has emerged.

We are beginning to see the human being not just as Freud's collection of repressed destructive urges, only barely restrained by learned moral constructs from destroying himself and others, but as a potentially autonomous being. The destructive tendencies we all have appear less the hidden truth of a personality than the results of a frustration in expression of that person—of life itself, in fact. Happiness and freedom from this frustration and from the negative thought patterns and behavior it engenders lie in letting your self-actualizing tendencies (which in most of us are weak or dormant) develop. Until they develop, one tends to regress into fear, frustration, or laziness. Once they become stronger, one's life becomes a process of permanent growth and unfolding of potential as well as, quite simply, much happier.

Although it may be difficult to grasp if you have not considered such an idea before, it is far more than an arbitrary value system imposed by Maslow and the rest. It is *not* just theory. It works. Becoming more self-actualizing, more fully functioning by making growth choices makes one happier, healthier, more beautiful, and more full of vitality. As Maslow says, "Clinical experience and also some experimental evidence teaches us that the consequences of making growth choices are 'better' in terms of the person's own biological values, e.g., better health, absence of pain, discomfort, anxiety, tension, insomnia, nightmares, indigestion, constipation; lack of fear, longevity, pleasure in fully functioning; beauty, sexual prowess, sexual attractiveness, good teeth, good hair, good feet; good pregnancy, good birth, good death; more fun, more pleasure, more happiness, more real experiences." In fact, self-actualization in Maslow's terms, or fully functioning in Rogers's, is not a *state* so much as a *process* —an uncovering of oneself that leads to the discovery of one's own identity, nature, and values. It also involves putting these things into practice.

A fully functioning woman is often radiant—more alive than most. She is someone who has access to her mental and physical powers and is able to use them wisely. As such, she has her own unconventional view of things but she is at the same time spontaneously more accepting of both herself and others. Her sense of satisfaction comes from *inside*, not from the "carrots" offered through advertisements and glamour. If she is glamorous in the way she dresses or behaves, this is because the glamour is fun—an amusing game, the kind a child would play. It is not because there is some need to validate her worth by wearing heavy blue eye shadow, bleached blond hair, or exotic clothes.

PUTTING THEORY INTO PRACTICE

Perhaps the most important question to ask then, if full functioning of self-actualization is so beneficial both physically and mentally, is how does one go about strengthening one's natural tendencies toward it? There are several helpers one can rely on. Here are some of the most useful.

1. Begin by letting yourself become aware of the fact that your self exists. That you are someone quite individual and quite different from everyone else in the world. To women who have never experienced this awareness before, such an idea can seem very strange at first. Others will

find it is something they have known all along without ever putting it into words. Still others will accept the notion as self-evident—with utter certainty.

One of the most successful ways to develop this awareness is through meditation or deep relaxation, and these techniques are discussed in "The Fourth Dimension: Stillness," in Chapter 14. When you are relaxed, nonproductive thought patterns and habits loosen their hold, as do common interfering emotions such as anxiety and fear, so you are better able to hear your *inner voice*. Listen to it. Let it be your guide in matters of taste and in decisions you have to make. As Maslow says, "Most of us listen not to ourselves but to Mummy's introjected voice or Daddy's voice or the voice of the Establishment, of the Elders, of authority or of tradition." Instead, begin to explore how *you* feel about something or what you really want.

2. Take a look at the ideas, behavior patterns, or assumptions about yourself and your life (they are called "belief systems"—more about them in the next chapter) that may impede your free expression. These mechanical patterns of thinking and behaving are usually unconscious. They come in many forms. They can be ideas you hold about yourself such as "I am physically weak," or "I can't wear my hair back because my nose is too big," or "I will never be slender," or "I am too old to change"; or they can be even more deeply embedded notions such as "I can never do anything right," or "I am *only* a woman." When you become aware of these notions and the power they hold over you, you will see that many of them are little more than habitual assumptions with no basis in fact, and you will gradually find them falling away so that you are more free to be whatever you want to be.

3. Whatever you are doing, try letting yourself experience it fully. Become really involved in an event, action, or project in the way a child would—wholeheartedly. Whether you are peeling potatoes, enjoying music, scrubbing floors, planning work, making love, or eating, let yourself be absorbed, forgetting everything else for the moment. Maslow describes these moments of experiencing as when "the person is wholly and fully human—the self is fully actualizing itself."

These are times which all of us experience, and there is a real delight in this kind of involvement. It silences the usually worried thoughts and concerns that tend to sap one's energy and make every event less interesting than it should be. This ability of complete involvement is a key to enormous vitality. At such times, little of you is wasted on anxiety about the past or future or meaningless and unproductive worry about yourself and others.

4. Consider new ways of doing things instead of mechanically following the same old patterns. Risk being different from the rest—your own natural way of living, thinking, dressing, working may be quite different from the way you have been trained to do these things. Your opinions of life may differ greatly from those of people around you. Be courageous about seeing things your own way and dare to be different in what you say and do when you feel different.

5. Be as honest as you can. Telling the truth has enormous power. Most of us lean far too much in the direction of being diplomatic and discreet. Many women tend too often to adjust their opinions and answers to fit in with the opinions of others. This leads to a sense of confusion where one is not really sure what one thinks. When you answer something honestly, when you do and say what you want instead of what you think is asked of you, it makes you aware that you are responsible for yourself. This in turn leads toward further self-actualization.

6. Be aware of peak experiences in which you perceive the world as a whole and everything as being *right*. Everyone has these occurrences but many people do not articulate them and so they happen and then are forgotten or ignored. The occurrence of these small moments of joy can be tremendously enriching, for you are temporarily set free from habitual ways of thinking and behaving that tend to stifle your creativity. Look for peak experiences and enjoy them when they come—they can be very useful as guidelines to decision making afterward.

7. Discover what you want and then go about getting it. Whatever you work for, work hard and wholeheartedly. This brings a sense of self-reliance and also frees a lot of otherwise frustrated energy for constructive use.

8. Take a look at the roles you play. There are dozens—the "intelligent woman," the "woman to be reckoned with," the "shy violet," the "sexy lady," and so forth. Some of them may be appropriate to what you want from other people, but most are not only irrelevant but also sap energy that could otherwise be used effectively.

The more you are aware of them the freer you will become from the hold they have over you, and the more you will be able to discover who you are and what you are about. The other thing about roles in relation to beauty is that no role that any woman plays (no matter how delightful) comes anywhere near being as exciting, vital, and fulfilling as the truth of what she is. And gradually beginning to peel away the roles by becoming aware of them is one way of discovering this. Ask yourself three questions:

Who Am I?

Here's a game to play that can help teach you a lot about yourself. Tear a dozen sheets from a small notebook. Now ask yourself the question, *Who am I?* twelve times, each time writing down an answer on one of the sheets. Your answers can be anything that you identify with yourself —something as concrete as your name, something as abstract as "I am light," or simply "I am a woman," "I am a teacher," or "I am a lover." When you have done this, put the papers in inverse order of importance with number one at the bottom of the pile and number twelve at the top.

Now go through each slip from twelve to one looking at each answer and considering what it represents to you. Is it a role? Is it an expression of yourself? Is it something you want to be? Or is it something that you feel is forced upon you? After you have looked at each label, lay it aside temporarily and consider what it would be like to live without it.

Usually, by the time you get to the last three or four, you have an awareness of a self quite apart from all the labels—of some part of you which is *primary*, which goes before all the symbols. This is also a useful way of beginning to discard the parts of you that are not essential and that hold you back or make you falsify yourself in relationships with other people. For, although in a sense you are all these labels, you are really none of them—not your profession, looks, ideas, political affiliations. You are *you*. These labels are only the tools you choose (or decide to reject) as expressions of yourself. They are your servants. The more aware of this you are, the easier it is to choose them wisely in the future.

What Do I Want?

This is another important question. Very often we tend not to ask it seriously, either because we assume that it is unimportant since we are really serious about fulfilling our obligations to others, or because we have become lost in the roles we play so that our sense of self and, therefore, our real values have become overshadowed and hidden. When this happens, a woman can think she *wants* nothing because really she believes she *is* nothing.

It may sound too obvious to be worth mentioning, but the question *What do I want?* has to be asked before there is any possibility of directing a change in one's life—whether the change be to lose weight, increase confidence, or improve vitality levels.

I have found from working with women in groups that it can be useful to keep a journal in which one records the answers to such questions as these (incidentally, the answers are constantly changing as your growth progresses) and also records desires, ideas, progress, and difficulties. Among other things, this kind of journal is an excellent way of uncovering the sense of purpose that is a crucial ingredient in guarding against stress damage and preventing illness. A journal in which you record your significant thoughts, observations, responses to new events or insights, as well as goals and progress, can also be a tool for expression that helps you, over a long period, to get to know yourself and to free you to be what you are.

Answering the question, *What do I want?* in a journal will give you specific goals to work for. They can be everything from "I want to be fitter . . . more vital . . . have clearer skin" to "I want to discover what kind of work I can do . . . find new ways of relating to other people . . . become direct and confident." Whatever your goals, when they are expressed clearly in a journal, and then later examined to see if they are real personal goals or simply things one thinks one should want, they become concrete aims you can easily pursue. Then it is easier to see the particular tools of action necessary to reach them.

What Is Stopping Me?

This is an equally important question, for what is stopping you is usually of your own making. Of course, it is impossible for a five-foot-one dark woman to become a six-foot blonde. But most of the things women want to be are not that farfetched—although sometimes they may seem virtually impossible from one's present standpoint. Most things in the way of change for the better are old habits, ideas, or belief systems which we let rule our lives although they may have little to do with reality. These ideas—like "I could never do that," or "It is impossible for me to lose weight," or "I am just naturally unhealthy," fall into this category. In the next chapter, we take a look at belief systems and how to make them work *for* rather than *against* you.

2

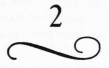

Self-creation

Whether you are aware of it or not, you are ceaselessly involved in the act of creating your life—your looks, attitudes, actions, and the quality of your relationships. You do it through image-making—a universal characteristic of the human mind which appears even to precede thinking in the brain. We see, worry, put together ideas, dream, speak, wonder, all through the use of images. We experience a continuous flow of mental pictures, both conscious and unconscious, every moment of our waking lives. In fact, the capacity to visualize—to "image"—is one of the miracles of the human organism, for through it we are able to organize reality, communicate with others, and make sense of the restrictions of time and space around which our lives are organized.

And images have tremendous potency. Your own images can be used for your good or they can be used against you.

BELIEF SYSTEMS

Each of us comes into the world with a particular set of genes that determine our skin color, sex, body type and, to a certain extent, our personality and intelligence. But by the time we are four or five, the form of what we were at birth has been altered physically and mentally so that we have become more complex and quite different in the way we respond and function, think and express ourselves. Some of these changes, such as physical growth, come from the same genetic inheritance that gave us our original form. Others, probably by far the largest number, come from what is commonly referred to as "behavioral programming" —the things we learn spontaneously through day-to-day living, such as motor control and speech, as well as the things we are taught, such as how to communicate with people, dress ourselves, use a pencil, and so forth. In all that we have learned from experience (things like if you touch a hot stove it hurts) and all we have been taught by our parents and other people, there are an enormous number of mental images that greatly affect our ideas and our lives ever after.

For instance, from our programming we get a notion of what in our behavior is considered good and what is called bad. We form innumerable impressions of what we are like and what others are like. And, finally, we come to have "sets" of knowledge about the world. All these things form our *belief systems*—conglomerates of images, ideas, and assumptions that make it possible for us to function from day to day.

Some of these belief systems are individual—they pertain to our inner world alone and are entirely personal. Others we share with the rest of humanity—for instance, together we "agree" that the brown-and-white, rather square-shaped animals with horns that graze in fields and give milk are "cows." We also agree in common with others that if you step in front of a moving bus you will be hurt. Such belief systems are important, for without them we would not be able to live or share our experiences with others.

INDIVIDUAL BELIEF SYSTEMS

Our own individual belief systems are somewhat different in character. They consist of the many unconscious notions and assumptions we hold about what we are and are not and can and cannot do. They influence whether we see life as exciting and challenging or rather as painful and hopeless. And although most people are not aware of it, these belief systems, formed gradually as we grow up, wield enormous power over us.

A child who grows up in a family where he is treated with respect tends to grow up believing that he is worthy of this respect. When his needs are frequently met, he comes to believe that they are likely to be met in a similar way in the future and, although he is probably completely unaware of this, he actually comes to expect it. Similarly, if someone is brought up in an environment where he is treated with disdain or carelessness or as if he were stupid, then he gradually forms more negative assumptions about himself and they become the "systems" by which he lives his life.

The whole creation and formation of our belief systems is a very complex process. It is largely an unconscious one, too, because the amount of sensory information fed into a human brain even in one day is immeasurably rich. We are continually responding to one perception, feeling, word, or sensory experience after another. Our belief systems, formed from these events, are therefore many-layered and extraordinarily elaborate. But they all have one thing in common: power.

The images we hold, consciously or unconsciously, about ourselves and our lives are *real* in the sense that they tend to reaffirm themselves over and over again in our experience.

Studies have been done in which a child's IQ, tested at school, is measured against his expectation of himself and his performance in the classroom. Almost invariably, the child whose belief systems include the idea or image of himself as not really very bright does badly in schoolwork regardless of what his IQ shows, and vice versa. In fact, there is also considerable evidence in older children that even IQ measurements soon come to reflect a child's basic intellectual self-esteem—or lack of it. All because of the belief systems he holds about himself.

SELF-FULFILLING BELIEF SYSTEMS

When it comes to health, relationships with other people, and creative functions, belief systems are particularly important in determining our success or lack of it.

If you take the time to sit down and look at a particular area in your life that you consider reasonably successful—say your work, or your relationship with a particular person—you will find that your ideas, feelings, and attitudes about it are generally of a positive nature: pleasing, charming, fun, interesting, and so forth. Similarly, if you look at an area of your life that doesn't work so well or with which you are not satisfied, you will find it is accompanied by negative images or visualizations. Most important of all, these negative images and the belief systems they create will then tend, when put to the test in real situations, to bring about exactly the effects you expect. If you feel you are uncreative when you paint a picture, it will turn out to be uninteresting. If you feel like a failure when you try to reach a goal, you will fail. Under even mildly stressful situations you become ill, and so on. And, of course, failures only further strengthen the negative belief systems you already hold. It is a vicious circle—that is, until you are able to become consciously aware of these negative belief systems you are unconsciously carrying around with you, examine them objectively, and then make a positive commitment to change them.

So long as they are unconscious, you are in their power and no real act of will is going to change them much. When they become conscious, you can begin working with them, looking at them, examining where they come from and their validity or lack of it, and decide on whether or not they are useful. Then gradually you can become free of them.

CREATIVE IMAGERY

Learning to harness this creative mechanism and to use it for your good rather than your detriment is perhaps the most important thing you can do for the sake of your health and beauty. It will give you the power to carry through the self-commitments in the areas of nutrition, exercise, relaxation, and self-care that make it possible for you to look after yourself wisely and well. It will also help create who you are in the future. Just what you want to create is up to you; this is where the art of creative imagery comes in.

Creative imagery is the deliberate, repeated use of specific mental images, while in a deeply relaxed state or meditative state, to bring about change for the better. Just how, in physical terms, creative imagery works is still uncertain. It does, however, appear that the images one chooses to focus on when repeatedly held in the mind are able to affect one's body, emotions, and mind through the autonomic nervous system. Some of the process, at least, is explainable in psychological terms.

When a thought or image is kept in the mind of someone in a state of deep relaxation, his brain shows neuronal activity in both right and left hemispheres. Nerve fibers leading from the cerebral hemisphere through the hypothalamus can directly affect the autonomic nervous system and the pituitary gland as well as the adrenal cortex. Everyone has had experience of this image-making to some extent in day-to-day life. For instance, if you keep a frightening image in your mind's eye—say of a ghost, a fantastic monster, or a situation you want at all costs to avoid— your body will respond via the autonomic nervous system with a racing heartbeat, perspiration, dryness in the mouth, or gooseflesh.

How strong your reactions are to the fearful thought depends entirely on how clear the image is. Similarly, when you hold a clear, relaxing image of perhaps a spring meadow or a person you love, your body responds with relaxed muscles, lowered heartbeat and blood pressure, and generally pleasant and passive bodily sensations. Researchers have found that through this mind-body connection we can exercise a great deal of control over our bodies and our behavior simply by choosing images to focus on and using them regularly. In fact, this kind of deliberate visualization is the technique behind the ability yogis demonstrate in raising and lowering their bodily temperature or heartbeat at will, going for long periods of time without food, and performing extrasensory tasks.

Time was when the use of creative imagery to heal illness, spur weight loss, or improve athletic performance would have caused many an eyebrow to raise among establishment psychologists. For although there has always been a vague belief that one's mind has some part to play in illness and health and that by "thinking positively" one can influence one's life for the better, until recently these notions were considered the province of evangelist preachers, success salesmen, and mystic philosophers. No self-respecting doctor would have considered such nonsense. Health and illness were considered *physical* phenomena dependent on only *physical* factors. And success? Success depended on hard work, privileges, and perhaps good luck!

The view is rapidly changing. A growing number of psychologists and physicians have been using specific mind techniques like hypnosis and meditation as part of the treatment for many serious illnesses, both mental and physical, with remarkable success. Not only have they been able to put them to practical use, they have also carefully studied and recorded the physiological changes of putting the mind to work in a specific way through biofeedback instruments.

American physiologist Edmund Jacobson, who has done some of the best work in relaxation (his technique for deep relaxation is given on pages 207–8), many years ago studied the effect of visualization or the deliberate use of specific mental images in muscular activity. He demonstrated what has now been confirmed many times over—namely, that the imagination has energy. He wired people up to equipment that could measure even minute changes in the electrical activity of their muscles and then asked them to visualize or "image" such things as lifting weights or running. He found that the muscles used in the activities they were imaging showed minute electrical changes, although no perceptible movement took place.

Recently this kind of imagery has been used by the Russians, Australians, and Americans to improve athletic performance of tennis players, runners, and other athletes. In addition to their normal training, athletes are asked to regularly imagine the successful movements and actions necessary for their sport. Trainers using such techniques claim the result from these sessions of creative imagery, where the athlete is doing nothing more than lying on a bed daydreaming, have been excellent in terms of performance on the playing field.

In medicine this kind of creative imagery is now being used for the successful treatment of so-called incurable diseases. For instance, radiation oncologist Carl Simonton and his psychologist wife Stephanie Matthews-Simonton, at the Cancer Counseling and Research Center in Fort Worth, Texas, have had very good results with medically incurable cancer patients. They ask patients to spend regular quiet periods in which they relax and then practice imaging in their mind's eye the symbolic destruction of the cancer cells in their body. How they do this doesn't matter much. Some patients see them as ugly black cells that are being mercilessly destroyed by the body's immune system in the form of white blood cells, others as hideous insects or rats being caught and killed by strong cats or birds. So long as the image fires the imagination of the patient along the lines of destroying cancer and restoring health, it doesn't matter what it is.

An interesting discovery of Simonton is that his patients' belief systems, that of their physicians, and even the belief systems of Simonton himself have to be brought to light and looked at for good progress in healing to take place. Most seriously ill patients (especially those who have been told that they have terminal cancer) have genuinely assumed that they are going to die. This assumption and all the images that make up the belief system of which it is a part wield tremendous power over the future of the patient. When so-called spontaneous remission or unexpectedly good response to visualization takes place in the patient, it is invariably due to the patient's ability to visualize himself as well.

Most patients Simonton sees also have to change another belief system in the process—they see themselves as victims of the disease they have and do not recognize the way in which they, through unconscious mental images and belief systems, have participated in its development. In patients who get well, all this changes—they find themselves taking responsibility not only for the conditions they are in at the moment but also for their healing.

Psychologists are also using creative imagery to help patients lose weight or give up negative habits such as smoking or drugs by showing them how to establish new and more workable belief systems—belief systems that can affect every area of their lives for the better.

PUTTING CREATIVE IMAGERY TO WORK

Although the mechanism of creative imagery appears to be highly complex, putting it to use is very simple indeed. For just as it is unnecessary for you to know how the nervous system, in conjunction with the brain and muscles, makes it possible for you to pick up an apple and take a bite out of it in order to perform the action, so it is not necessary to understand biological theories about creative imagery in order to practice it to your benefit. The imaging mechanism of your brain works automatically; all you have to do is provide it with images that are useful to you and let it do its job.

Nor do you have to worry about whether or not you believe in creative imagery or whether or not you can do it well enough for it to work for you. If there is a goal that you want to achieve, you need simply to visualize it—again and again, at least twice a day; the rest is automatic, as long as your goal is something you consciously consider to be *feasible*. It would be absurd, for instance, to lie down for ten minutes each morning and afternoon and visualize yourself as an eagle. You might improve your imagination no end, you might also develop a great empathy for eagles, but it is unlikely that you would develop wings or a beak.

You also need not worry about success or failure. As Maxwell Maltz says in his book *Psycho-Cybernetics*, "You must learn to *trust* your creative mechanism to do its work and not 'jam it' by becoming too concerned or too anxious as to whether it will work or not, or by attempting to force it too much by conscious effort. You must *let* it work, rather than *make* it work. This trust is necessary because your creative mechanism operates below the level of consciousness."

It has been my experience and is the experience of others I have spoken to who use the techniques of creative visualization that the only real "trust" necessary for it to work is that which makes it possible for you to spend time repeatedly practicing creative imagery. You do this by letting yourself go into a state of deep relaxation or meditation and then repeating your chosen image again and again over a sufficient length of time for it to take hold in your unconscious and begin producing results. You certainly don't have to trust it in the sense of believing in it for it to work. It will work whether you believe it or not. Just be consistent in using the technique regularly.

HOW TO GO ABOUT IT

Creative imagery is an inner state of mind. To visualize effectively you need to put yourself into a calm, relaxed state in which mental images flow easily. Generally the more relaxed you are, the more successful your visualizations will be. But this kind of relaxation is something that is learned gradually by practice. Even if you feel in the beginning that you are hardly relaxed at all, you will get benefits from your imaging and this will become progressively more true as you repeatedly practice visualization.

Begin by lying down, or sitting in a comfortable chair with your back well supported. Use one of the meditation or relaxation techniques in Chapter 14 to relax deeply. When you are deeply relaxed in your inner space, there are several things you can do:

1. In this space, you can examine in a new light any question that has been bothering you. You will have access to the deeper layers of your mind where many answers can be found, provided you are willing to ask the questions simply and then just wait in stillness for the answer to come.

2. This place is one in which you can become aware of your belief systems and bring them to consciousness so that you can examine them in a detached, objective way and see whether they are working for you or not. You can then decide what you want to keep and what to let go.

3. It is a place where you can learn to listen to the sound of your inner voice. The more you do this, the easier it becomes. This inner voice can guide you to where you are going next and tell you what you are about.

4. It is a place where you can come to know yourself for who you really are, quite apart from roles and habitual assumptions you have always had about yourself.

5. Most important of all in bringing about change, you can use this inner space to practice creative imagery.

Before you begin, here is an exercise that is useful as a preliminary to creative imagery or visualization, which is particularly relevant to a woman's health and beauty and to developing an awareness of one's own identity. Even if you practice this exercise again and again, you will probably find that each time your visualization increases in vividness and you will get images that are different from those you had last time.

Close your eyes and go through the process of relaxation. When you are in your inner space, take a look at yourself as if you were looking into a mirror. Look at your face, your hair, the color of your eyes, the shape of your cheekbones and your jaw, the texture of your lips.

Now look at your body, your breasts, your chest, your shoulders and waist, the curve of your hips and the color of your skin. Is it soft and smooth, pink or white, copper-colored, black, or golden? Look at your feet and the shape of your legs and ankles. Now watch yourself move in your imagination. How do you walk, speak, gesticulate, sit? What are you like? How do you *see* yourself? Also how do you *feel* about the face and body, the movements and the voice you are hearing? Notice how vivid the images are that you get.

Then, after five minutes of watching yourself, come out of the state of relaxation. Simply tell yourself, "I am now going to come out of my inner space . . . I am going to count backward from three and as I count I will come closer and closer to the surface so by the time I am finished I will open my eyes and find I feel very well, alert and alive." Now count to yourself, "Three . . . two . . . one . . . ," and open your eyes. Spend a few minutes now looking at yourself in a mirror. How much did you miss?

When they first begin with this exercise in visualization, many women are quite surprised to find their images of themselves are not very concrete—that is, they don't find it easy to see themselves clearly.

Go back to your journal or to the notes you made in answer to the question, *What do I want?* What did you write? Do you want to be thinner? Healthier? Have beautiful, clear skin? Walk with more grace? Speak more articulately? Be more yourself? Have more vitality? Relate better to others?

Pick one goal you would like to achieve. Make it *concrete*—something you can express simply in a few words such as "I want to have more energy," or "I want to have a beautiful smooth skin," or "I want to be lean and lithe."

Go through your relaxation technique until you enter your inner space. Now you are ready to begin visualizing. You can do this in two ways: *verbally*, by simply repeating over and over a few words that describe the image, or *visually*, by simply seeing yourself as already having become what you want to be.

For some women, who at first experience difficulty in visualizing, the verbal method works better; for others, the visual method is more successful. Try them both and see which you prefer. Later on, after you are familiar with the use of creative imagery, you will probably want to use both.

VERBAL IMAGERY

Let's say you pick as your goal the desire, *"I want to have more energy."* Using the verbal method, turn the wish into a positive statement. It becomes *"Every day I am more and more energetic and well."* It is important that your goal be phrased in this way. It has to be in the *present* tense—not "One day I will be better" or "I hope that I will be more energetic," but Every day *I am* more and more energetic and well. It is happening *now.* Your subconscious mind, which holds the power to bring about change, does not function in terms of time and space as your conscious mind does. It understands only the simplest and most direct instructions, and when they are given it works as if they had already occurred or are occurring now.

The words you have chosen become your image. You put them to work by simply repeating the words over and over again silently to yourself while you are in the deeply relaxed state in your inner space. It is the constant replaying of the message day after day twice a day that works best, not how long you do it each time you relax. One convenient way of doing it is to repeat the direction ten times in each session, moving one of your fingers with each repetition until you have been through all ten. Then you simply say to yourself the same, "I am now going to come out of my inner space . . ." (by counting backward from three, etc.), and open your eyes.

The best time for most women to practice creative visualization is in bed at night just before they fall asleep, and then again in the morning just before they get up. But really you can do it anytime—whenever you can find ten minutes to yourself in the middle of the day, or in the middle of the night if you awaken, or during meditation. The important thing is to do it regularly twice a day every day. You needn't worry about doing it wrong, either. Because, in truth, there is no wrong way, and every supposed wrong in the way you are doing the technique will gradually put itself right with practice.

SEEING INSTEAD OF SAYING

If you prefer, you can use a *visual* way instead, or you can use a combination of both. Picking the same goal, *I want to have more energy*, go through your relaxation technique. When you are at the inner space, instead of repeating words let your mind play with the image of your goal as if it had actually come about already, almost like a daydream. In other words, see yourself moving through your day, relating to people, doing your work, playing games, all the while full of vitality and bounce.

Watch yourself in your imagination and enjoy the ease with which you do things that once seemed difficult or tiring. Notice the glow of your skin, how well you look; see the vivacity in the way you speak and move. Watch yourself and *enjoy* it. The more of it you let yourself imagine and the more you enjoy your imaginings, the stronger will be the images you are creating and the more quickly they will become reality. But as with the verbal instructions, always keep your images in the *present* as if they are actually happening now and not as if they might happen in the future or are something you would like to see happen.

You may find at some point that something or someone is interfering with your image. For instance, you might find that as you watch yourself moving about energetically through the day in your mind's eyes, another figure appears—say an old woman—who speaks to you. Perhaps she says something like, "You silly girl, if you don't slow down you know you will exhaust yourself or get sick." Or, "Why are you pretending to be full of energy when you know that you are really tired?" and so on. Pause for a moment and take a look at the figure.

Who is she? Your mother? A friend who tends to be negative about everything you try? The voice of a belief system from inside you which, without your being aware of it, has been telling you for years that you are tired?

Answer the figure back. Tell her quietly but firmly in your mind, "No, you are wrong. I am well and I have lots of energy. I also know how to use it wisely. I will rest and look after myself when I need to, I will eat well, I will enjoy what I do. I will be happy with my vitality." Then go with your visualization. Unexpected intrusions like this while you are visualizing are often very useful, for they help make you aware of belief systems and notions that may have been unconsciously impeding your progress toward a goal.

Then, when you have practiced your visualization for, say, five or ten minutes, tell yourself you are going to count backward from three and open your eyes.

SOME TRICKS TO HELP YOU

1. In the beginning, when you are just starting to explore the power of creative imagery, it is a good idea to pick only one goal at a time and work on it for several weeks or months until it is being progressively realized before taking on another thing you would like to change.

2. The technique of keeping a journal is very useful in recording your progress, but even more important is keeping a record of insights and experiences you come upon while practicing the deep relaxation and visualization techniques. The information and insights they turn up for everyone are invariably rich. Many times something you record today which seems not particularly useful now will have a message of immediate importance to you three months from now.

3. There is one very simple goal that I find particularly useful because it covers all areas of one's life and you can use it over and over again, year after year, with benefit. It is, "*Every day I am more and more myself and my life is richer and richer.*"

4. Finally there is another technique which, although it is not really a visualization, is particularly useful in helping you become aware of the inner self. In a way it is a kind of game of peeling away the unnecessary or the superficial little by little like the layers of an onion. In fact, it is really a Sufi meditation although it can be found in the spiritual practices of Hinduism, Buddhism, and other Eastern traditions too. It is simply a verse that you repeat slowly to yourself while in a state of deep relaxation in your inner space. It tends gradually to peel away the belief systems and the unnecessary notions, to clarify your thoughts and to free you when you use it often. I took this particular form from F. C. Happold's book *Prayer and Meditation* (Penguin). It goes like this:

> I am not the body
> I am not the senses

I am not the mind
I am not this
I am not that.
What then am I? What is the self?
It is in the body
It is in every body
It is everywhere
It is the All.
It is self. I am It. Absolute Oneness.

3

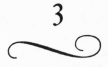

Self-responsibility

The way you look and feel, how effective your behavior and your life are, and how all of these things will be in the future depend primarily on *you*, not anything else. But unless you are aware of this fact, and unless you have an active sense of participating in and being responsible for your own well-being, you will not have the motivation you need to put into practice all of the information in this book and elsewhere about nutrition and exercise, stress control, and self-awareness which can help you make the best of your potential for health and beauty.

Self-responsibility is the key. But for most of us the idea of taking responsibility for ourselves is not always easy to accept, no matter how attractive it seems in the abstract. In part, this is because to a large extent our society tends to support behavior and standards that encourage dependence rather than autonomy. The woman who spends half an hour a day jogging, who goes away for a weekend retreat of meditation, or who insists on eating a really good diet is often treated like some kind of nut —joked about, teased, or simply undermined in her behavior by others who are "regular" people. For the status quo and all it implies—including a life which accepts all illness as inevitable and all misfortune as something beyond one's control to which one falls an innocent victim—are powerfully self-perpetuating. The values of wellness and self-responsibility, which are necessary for long-term health and beauty, are a direct challenge to the status quo.

This means that you may have to go to special lengths to assert your more ambitious and healthier way of life. For instance, you not only may have to put up with a bit of contempt from others, you also may sometimes have to go out of your way to pursue optimum health and beauty —to buy special food instead of opting for the usual overprocessed supermarket fare, or to excuse yourself from various social commitments in order to do what is best for you.

Luckily, at this time there seems to be developing a strong current of awareness of the power and the importance of self-responsibility, wholeness, and health. This makes it all the easier than it would have been, say twenty years ago. For there are a lot of men and women who have become interested in living in a way that makes it possible for them to realize their potential for optimum health, both physical and emotional. So there is more support around than there was before. Also there are now available a great many good books that give useful information about nutrition, meditation, exercise, and self-awareness. Finally there are a number of interesting programs and techniques that foster self-responsibility and personal growth. Some of the best-known include EST, bioenergetics, Transactional Analysis, and ARICA. None of them gives any final answers, but all offer modalities and techniques that can be useful in breaking up old, inappropriate belief systems and behavior patterns and in pointing the way toward greater autonomy. I personally tend to steer clear of organizations and programs because I mistrust the personality cults that often surround their leaders, but I know these four programs in particular have been of great help to many people. It would be worthwhile investigating what they might offer you.

SELF-RESPONSIBILITY IS A HABIT

Just as regressive choices and negative behavior patterns tend to reinforce themselves, so growth choices or choices for wellness tend to encourage further self-responsibility and make it progressively easier to make more growth choices.

For instance, what in the beginning may seem a bit difficult—say, turning aside from eating something that looks delicious but does nothing to contribute to your health and beauty—gets progressively easier each time you do it. For the rewards these growth choices bring of well-being, good looks, and a steadily increasing sense of personal strength are more satisfying in the long run than the former unproductive behavior patterns whatever they may have been—drinking too much, smoking, or eating those irresistible goodies you are better off without.

In a way, building self-responsibility simply depends on acting on the conviction that *you* are in control, not the cake or the cigarettes, pills, or alcohol, or the tendency to lie around instead of getting physical exercise. And acting as if you are in control by accepting personal accountability for your health and your life is the simple thing that makes it all happen. It steadily brings the control you seek.

There are some other things which I and others have found particularly helpful in building self-responsibility. Here are a few:

1. Assume that you are worthwhile and accept yourself as you are right now. It is interesting that people who are chronically ill or dependent on drugs, alcohol, excessive eating, or nonproductive behavior patterns tend to have very little self-esteem. And self-esteem is not something that comes only *after* one has made the changes in one's life that one feels should be made. Making the changes is much easier if you already accept yourself and have respect for who you are. OK, so you are not perfect, but you are all right and you are well on your way to being still better.

2. Assume that you are in control of your own life. For although you may be influenced by other people's ideas, by what you read, hear, or see, ultimately it is you who make the choices that are responsible for your well-being.

Where you are right now is the result of past choices you have made, and where you will be in the future depends on the choices you make now. When you accept this responsibility both emotionally and intellectually, you will find that you are free of a lot of excuse-making. You will also find you are no longer blaming other people or fate for your situation. And when these scapegoats are cleared away you will find it easier to see that it is you who are the cause of what happens, not something outside yourself. You will then no longer see yourself as a victim nor will you consider yourself impotent or inadequate.

3. Accept that you have a right to be happy, healthy, and beautiful. And know that it is a good thing to fulfill this right. It is not selfish, nor is it disregarding other people's happiness. For when you are happy and healthy, you are free to share yourself, your abilities, and your beauty—both external and of the spirit—with those around you. And the better you feel about yourself and your life the easier you will find it to make choices that are good for you and ultimately good for others too.

4. Set yourself goals. They are important, both little goals and large ones. Not only are they ways of accomplishing things you would like to achieve, but also they are helpful in protecting you from falling into habit patterns that are not beneficial. The goals you choose should be real ones too—goals that you really want to achieve, not goals someone else is creating for you or goals you believe you *should* want to accomplish. Goals and a sense of purpose help one remain well-grounded, which is fundamental to optimal health. It is good to know where you are going.

5. Be aware of your choices. Notice the belief systems or habits or assumptions behind different decisions you make. Are they appropriate to

you now? To your goals? To your idea of yourself? Or are they out-dated? When you choose something, is it a choice you make because you believe it will bring you greater happiness, independence, and better health and creativity—or are you merely choosing second-best?

Only you can answer this. Only you can know whether you are play-ing for the success of your goals or for the sympathy that comes with failure. The more aware you are of why you make choices, the more free you will be to make growth choices instead of regressive ones. For sympathy or the temporary gratification of smoking, excess eating, and other negative habits is of little worth next to the joy and happiness which are the prize from growth choices. Sometimes it is uncomfortable to face old habits of thinking and behaving and then discard them. With practice, though, it quickly becomes much easier to discard them.

6. Reach out for self-actualization. Determine to become everything that you can be. See yourself being it when you practice relaxation or medi-tation. Enjoy the vision—the more clearly you imagine it, the sooner it will become a reality.

Periodically ask yourself questions about your life, such as "Do my lifestyle, the people I spend time with, the activities I take part in con-tribute to my goal of becoming a fully functioning person or are there some things that need to be eliminated?" "Am I choosing consciously to do this particular thing, or is it the result of unconscious fears or old be-lief systems?"

7. Keep a sense of fun and humor about everything. Self-actualization is valuable but not when carried to extremes. Occasionally someone be-comes truly self-obsessed and in the process cuts himself off from the richness of experience behind him. The only reason to become more healthy and more beautiful is to enjoy your life more. Pursued as narcissistic ends, they lead nowhere for they are nothing themselves. But they can be a wonderful help to being more alive—and that is where the fun is.

The Second Dimension

Fuel for Health and Beauty

Introduction

Your skin and your hair, your body and your brain are all physically made out of what you eat. That is why fuel—good nutrition—is the second dimension of health and beauty. If the food you use to fuel your body and mind is all that it should be and if it is right for you and your individual metabolism, then you will have a good chance of remaining full of vitality and mentally clear. You will also have gone a long way toward making the most of your potential for fitness and good looks. If it is not, you will age more rapidly than you should, be prone to illness, frequently suffer fatigue, and have to put up with less than glowing skin and shiny hair.

Most information available to women about how nutrition affects beauty is superficial and inaccurate. Much excellent information about the relationship between health and nutrition can be found, but it is sometimes hard to apply to specific beauty problems, such as: How does one use diet to help prevent premature aging and wrinkling of the skin? What effect does diet have on your hair and nails? What can specific trace minerals do to correct hormonal imbalances that result from taking estrogen in the Pill or hormone replacement therapy and so eliminate the falling hair and splitting nails that many women are plagued by? These are a few of the questions we will be looking at in this section.

Perhaps even more important, we will be looking at how ways of eating can help rejuvenate a body and mind—the powers of raw foods, juice, fasting, and water. We will also examine the best long-term way of eating to preserve youth and health. We will consider the effects of air and water pollution on beauty, and how nutrition can help protect you from them. We will look into the relationship between nutrition and one's mental and emotional states. Finally we will examine in detail the actions and interactions of different vitamins and minerals on health and beauty, and touch on the megadoses of each for use with specific problems.

I first learned about the effect that diet has on health and beauty from a British physician who made it his business to treat as many illnesses as possible through improved nutrition. When we met he had, for over forty years, successfully treated resistant cases of migraine, arthritis, and other chronic ailments by putting patients on diets which (with slight variations depending on the condition he was treating) were all high in raw foods, low in fats and protein, high in complex carbohydrates, and which completely eliminated sugar and refined or overprocessed foods.

He taught me a lot. "You want to know how much nutrition affects a woman's good looks?" he said to me. "Just take a look at the body of the average thirty-year-old woman. It is clogged with drugs, preservatives, poisons, artificial sweeteners, artificial hormones from meat and poultry, chemical dyes, emulsifiers, artificial softeners, hydrogenators, alkalizers, acidifiers, and a host of other substances that are anything but natural to the human body. These things rob the system of nutrients needed for vitality and tissue repair. They encourage the buildup of wastes in the tissues, and put strain on all the cells of the body, encouraging them to age quickly. The woman looks in the mirror and is disappointed by lackluster hair and dull, lifeless skin. When she heads for the tennis courts she can't figure out why she gets tired so much faster than she did a few years earlier—little wonder!"

Then he continued, "But that is only half the truth. Get rid of all this rubbish by changing her diet to make sure she gets really adequate supplies of vitamins, minerals, and enzymes in a proper balance and six months later you will have a new woman . . . younger, more vital, more beautiful."

At first his statement shocked me. I had been brought up to believe that so long as you ate a well-balanced diet with a little bit of everything for variety you would get all the nutrition you need. Then I began to think. I looked around me and saw that women did seem to age a lot faster than I thought they should. And surely the women I knew weren't *meant* to age that rapidly. After all, they had every privilege—good food, money, and plenty of time to look after themselves—and yet at thirty-five most of them were beginning to look middle-aged. Why?

I decided to find out, for I was determined not to become one of them. I went to medical conferences and listened to eminent physicians speak about prevention of illness, emotional troubles, and early aging through optimum nutrition. I read books and medical papers. I learned about vitamins and minerals, the practice of orthomolecular medicine,* food allergies, hypoglycemia,† and theories about the aging process. I sorted through a tremendous volume of information and facts, many of them conflicting, but most of them fascinating. Gradually the pieces of the puzzle began to come together.

But I am never able to accept anything unless I try it myself, so I quickly became a guinea pig: one month fasting on water for three weeks; another eating a high protein or high fat diet; still another on the average Western fare (as average as nutritionists could describe for me). I wrote about what I had learned and about how different diets had affected me and other women who tried them for me. In time the information I had gleaned and my makeshift practical experiments began to jell. A picture emerged of basic principles for a long-term nutrition plan capable of keeping me and others well and fit.

I found, reassuringly, that most of my "discoveries" corresponded with the most avant-garde nutritional work of medical and biochemical experts as well as established naturopathic principles. Some, though, were my own intuition. For instance, I found from experience that raw food improves overall physical appearance and vitality faster than anything else. But although a few physicians have published work on the use of raw food in the treatment of medical conditions such as diabetes and osteoarthritis, none of them was really concerned about what it could do for cellulite-prone thighs, brittle nails, or the fatigue that robs women of their free-flowing boldness of movement and their enthusiasm for life. Yet I had tried a diet that was largely raw and so had other women (even a few men too) and we found that it worked. From my point of view, if it helped diabetics and lowered cholesterol levels, then who was I to complain?

---

* Orthomolecular medicine is essentially the treatment and prevention of disease by the expert adjustment of the natural constituents of our bodies. The word was coined by Nobel Prize winner Linus Pauling. The practice involves nutrition and the use of vitamins, minerals, and enzymes and amino acids, sometimes in high concentration.
† Hypoglycemia is reactive abnormally low blood sugar—that is, low levels of glucose in the blood, caused by too much sugar in the diet or disorders of the liver interfering with the storage and release of sugar. It is a common complaint, particularly in women who eat poorly and then feel they need a sticky bun or candy bar or cup of coffee to give them energy.

So what follows is a considered mixture of well-substantiated scientific fact taken from research into the effects of nutrition on health, and some practical information that I, and others who have helped me, have found to work.

Of course, as the science of nutrition develops, some things will change; there are likely to be additions here, a correction or two there, but the basic principles, I believe, will stand. These are principles that any woman can follow to make the most of her fitness and vitality, her hair and skin. They will carry you through the years, preserving your good looks, guarding your face and body from premature aging, and keeping your energy level high.

The role nutrition plays in beauty is so vast that it is impossible to cover every aspect of it, but all the basics are here for building a lifestyle that will keep you young, well, and brimming with good looks and vitality. But theory is only part of it; to make fuel for beauty work for you, you have to put it all into practice. For me that has been just as much fun as learning about it all in the first place. I hope it will be for you too.

4

Spring-cleaning Your Body

The first step on the road to total beauty is detoxifying yourself. In fact, it is just this principle that keeps the luxurious and expensive health farms and beauty spas all over the world earning money hand over fist. When you eliminate foreign substances from your blood, organs, glands, and tissues (which is the prime purpose behind the diets they prescribe) you feel amazingly well very quickly. The look of your skin improves, lines in your face are softened and smoothed, and your body starts to return to its own perfect form. It is as simple as that—no magic, and no necessity to pay a fortune for it.

The second step to total beauty is just as important. After your body has been internally cleansed, if you are to maintain the feeling of well-being and new glowing looks, you have to see that you never go back to the old careless eating habits that polluted it in the first place. You need to form new ones that provide your body with everything it needs for optimum health, and very little of what it *doesn't* need. Excess is very destructive to long-term health and beauty.

RAW FOODS HAVE SPECIAL QUALITIES

The basis of any spring-cleaning or elimination diet is raw food. Raw food should make up at least 50 percent of your maintenance diet for beauty, year in, year out. For fresh foods grown in healthy soil and eaten raw have the highest concentration of vitamins and minerals in easily usable form of any foods you can eat.

Physicians and biochemists have found that raw food diets have curative properties which no one yet can fully explain. In 1972 a Swedish scientist discovered that apparently unknown health-giving substances occur in raw foods which he believes may even be capable of enhancing the genes passed on from parents to children. Another researcher named these substances "auxones" and insists that the absence of them in a diet results in mesotrophy, "half-nutrition" or "half-health."

But the notion that a diet of raw food can significantly improve health is not a new one. Ancient physicians used raw food diets for healing as did some pioneers in twentieth-century medicine. American researcher Dr. S. M. Pottenger in California experimented for several years with 900 cats. He put some on a diet of raw food, others on cooked food, and monitored their health and reproductive capacities from generation to generation. He discovered that while those on raw foods fared very well, those on cooked food suffered from degenerative illnesses such as bone abnormalities, teeth problems, and malformation of the jaw. He also found that by changing the diets of those on cooked food and giving them raw food instead, plus cod liver oil, he could greatly improve their condition and reverse or retard the degeneration. Then he tried the same thinking on human patients, treating a great many illnesses with a diet of raw fruit and vegetables and unpasteurized milk. He even went so far as to give his patients a raw liver "cocktail" made in a blender and seasoned with fresh herbs. The mixture was revolting (according to many who have been treated at the Pottenger Clinic in Southern California) but the results were superb. People got well.

Another experiment took place many years ago at the Royal Free Hospital in London. Twelve arthritic patients were put on a diet of raw fruit and vegetables for a short period (between one and four weeks) and given no other treatment. Then they were monitored for improvement. Eight were significantly better, two measurably improved, and two remained unchanged. All of them got slimmer during the treatment. This weight loss—which appears to have nothing to do with calorie counting —often occurs naturally on a diet entirely of raw food and is another of the beauty benefits that you can glean from going on such a regimen.

At about the same time, the Swiss physician Max Bircher-Benner (famed for advocating fruit muesli, which still carries his name) was using raw food to cure patients in his Zurich clinic. He found that raw food has an ability to prevent "digestive leucosis"—the mobilization of white blood corpuscles which concentrate on the walls of the intestines when one eats a cooked meal. Bircher-Benner claimed (and his claim has since been supported by others) that eating raw food leaves the white corpuscles free for other tasks, saving your body the effort of nonessential defensive action and helping to strengthen its overall resistance to disease.

Erwin Schrödinger, an Austrian physicist working in Dublin at the Institute for Advanced Studies, winner of the Nobel Prize with Dirac in 1933, believed that raw food had unequaled health-promoting properties.

Meanwhile Professor Eppinger at the University of Vienna was also working to try to describe why raw food seemed to do so much for so many. Eppinger discovered that fresh raw foods raise the microelectrical potential of living cells. This, he said, stimulates cell metabolism and increases the cell's resistance to damage and its reproductive powers. Eppinger also showed that enzymes that occur in raw food encourage the full assimilation of some vitamins and minerals. Without them, the nutrients may be present in your diet but your body may be unable to make use of them—particularly if its own enzyme systems do not function as well as they should because of aging or chronic illness.

Then, for many years, the value of raw food in contributing to health was upstaged by our very elaborate and somewhat mechanistic approach to nutrition, which assumed that if you count calories, grams of fat, protein, and carbohydrates and take pills to make sure you get all your "minimum daily requirement" of minerals and vitamins, it does not matter what else you eat. Recently though, this old-fashioned approach to nutrition has given way to a more sophisticated awareness of what's involved in good nutrition, and scientific interest in raw food has started to blossom.

Recently an American doctor, John Douglas, found that a raw diet can be used to treat diabetics, eliminating their need for insulin in some cases and reducing it significantly in others. He has also used raw diets successfully to treat high blood pressure and resistant obesity. His reasoning for turning to a raw diet for help was simple: since early man lived entirely on raw food, a raw food diet might be less stressful on the human body and less conducive to diabetes than a regimen of cooked foods. So he tried it and had good results. The diet he uses includes seeds, nuts, vegetables, fruits, egg yolks, honey, oils, and goat's milk.

Curiously, one of the things that occurs when you go on a diet of raw foods for any length of time (noted by Douglas and others) is that before long you can no longer tolerate poisons as well as you did. For instance, alcohol and cigarettes, which form such a large part of social life for many people, no longer hold the same fascination. In fact, on a raw food regimen some people are even made positively ill by them, with headaches and other unpleasant physical symptoms. This is something that has also been noticed by Russian scientists who have used fasting as a cure for various mental illnesses, among them schizophrenia. When, after a fast of several weeks, the patient is completely free of his symptoms, his system will no longer tolerate poisons such as those in alcohol or bad food. When he takes them his body rapidly eliminates them from his system, sometimes with temporary adverse reactions in the process. It seems that the cleaner your body becomes, the more alive it is and the less it will put up with anything that interferes with that aliveness. This aliveness is one of the most important aspects of true beauty.

It is an established fact that a number of chemical and physical properties of food are changed by heat. For instance, important water-soluble
vitamins such as Vitamin C and folic acid are destroyed. Others are lost
in cooking or simply thrown away with the cooking water. These nutrients are essential for the healthy function of endocrine glands, for your
digestion, to preserve healthy blood vessels, and to produce well-func-
tioning cells and mucous membrane in the body. Establishment science
also knows that heat can lower the quality of proteins considerably and
that when food is fried in fats or oils at high temperatures, this not only
destroys nutrients, it can also result in the formation of substances that
are toxic to the body—especially when fat from deep frying is kept and
used over and over again, for instance when making french-fried potatoes.

Raw vegetables and fruits are also acknowledged as an excellent source
of fiber or roughage because of all the cellulose they contain. Fiber has
recently been shown to play a vital part in helping to keep people
healthy. One scientist who has researched the healing properties of raw
foods, Dr. Garfield H. Pickell in Nova Scotia, even attributes their
beneficial properties to the fiber content of these foods. He believes that
raw foods offer the intestinal tract the opportunity to do the work it was
designed to do, separating the wheat from the chaff. By cooking foods,
he says, we are depriving the digestive system of one of its important
functions and, like most other parts of the body, when it is no longer put
to proper use it may atrophy so that it no longer works efficiently in ex-
tracting nutrients from food and absorbing them into the bloodstream.
Another plus for raw foods is the fact that they demand a lot of chew-
ing, more than cooked foods do. This means that insalivation in the
mouth (the first step in the digestion of carbohydrates) is more complete
so foods eaten tend to be more thoroughly digested and nutrients absorbed.

Another interesting thing about eating raw foods is that you appear to
need less of them than of cooked foods to remain healthy. A Japanese
researcher not long ago experimented on himself to confirm what he had
observed—namely, that a little raw food offered far greater nutritional
power than the same quantity of cooked food. He ate a diet of uncooked
whole-grain rice, raw radishes, spinach, kale, and grated raw potatoes
and found that he maintained good blood quality and excellent health,
although by conventional nutritional standards his diet was low both
in protein and in calories. Then he switched to the exact same diet,
both in quantity and quality of foods but this time the food was cooked.
He soon developed symptoms of edema (water retention) and anemia.

Most of the speculative research into the benefits of a raw food diet
centers about two main areas: the nature and purpose of enzymes contained in raw food (which appear to lend support to the body's own enzyme system) and the possibility that, in addition to its chemical and

physical properties—vitamins, minerals, carbohydrates, fats, and so forth —which we are able to measure in the laboratory, raw food may have other characteristics such as electromagnetic energy derived from sunlight which is beneficial to human health but which as yet eludes scientific measurement and definition.

ENZYMES MAY HOLD A KEY

Enzymes, which act like catalysts, are complex substances that make it possible for the chemical reactions on which life processes depend to take place. Some scientists have even called them the "keys to life." They are living substances which are sensitive to temperatures above 118 degrees Fahrenheit (48 C). At 120 degrees Fahrenheit (49 C) they get sluggish, rather like a human body immersed in a hot bath. Above 130 degrees Fahrenheit (54 C) they are destroyed completely.

Without enzymes life could not exist. We have our own enzymes, as do all animals and plants. Enzymes contain enormous potential. In a seed, for instance, they stay in a dormant state until conditions for growth are just right and then they activate to create a tiny plant. The human body is full of enzymes that perform such functions as converting starch into sugar, breaking down proteins into amino acids, and releasing energy for cell use.

Biologists have long emphasized the importance of enzymes in all the chemical processes that take place in cells and in the human system as a whole, but until recently the possibility that the enzymes in foods may be important to human nutrition and health has mostly been ignored.

Enzymes are naturally present in raw foods. But anything cooked is completely devoid of them. The commonly accepted belief has always been that since the human body makes its own enzymes, any we take in through foods are probably superfluous. Now, some researchers believe that the enzymes in raw food may work together with the body's digestive system to ensure that our foods are thoroughly digested and assimilated. This complete digestion and assimilation is vital to full health because without it you can eat the most superb diet and still not be truly healthy, since the nutrients you need are not efficiently making their way to the cells where they are most needed.

ENERGY FROM THE SUN?

Scientists who, like Dr. Ralph Bircher in Zurich, are interested in the electromagnetic potential of foods, speculate that when we eat raw food we may also be absorbing unaltered solar energy from plant life which may be vital to health in electromagnetic terms, and that although a cooked diet is capable of sustaining life it may not be as good as raw food at regenerating life forces in the body.

This is an aspect of raw food that as yet has been little investigated scientifically. The changes in the electrical potential of cells, for instance, that come as a result of eating something cooked as compared to something raw, have only begun to be looked at and there are few scientific papers yet published on it. But generations of physicians have found that the regenerative capacity of a raw diet is so great that in many cases it alone is capable of restoring health to many a body seriously ill with chronic disease. Also yogic tradition has long insisted that raw food does indeed have special energetic powers which will not only improve one's physical health but will also increase one's mental and emotional clarity.

WHAT RAW FOODS CAN DO FOR YOU

I speak from personal experience when I say that although—in spite of all this research—science does not as yet appear to be able to analyze fully what the powers of a raw diet are due to, there is no doubt that it works. A raw food regimen for two weeks (or even a few days) will literally do wonders to revitalize your whole being mentally and physically. It will also begin the process of elimination of stored wastes (which contribute to early aging), banish chronic fatigue, and leave you feeling lighter and more joyous than you do now. I would never have believed this if I had not found it out for myself by trying it for several weeks. At that point I became a terrible bore for whenever anyone would say to me, "You look radiant," I would launch into my diatribe about the virtues of my raw diet. Some of my friends bore my enthusiasm with patience and long-suffering, others became intrigued and decided (sometimes openly with my help in designing their diet, sometimes surreptitiously so I would not know until after the fact) to try it. Without exception, every one of them reported exactly the same results that I'd had although in different words: "I feel great"; "I look younger"; "I am full of energy"; "The flab on my thighs seems to be disappearing and I haven't been doing any exercise"; "I feel happy—all the emotional ups and downs seem to have calmed"; "I've lost weight I could never lose before and I've been eating like a horse," and so on.

When I voiced my discovery to various British and European physicians who worked with nutrition, many of them just smiled patronizingly. They *knew*. I was just finding out.

A detoxifying raw food regimen for two weeks is the first step on the road to lasting health and beauty. It is also the only way you will find out for yourself how much greater your potential for good looks, energy and emotional enthusiasm is than you probably believe. Finally, it is an excellent introduction to a better way of eating for life. For it can lead you on to a new, less restricted way of eating that will keep you permanently fit and well. You can use a raw food regimen in another way too: every few months you can always go back to it for a few days to revitalize yourself whenever you feel you need it, particularly at the end of each winter and at the beginning of the autumn—the changes of the seasons. You can also spend beneficial weekends on this regimen whenever you have overindulged—at holiday times, for instance. It will straighten you out faster than anything else I know. But there is only one way you can find out what raw food can do for you: try it.

RAW ENERGY DIET

Raw vegetables (all sorts), uncooked fresh nuts such as hazelnuts, brazils, almonds, and cashews (mixed together, they become a first-quality protein giving an excellent balance of all the essential amino acids), uncooked seeds (sunflower, sesame, pumpkin), raw fruit, raw grains such as oats and wheat, raw egg yolks (avoid raw whites—they contain a substance that can block the absorption of biotin, one of the B-complex vitamins), raw fruit and vegetable juices, fresh herbs, raw honey and dried fruit, yogurt if you like. Nothing else. No alcohol, nothing cooked, no meat, fish, poultry, or heat-treated dairy produce (no pasteurized milk, cheese or cream).

If all this sounds restrictive, it is only because you have not yet begun to explore the delightful possibilities of such a regimen—particularly in spring and summer when the days are warmer and raw vegetables are available in great variety.

Sample Menu

BREAKFAST

Fresh squeezed orange or grapefruit juice
Muesli (see recipe section—Chapter 7)
Fresh fruit, if desired
Herb tea, or coffee substitute with honey (no milk, sugar, or synthetic cream)

LUNCH

Large raw salad, preferably with grain or seed sprouts, sprinkled with a
few sunflower seeds or mixed ground nuts (hazelnuts, cashews, brazils,
almonds etc.—not more than 2 tablespoons per salad)
A slice of melon, or bowl of fresh berries, or piece of fresh fruit for dessert

DINNER

A bowl of natural yogurt sweetened with honey, or uncooked soup
A salad as at lunch
Dried or fresh fruit

BETWEEN MEALS

A drink (see Fresh Juice Drinks) or a piece of fruit

This is just a general outline. In fact, you can eat any fruit or vegetable so long as it is raw. If you eat in a restaurant, order a salad of raw
vegetables as a main course, some mineral water or a glass of fresh
squeezed orange juice and some fruit for dessert, then have the nuts at
another meal. Most restaurants are more than willing to make whatever
you want. Eat only as much as you want, and never eat if you are not
hungry. If you are overweight, go lightly on the nuts and use lots of
fresh seed and grain sprouts for your protein. If you ordinarily take supplements of vitamins and minerals, continue as usual even though you
will probably need much smaller quantities of them on raw food. For
salads and other recipes suitable for the Raw Energy Diet, see the
recipes in Chapter 7.

THE *ROHSÄFTE-KUR*

There is a spring cleaning regimen which I think is the best contribution
the Germans ever made to the renewal of beauty and vitality. It is called
the *Rohsäfte-Kur*. I use it to revitalize myself after the long winter when
I tend to eat too much, exercise too little, and spend far too much time in
centrally heated offices and houses. You can also use it when you find
yourself feeling "dead" because of too much stress, too little sleep, or fatigue. (Of course, you should always get your doctor's OK before beginning any new regimen.)

The *Rohsäfte-Kur* is a raw juice fast which many nature-cure specialists believe is even superior to the water fast. On it you eat *nothing*, but you drink plenty of freshly made raw fruit and vegetable juices. The juices have remarkable properties, probably due to the enzymes they contain in relatively high concentrations. They make you feel super-alive —mentally clear and beautifully receptive to things around you. They also make skin glow and quickly trim away excess pounds. The *Rohsäfte-Kur* can literally make you look years younger.

Besides their enzyme content, raw juices are rich in vitamins, minerals, and trace elements useful in restoring biochemical balance to the cells of your skin and muscles and in revitalizing all the tissues of your body. And in contrast to when one is on an ordinary diet, while one is on a juice fast the assimilation of these nutrients is almost total.

According to authorities on the *Rohsäfte-Kur*, raw fruit and vegetable juices (like those in the Raw Energy Diet) accelerate the burning up and elimination of accumulated wastes, but they do it even faster. This is why the regimen has become the cornerstone of rejuvenation treatment at many expensive European health resorts. You can do the same thing for yourself at home for practically nothing.

To do a *Rohsäfte-Kur* properly, you need a juice extractor (sometimes called a centrifuge)—an excellent investment for long-lasting health and beauty in general. Some juicers have attachments so they can be used as a blender and shredder for vegetables as well. Nowhere will you find a more concentrated course of nutrition for health and beauty than in raw juice made fresh and drunk immediately.

Here Is How to Go About It

The day before, eat lightly. Have fruit for breakfast and a salad for lunch and dinner, perhaps with a little cottage cheese or some yogurt. This helps prepare your body for the juice fast. You can also take a mild laxative the night before if you like.

FIRST THING

A tisane: take a cup of herb or flower tea such as peppermint, camomile, rose-hip or solidago (goldenrod—particularly good for eliminating excess water from the tissues if you tend to retain it).

BREAKFAST

Prepare a large glass of fresh fruit juice such as orange, grapefruit, apple, pear, grape, diluted with enough spring water to make two glasses. Sip slowly until you've drunk both glasses.

MIDMORNING

Another glass of diluted fresh fruit juice if desired, or a tisane.

LUNCH

A large glass of fresh vegetable juice such as carrot, celery, tomato or cucumber, or a mixture of these, again diluted with half water to make two glasses and drunk slowly.

MIDAFTERNOON

Another glass of freshly made fruit or vegetable juice, undiluted.

DINNER

A glass of freshly made fruit or vegetable juice, undiluted.

BEFORE BED

If you are hungry, a few raisins (not more than a dozen) chewed slowly, and another tisane, or glass of spring water if you prefer.

In other words, throughout the day you should drink between one and a half and three pints of juice, depending on how much you feel you want. It is best for half of the juices to be vegetable and half of them fruit, since the fruits are the natural cleansers of the system and the vegetables are the revitalizers. As with a true fast, if you experience any feelings of discomfort such as headache (a sign that you are quickly eliminating wastes, tuck yourself away in a dark room and drink only herb tea or water until it passes. If you take a lukewarm bath (*not* hot) in the evening, it will help you to sleep well.

It is important that all the juices you drink be freshly made and drunk right away. If they are allowed to stand in a room for a few minutes they oxidize and lose much of their therapeutic and nutritional value. When you choose your vegetables and fruit, make sure they are fresh and carefully washed in running water.

Provided you are generally healthy, you can continue on this regimen for between three and five days, making sure all the while that you get plenty of rest and that you get out and walk in the fresh air for exercise. Try also to rest for fifteen to twenty minutes a couple of times each day during which you can practice some form of deep relaxation or meditation technique (see Chapter 14). When you come to break your fast and go back to normal eating, eat only raw food the first day and do not overeat. Be sure to favor raw vegetables and fruits the first three days after your *Rohsäfte-Kur,* and eat no meat until the third day after breaking the juice regimen.

GET TO KNOW THE FRUITS AND VEGETABLES

Each fruit and vegetable has its own complement of minerals, trace elements, vitamins, and enzymes, and is particularly useful for certain things. For instance, cucumber juice is a natural diuretic—it helps eliminate excess water from the body. Beets, red grapes, black currants, spinach, and carrots are often used for skin problems and insomnia. Tension and stress problems are often helped by apple, carrot, orange, and celery.

I find carrot juice is the best to use as a base for most mixtures of vegetable juices because of its sweet and mild taste. It mixes well with just about every other kind of juice, even fruit juices. Some of the others such as watercress (which is useful for women who are prone to anemia) and nettle (a natural diuretic) are bitter-tasting and should only be used in small quantities mixed with carrot, apple, or other mild juices. Here are some of the more common vegetable and fruit juices and the reasons they are valued in the *Rohsäfte-Kur*. But do experiment with them and make up your own mixtures:

BEETS

Beet juice is an excellent cleanser of the body, particularly the liver, kidneys, and gallbladder. It is also useful in building up the red corpuscles of the blood and improving blood quality generally. It is particularly good when taken in a ratio of one part beet juice to two parts carrot juice.

CARROT

Considered the best alkalinizer for a system that is too acid from excess food, alcohol, or sugar. Carrot juice contains B-complex vitamins and vitamins A, C, D, E, and K. Combined with lettuce, turnip, and beet juice, it is also useful as a rebuilder of healthy tissue. It is particularly good for treating skin problems.

CUCUMBER

A natural diuretic. It is considered an aid in promoting hair growth because of its high sulfur and silicon content.

CABBAGE

When mixed with carrot juice (two parts carrot to three of cabbage), cabbage is an effective cleanser of the digestive tract and is useful in readjusting the appetite in people who tend to eat too much.

LETTUCE

Contains good quantities of iron and magnesium. It is valued for its calming effect on muscles and nerves. Taken together with beet and carrot juice, it is also considered excellent for improving the texture and appearance of skin and hair.

WATERCRESS

Is high in sulfur and iodine and is considered a powerful cleanser. But it is very bitter in juice form and so should be used only in small amounts combined with milder juices.

You can mix juices in delightful ways, and as a final addition, try a teaspoonful of fresh lemon juice or fresh cream added to each glass. Fresh finely minced herbs such as basil or chives sprinkled in also add something special.

Supplements

Certain vitamin, mineral, and herb supplements can be very useful on a raw food diet, a *Rohsäfte-Kur*, or a water fast. They help to aid elimination and rebalance the system so that you are spared many of the temporary problems of excess acidity such as headache and fatigue while you are rapidly eliminating wastes. An extraordinarily knowledgeable nutrition-oriented psychologist, Celia Wright, taught me most of these. I find them very beneficial.

EACH DAY

Vitamin C—1,000 mg taken three times a day (sustained-release tablets are best, but cost more)

B_6—100 mg taken twice a day

Niacin—100 mg taken three times a day

Manganese—50 mg taken three times a day

6 kelp tablets taken morning and evening and 8 tablets of brewer's yeast taken three times a day

A blood-cleansing herb mixture, for instance, one containing some of these herbs: sarsaparilla, dandelion, burdock and yellow dock (all roots), and sassafras bark.

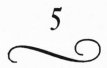

5

Water:
Take a Look at What You Drink

Water is probably the most ignored nutritional factor of all when it comes to health and beauty. Yet after oxygen it is the most important thing you consume—more important, even, than your foods, although they contain some of the most beneficial water you will ever take into your body. Besides helping to regulate your body temperature, it is the perfect solvent for nutrients and the best dissolvent of wastes stored in your tissues—which it can help eliminate quickly and easily. Like the spring cleaning diet and the *Rohsäfte-Kur*, a water fast can be an excellent way of detoxifying the body so it helps keep skin clear and beautiful. In Europe, the healing properties of water have long been known. So has the fact that different waters have different qualities and ways of acting on the body. To make the best use of water, there is a lot you need to know about it. Unfortunately, not all the news is good.

THE TROUBLE WITH TAP WATER

Natural spring water, laboratory-tested for quality as it is in France and uncontaminated by chemical additives, is one thing; the water that flows from your taps is quite another. Far from promoting your good health, it may actually be damaging it. Recent studies show that even relatively low levels of the some 1,500 chemical pollutants commonly found in British tap water may be cancer-causing when imbibed day after day over many years. In some geographical areas water has been linked to a high incidence of death from heart attack, and the presence of lead in drinking water is now considered responsible for many behavioral problems and cases of low intelligence rating in both children and adults.

Like our toxicological methods used for testing food additives, the water purification systems we commonly use are based on late nineteenth-century science and technology. They will remove visible pollutants such as sand and they will destroy germs. To kill dangerous organisms, they depend on the addition of large quantities of chlorine which was once so effective in eliminating typhoid epidemics and other water-carried illnesses in the early twentieth century.

Chlorine is an excellent germ destroyer, but it can do nothing to remove the kind of chemical pollutants that are now widespread in the water of industrialized nations. In fact, according to recent findings, it probably does *worse* than nothing because it reacts with many of the pollutants in water to form a great many chemical compounds that have been shown to increase the risk of bladder cancer, and that may well be the culprits behind the significantly higher levels of all types of cancer recorded in some cities.

Another worrisome chemical commonly found in our tap water is arsenic. Arsenic, used in the manufacture of insecticides, tends to accumulate in the bones, muscles, and skin where it can cause slow poisoning to the whole body. Nitrates, other common pollutants, are particularly dangerous to babies because they change to nitrites in the body where they react with hemoglobin in the blood and interfere with the carrying of oxygen to the cells. This has been known to cause death in infants under three months old. Nitrates can appear in water that has flowed through agricultural areas where lots of artificial fertilizers have been used.

A number of organic chemical pollutants are also suspected or confirmed carcinogens or mutagens. (Carcinogens are capable of causing cancer; mutagens are known to cause genetic changes in cells, which not only contribute to the aging process but also can result in birth defects when passed on to offspring.) Carbon tetrachloride, for example, has been shown to cause liver cancer in laboratory animals; vinyl chloride can be responsible for lung diseases, cancer of the liver, and miscarriages.

There are literally hundreds of other contaminators. According to World Health Organization (WHO) studies, the Thames, which currently supplies two thirds of Greater London with water, is contaminated with about 14 percent sewage, and one expert describes ordinary British tap water as a veritable treasurehouse of substances that shouldn't be there: traces of weed killer, fertilizers, pesticides, industrial effluent dissolved in gases, gasoline and oil from boats on reservoirs, copper sulfate (used to kill algae), fungi which grow on the main conduits (plus the chemicals used to destroy them), and metals such as iron, copper and lead, from the pipes used to carry the water.

SOFT WATER IS NOT ALWAYS GOOD

The fact that deaths from stroke and heart attack occur more frequently in areas where water is soft is now widely known. By now, researchers in Britain, Canada, and the United States have confirmed the original Japanese finding many times. Examination of the cause of death in towns with soft water and comparison with towns with hard water show that deaths from heart disease are significantly higher in the soft water areas.

Soft water has relatively low concentrations of minerals, particularly magnesium. This is something which, because it may affect the activity of magnesium-activated heart enzymes, can, according to recent research, increase the risk of death when a heart attack occurs. (The magnesium concentration in the heart of someone who has died of a coronary thrombosis is very low compared to that of people dying from other causes.) Magnesium also appears to be helpful in reducing high blood pressure, and calcium—another constituent of hard waters—is useful in the prevention of osteoporosis, a softening of the bones to which many postmenopausal women are prone. So soft water, admired as it is for the beautiful way in which it washes hair, is a less attractive substance when it comes to preserving your health and life.

Soft water is thought to be dangerous in other ways too. This is because of the kind of plumbing it passes through to reach your tap. When water is soft, and particularly when it is acidic, it is capable of dissolving small quantities of the copper, lead, zinc, or asbestos pipes it travels through. These pass into the water either in solution or as minute particles, and are taken into the body when you drink it. This can have serious consequences for health, for even small concentrations of such substances as lead and copper have been known to disturb brain chemistry severely and to produce intellectual disturbances such as hyperactivity in children. Copper, for instance, although necessary to health in minute quantities, can in larger amounts cause nervousness, increased blood pressure, and insomnia. It has also been found in excess in the bodies of schizophrenic patients and in their water supplies.

Cadmium, an element that occurs in zinc as an impurity, is also stored in the body's tissues, and can contribute to arteriosclerosis, to loss of minerals from bones, and high blood pressure—especially if you happen to be deficient in either calcium or zinc. Lead, from which many pipes used to be made, accumulates in the tissues over a long period of time and is very difficult—sometimes even impossible—to get rid of. It has been shown to cause liver and kidney ailments, mental illness, anemia, and irreversible brain damage in children. It may even affect the unborn fetus in the mother's body. Research among groups of underprivileged children with low IQ's and high levels of lead in the blood and urine show a direct correlation between the two. Researchers warn that most people in Britain may be drinking water containing lead in excess of the amount considered generally safe by WHO. And in some places where the water is soft and there is a predominance of lead piping, the concentration of lead can be *fifteen times* that considered by WHO to be hazardous to health.

CANCER DANGERS?

The most recent findings about water dangers concentrate on the possible relationship between some substances in water and the incidence of cancer in the population drinking it. This research is still young, but there has been enough hard evidence to make the National Cancer Institute in the United States announce that there is an indisputable link between the quality of water in different cities and deaths from cancer among their populations. Every year more evidence turns up that some things in various water supplies appear to be cancer-provoking. It is still a question of finding out what they are and, even more important, what one can do to ensure a pure water supply that is conducive to optimum human health rather than detrimental to it. Meanwhile, if you are concerned for your own health and good looks, you need to take a long look at the water question and investigate alternatives to tap water for drinking.

Because the best long-term diet for health and beauty (see next chapter) contains so much in the way of fresh vegetables, fruit, and juices, when you follow it you will probably find you don't feel a need to drink much extra except perhaps when the weather is particularly hot. Then, opt for the mineral waters (you can even make your herb tea with them), chilled, with a twist of lemon or lime.

THE GOOD WATERS

French mineral waters are the best in the world simply because the French have always taken the quality and the purity of water very seriously. They developed a strict grading system for bottled waters, and standards for purity and mineral content, acidity and alkalinity are monitored by their ministry of public health. There are over 1,200 natural springs in France. Bottled water comes from fifty of them. The largest springs are well known: Vichy, Perrier, Évian, Vittel, Volvic, and Badoit. Each of these has been granted the designation Eau Minérale Naturelle. This means it maintains a constant mineral content. It also means that each has a reputation for specific therapeutic properties. These waters will always be safe from bacteriological or chemical contamination, and they cannot be mixed with any foreign substances (including gas, except from their own spring) when they are bottled.

Some Eaux Minérales Naturelles such as Évian and Volvic are lightly mineralized. Others such as Vichy and Contrexéville have a higher mineral content. Vittel, Vichy, and the Italian San Pellegrino contain fluoride. Most mineral waters contain a good proportion of the natural minerals necessary for good health such as potassium, calcium and magnesium as well as trace elements which we need only in very small quantities such as iodine, copper, and iron. And drinking these waters is one of the best ways of ensuring that your body gets the minerals it needs in an easily assimilable form.

The fizzy waters are full of carbon dioxide, either because they come from the ground that way or because it is artificially added when the water is bottled. The bubbles do not affect the mineral content of the water. Fizzy waters are absorbed into your body faster and you can usually drink more of them without feeling unpleasantly bloated. Each water has its own special taste and qualities. Experiment with them and you will develop an awareness of flavor and a selectivity that will rival any wine drinker's palate. Here are some of the best.

A Connoisseur's Guide to Water

VOLVIC

This is my favorite. It is an exceptionally pure still water from the Auvergne Mountains in central France. It pours forth from a spring surrounded by seventeen square miles of countryside completely free from industry, intensive farming, or other possible sources of pollution. It is lightly mineralized and, like Évian, it is very useful on a detoxifying cure or fast, as well as being a delightful everyday drink. Its taste has more character than Évian's and a vibrant quality that seems to set it apart from other waters; perhaps that is why it is often preferred for fasting and cures.

ÉVIAN

The lightest and softest of the French waters, Évian comes from a subterranean water table at Évian-les-Bains on Lake Geneva at the foot of Mont Blanc. Because it is low in minerals and exceptionally light in taste, it is recommended by pediatricians in France for baby formulas. It is slightly alkaline, and easily assimilated and diffused into the blood and tissues of the body. It is said to be able to detoxify without causing fatigue and is often drunk by people taking detoxifying cures or following diets such as the *Rohsäfte-Kur* for rejuvenation.

VITTEL

From the Vosges Mountains in France, Vittel is a highly mineralized water whose stimulating properties are attributed to its calcium, magnesium, and sulfur content. It has a good, full-bodied, slightly heavy taste.

PERRIER

This sparkling water, which has recently become almost a status symbol among the fit and privileged, pours forth already carbonated from a spring at Vergèze in southern France at a rate of 21,000 gallons an hour. The company collects it, removes the carbon dioxide, and then puts the same gas back in at a controlled level. It is a refreshing drink, popular with athletes and recommended by French doctors to be taken after strenuous exercise. It is also a favorite cure for liver upset when mixed with three grams of vitamin C and a tablespoonful of honey.

VICHY

A slightly salty, lightly carbonated water from the Vichy spa, which has been used since Roman times. It contains a large number of mineral elements reputed to have the properties of regenerating the blood and encouraging healing. It is very high in iron, which is removed by the bottlers because it would leave black deposits around the bottles and make the water cloudy. It is recommended to build up strength and as a general tonic. I personally do not like the taste, but they say you get used to it after a while.

CONTREXÉVILLE

Another water with the earthy taste that you usually have to get used to. From Contrexéville in northeastern France, it is heavily ionized and has a high calcium sulfate content that gives it diuretic properties. It is used by French women for whom fluid retention is a problem, by people who need to lower their blood cholesterol level, and those on weight-reducing regimens. French doctors also advise it for old people and for anyone with urinary problems.

THE WONDERFUL WATER CURE

The most profound and drastic way of spring-cleaning your body is with a fast—where you take nothing except water for one to three days. If you have never gone a day or two without food, you will probably be surprised to find out how much it can do for you. But you must try it only under controlled circumstances, making sure that you begin and break the fast properly and that you have your physician's approval.

Thirst appears to be regulated by the hypothalamus in the brain. Animals in whom this area is destroyed lose all desire to drink and eventually die of dehydration. Some women who worry about their weight wrongly restrict their water intake. Others mistake signals of thirst for signals of hunger (also partly regulated by the hypothalamus) and so eat too much and drink far too little water each day. One of the things a short fast can do for you is make you aware of the difference in the two signals. But there are a lot of other things it can do too.

Fasting can be a tremendously powerful tool for rejuvenation and clearing your mind and body of whatever seems to be impeding their functioning at top peak. Physicians who advocate and use fasting themselves, such as Dr. Allan Cott in the United States, find that fasting is also useful in the treatment of many physical ailments from migraine and osteoarthritis to high blood pressure and anemia. In the U.S.S.R., Dr. Yuri Nikolayev has used fasting successfully to treat schizophrenia and other mental illnesses. Both Cott and Nikolayev say that fasting helps the body mobilize against many ills and also gives it a chance to catch up with elimination by forcing it to draw off stored waste from the tissues and then excrete them. This way gradually the whole body is biochemically rebalanced.

Nikolayev goes even further. He believes that fasting is a means of purifying every cell in the body. He also claims that 99 percent of sick people suffer because of improper nourishment due to littering their bodies with unnatural foodstuffs and, as a result, collecting poisonous substances in the body. Fasting can help clear all this.

WHAT HAPPENS ON A FAST?

When you stop eating (and to a lesser degree, when you go on the *Rohsäfte-Kur* regimen or even on an all raw food diet), your body begins to throw off its stored wastes at an incredible rate. This can lead to a coating of the tongue and teeth with a most unpleasant-tasting stuff, a headache, a feeling of being unwell for a few hours or, in the case of those who have been heavy drinkers or who have long polluted their bodies through poor nutrition, even temporary nausea or diarrhea. There is also often a marked increase in temperature which, experts on fasting claim, comes as a result of the toxin-burning processes. These unpleasant symptoms (and they by no means occur in every case) are simply a sign that the fast is working; they need no special treatment, just patience, for they usually pass quickly.

As stored wastes are eliminated from your body by a fast, your skin takes on a new glow and translucence. Lines on the face are softened and your eyes become clear and bright. This has been reported over and over again by people who have tried fasting and know its benefits. In addition, your mind becomes clearer so that thinking is easier. Many writers and artists use fasting because it can improve creativity, and it is no accident that throughout history saints and philosophers have turned to abstinence from food as a way of increasing spiritual awareness and improving mental clarity. In ancient times too, Persian and Greek physicians used it to cure illnesses, from syphilis to general debility.

HOW TO GO ABOUT IT

Going on a fast is simple. You simply stop eating. Then you take only water until you are ready to break the fast, which you do gradually by introducing first only fruit and vegetable juices and then salads and fruits, and simple foods such as yogurt. All the while you drink only water, with or without whatever vitamins and mineral supplements you may regularly take.

There is some dispute between physicians who advocate fasting as to whether supplements are necessary. Certainly on a two- or three-day fast one need not be concerned about developing any nutritional deficiencies, as they will quickly be remedied as soon as one begins eating again. On a longer fast there is always the danger that one could become deficient in zinc (one of the minerals necessary for maintaining a calm state of mind) as well as in the water-soluble vitamins such as C and some of the B complex, which are not stored in the body as are vitamins A, D, and E. One woman physician, who has successfully used fasting for many years, advocates that fasters take tablets of dried kelp, an excellent source of minerals and trace elements, in addition to pure water. Most physicians give nothing but water.

A properly conducted fast is not dangerous. And anyone who is generally healthy can safely fast for a few days a month or even one day a week with nothing but benefits from the experience. If you are very slim, then you should not fast for more than a day at a time because you don't have the reserves to support a longer abstinence from food. If you are normal to overweight, then you can fast from a few days to a few weeks, provided you are under medical supervision by a doctor who knows about fasting and understands the processes involved (unfortunately, most don't). On your own you should not attempt a fast of more than a few days—preferably two or three. Some people should never fast at all. This includes anyone with kidney disease, bleeding ulcer, cancer, heart disease, juvenile diabetes, or a cerebral disease.

If you decide to fast for a day or a weekend, here is how:

1. Start by eating only raw fruits and vegetables the day before you begin your fast, to help clear wastes in the digestive system out of your body.

2. Spend your two or three days on water, with or without mineral and vitamin supplements, eating nothing but drinking as much water as is comfortable for you. You must have nothing else—no coffee, tea, soft drinks, or alcohol.

3. Try to spend as much time as possible during the fast on your own doing something quietly enjoyable such as listening to music or reading a book. It will give you an opportunity to experience fully the mental and physical awakening that comes as a result of clearing out the system.

4. If you have any trouble with headaches or feelings of not being well, do not worry; simply relax and they will pass quickly.

5. Always be sure you break a fast properly, or you can quickly undo all the good that the period of abstinence has done for you.

The first day after a two- or three-day fast, drink only fruit juice to begin with and then eat some raw vegetables later in the day. Do not return to your full normal diet, including cooked food, bread, and meat, until the third day after you have broken your abstinence.

6

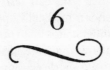

The Lifestyle Diet
for Lasting Health and Beauty

So you've been through a spring-cleaning diet, perhaps the *Rohsäfte-Kur* or maybe even a short fast; you've eliminated much of the accumulated wastes from your system and you've started to drink pure spring water. You look and feel better—now what kind of eating do you follow permanently to maintain the benefits? The answer may surprise you, especially after reading for years how important things like polyunsaturated fats and vast quantities of protein are supposed to be for skin and hair. For the perfect diet for lasting health and beauty, as close as one can come to it, is a way of eating that is *low* in fat, *low* in protein, and *high* in fresh raw foods and unrefined complex carbohydrates complete with their natural fiber. The ideal diet for health and beauty is a way of eating that excludes sugar and refined carbohydrates such as white flour and bread. It also excludes coffee and includes only small quantities of alcohol. Finally, it is low in calories, not only because this will help keep you slim but because it will also help preserve your youth and your energy. Little robs your body and mind of its vitality like overeating, especially when the foods eaten are overcooked, overprocessed convenience foods like those of the average Western diet complete with all its chemical additives. For long-term health and beauty you need to return to a more primitive way of eating—call it the Lifestyle Diet—and stay away from them.

A Typical Day's Food on the Lifestyle Diet

To give you an idea of what I mean, here is a sample menu for a day's fare:

FIRST THING

The juice of half a fresh lemon squeezed into a glass of hot or cold spring water

BREAKFAST

Yogurt breakfast: 8 to 10 ounces (225–275 g) of unsweetened natural yogurt mixed with a sliced banana, 2 tablespoons of mixed ground sunflower, sesame and pumpkin seeds, 2 tablespoons of wheat germ and 2 tablespoons of lecithin

OR

Mixed dried fruit, soaked overnight in spring water with the same toppings except the banana

OR

Banana yogshake: blend 10 ounces (275 g) of natural yogurt with a banana and a dash of real vanilla extract

OR

Bowl of homemade Birchermuesli made from a tablespoonful of mixed grain flakes plus 4 to 6 ounces (110–175 g) of yogurt, chopped fruit, nuts, and raisins

OR

Bowl of hot oatmeal sprinkled with bran and cinnamon and served with skimmed milk and a sliced banana

AND

Herb tea such as rose-hip or lemon verbena or lime-blossom with a teaspoon of honey, if desired

OR

Coffee substitute such as dandelion coffee served without milk or sugar

MIDMORNING

Herb tea

OR

Glass of fresh vegetable juice or low-salt bottled vegetable juice

OR

Some sticks of raw vegetables such as carrots and celery

OR

A slice or two of whole-grain bread or crispbread, spread with nonfat cottage cheese and sprinkled with cayenne pepper

LUNCH

Salad: choose from a mixture of raw vegetables such as lettuce, cucumber, endive, chicory, green pepper, onion, celery, Chinese cabbage, sprouted seeds or grains, mushrooms, watercress, served with a non-oil dressing

AND

Bowl of split-pea soup, if desired

OR

Bowl of vegetable soup, if desired

OR

Baked egg soufflé if desired

AND

Slice of whole-grain bread or crispbread spread with low-fat cheese or
    fruit

OR

Baked potato with skin, topped with low-fat cheese or herbs but no butter and no salt

OR

3 ounces of ricotta or low-fat cottage cheese (75 g) sprinkled with
ground sesame, pumpkin, and sunflower seeds

AND

Fresh fruit or fresh fruit salad (unsweetened) if desired

AND

Herb tea or coffee substitute, if desired

MIDAFTERNOON

Same as midmorning

OR

Piece of fruit

DINNER

Glass of fresh vegetable juice or low-salt bottled vegetable juice, if desired

AND

Salad: as for lunch

AND

Steamed vegetables, if desired, cooked without salt and served without
oil or butter

AND

Baked potato with skin

OR

Brown rice

OR

Slice of whole-grain bread

AND

        (if protein allowance for the day has not been reached)
4 ounces (110 g) of chicken roasted without the skin

OR

4 ounces (110 g) of poached or broiled fish

OR

4 ounces (110 g) of lean meat, preferably organ meat such as liver or kidneys

OR

Casserole of lentils, beans, peas, or other vegetables, eaten with whole-grain bread

OR

3 ounces (75 g) of low-fat cheese sprinkled with the three seeds

AND

Dessert of fruit, if desired

AND

Glass of good wine, if desired

AND

Cup of herb tea or coffee substitute, if desired

Of course there is far more food here than you would want to eat in a day. This only gives you an idea of the kinds of foods you may choose from. You needn't eat everything. The essentials in the Lifestyle Diet are the salads (50 percent of your foods should be taken raw), a little but not too much protein in the form of animal protein (meat, fish, or chicken) or the three seeds—sunflower, sesame, and pumpkin—or low-fat cheese or vegetable soups and casseroles taken together with whole-grain breads to make a complete protein, and nonfat yogurt, which is a wonderful alkaline-reacting protein that encourages the growth of the beneficial intestinal bacteria. The rest is a matter of simple pleasure—you can pretty much take it or leave it.

WHY FIBER MATTERS

For a healthy diet, more than forty nutrients are necessary. They include protein, carbohydrates, fats, vitamins, minerals, and trace elements plus something that your body can't even digest: fiber. Only recently has the importance of fiber been recognized.

Fiber—roughage—occurs naturally in plant foods as they come out of the ground and off the trees. It is an important constituent of grains such as whole wheat and brown rice, and it occurs as cellulose in raw vegetables and fruits. Epidemiological studies have shown that many of the problems of human degeneration once thought to be the result of natural aging are instead due to a process of physical deterioration that occurs as a result of poor nutrition. And the missing element most frequently associated with these degenerative changes is fiber. Such diverse illnesses as diabetes, coronary heart disease, dental caries, ulcers, and even varicose veins have been linked with an overrefined diet lacking fiber, such as the average Western fare—complete with fast foods, white bread, and sugary goodies from which nearly all natural fiber has been removed.

These illnesses, which many researchers have come to refer to as "diseases of Western civilization," have four things in common. First, they are virtually unknown outside the "civilized" world. (The exception is a high incidence of peptic ulcer among Asians who eat polished rice.) Second, when people from other ethnic groups come to live in "civilized" society, or when modern food technology finds its way to them, as it has in many parts of Africa, they *do* begin to develop these diseases. Third, the diseases tend to occur either in sequence or together, two or more at the same time in the same patient. Finally, the incidence of these illnesses has increased greatly in the Western world in the past fifty years. (Coronary deaths, for instance, are up 800 percent since World War II.) Although explanation of this phenomenon varies somewhat from one researcher to another, there is general agreement that the relatively sudden change in our eating habits since the 1870s—when roller mills were introduced, making it possible to mass-produce white flour—is one of the most important contributory factors.

A CASE OF MALADAPTATION

As Darwin showed, human beings, like all other life forms, have an astounding capacity for adapting over a period of generations to suit their geographical, climatic, and social conditions. From a nutritional point of view, the human race has made many adaptations in the course of its existence on this planet. For the last 40,000 years, for instance, people have been eating cooked as well as raw food. And for the last 8,000 years humans have been altering their agriculture by developing new grains and cereals from which to make bread. But these changes have been exceedingly slow—minimal, in fact, compared with the near revolution in food production and processing technology and the resulting alterations in our diet since the last century. Since then our consumption of refined sugars and starches has shot up. In 1810 we consumed ten pounds of sugar per person per year. Now it is nearly 120 pounds, which means that on average each of us eats five ounces of sugar every day of our life.

When roller milling was introduced, millers no longer had to stone-grind wheat. Flour could be made faster, more efficiently, and more cheaply. The method offered two further advantages. First, millers could produce more of the refined white flour that until then had only graced the tables of the privileged. Second, they could profitably sell the chaff— the outer coating of bran—and the germ, which contains all the precious vitamin E, to farmers for animal fodder. All well and good, except that these by-products contained most of the vitamins and minerals and much of the wheat protein as well as the indigestible roughage, while the flour that went into the new white loaves was mostly denatured starch.

Then evidence started to appear showing that when we refine our carbohydrates to such an extent (70 percent in the case of flour, 100 percent in the case of sugar), we create a carbohydrate of such concentration that, if we eat it regularly over a long period, our bodies are unable to cope until they gradually break down and chronic illness results. It appears that the human body has simply not had time to adjust as it did in the long period of evolutionary adaptation we went through, when our previous nutritional habits changed gradually.

FIBER PROTECTS YOU

Fiber helps protect your body from degenerative illness in a number of different ways, but probably the most important is the fact that it encourages the full and rapid removal of wastes from the intestinal tract. Food from which the indigestible fiber has been removed does not satisfy the colon and does not encourage it to work efficiently. It slows down elimination. And when elimination is slowed down, chronic constipation results. It is interesting to note that a person may be having a bowel movement every day and still have hidden constipation because the passage time for refined foods through the digestive system is long, sometimes three to four days, where the average time on a primitive diet of unrefined foods is merely a few hours. There is now every reason to believe that constipation—or, more properly, "colonic stasis"—is largely responsible for the high rate of cancer of the colon in the West. It is also a forerunner of diverticulosis and varicose veins and probably many other degenerative problems as well.

In ethnic groups that live on unrefined carbohydrates many of our most common degenerative diseases are virtually unknown. At one African hospital, for instance, out of every 10,000 patients examined over a three-year period, only three cases of varicose veins were discovered. In Europe and in America, varicose veins have become a common surgical complaint, with some 10 percent of the population affected by them. In recent years, with the growing awareness of the importance of fiber in the diet, surgeons and physicians have been recommending adding a couple of tablespoons of bran to a wide variety of foods to combat the problem, and there has been an encouraging trend to return to the kind of eating that includes whole-grain breads and excludes highly refined, sugar-filled breakfast cereals, biscuits, cookies, and cakes.

Colonic stasis is not only detrimental to overall health, it directly affects external beauty. When wastes are not properly and efficiently eliminated from your system, they build up in the tissues and damage the genetic material of the cells, which may encourage early aging. Returned toxic wastes also encourage the formation of cellulite, a kind of tissue sludge that creates puckered thighs even on the slimmest legs. Finally, when wastes are not eliminated through the alimentary canal they seek other outlets. This can result in bad breath, skin eruptions, lackluster hair, black rings under the eyes, and many other external manifestations that things are not as they should be which directly affect the way you look. So fiber is important. The Lifestyle Diet, made up of foods eaten in much the same form as they are taken out of the earth, is high in fiber. It is also high in complex carbohydrates. And there are some very important reasons for this.

THE MISUNDERSTOOD CARBOHYDRATES: FIRST-RATE FOODS

Carbohydrates have a terrible reputation. So many diets in recent years have emphasized the importance of protein and discredited the value of carbohydrate. And to some extent they are right, for most of our carbohydrates in the West are so refined or so concentrated (basic monosaccharides and disaccharides such as refined sugars, syrups, and so forth) that they are virtually empty foods, stripped of vitamins, minerals, and fiber. These simple carbohydrates require no digestion. They are rapidly assimilated into the system where they raise the level of cholesterol and other blood fats and contribute to the development of arteriosclerosis. Refined carbohydrates also overstimulate the pancreas; this can lead to blood sugar disorders such as hypoglycemia with all its unpleasant symptoms—fatigue, depression, and mental confusion.

Unrefined complex carbohydrates such as vegetables, fruits, and whole grain are different. They are the best foods you can eat. They supply essential vitamins, minerals, and trace elements plus dietary fiber in excellent natural balance. For unlike the monosaccharides and disaccharides, which rapidly flood the system with glucose, complex carbohydrates are metabolized much more slowly, releasing a steady stream of glucose into your bloodstream at the rate of only a few calories a minute, which is ideal for maintaining energy levels and health in the human body. This slow, steady stream of glucose is important not only for creating continuous energy for physical activity but also for the proper functioning of your brain, which on its own uses about 25 percent of all the glucose in your body. Without a slow, steady release of energy you can develop feelings of discouragement and chronic fatigue as well as far more serious problems.

When carbohydrates are metabolized in the body they oxidize completely. Unlike both proteins and fats, they leave no chemical residues which then need to be eliminated as wastes. The burning of carbohydrates produces only simple water, which is excreted, and carbon dioxide, which is breathed out. This is one of the reasons the Lifestyle Diet with its 70 to 80 percent unrefined carbohydrate content is able to supply your system with a constant stream of energy without ever producing toxins in the way in which high fat or high protein diets will. The toxic residues from a high fat, high protein diet can not only result in tissue sludge and contribute to premature aging, they can also make you feel fatigued and encourage the development of many chronic conditions, from simple cellulite to arthritis. The Lifestyle Diet helps guard against this. It can also reduce excess weight slowly and then keep it off, without dieting.

Raw foods play an important part in the Lifestyle Diet too—fruits and vegetables and two mixed raw salads a day. Not only do raw foods provide the highest complement of vitamins, minerals, and enzymes you can eat, plus lots of natural fiber, they also have a detoxifying ability outlined in the last chapter.

WHY IS THE LIFESTYLE DIET LOW IN FATS?

Fats in any amount that is more than you actually need cause damage. They interfere with efficient carbohydrate metabolism and encourage the development of diabetes. They raise fat and cholesterol levels in your blood and the level of uric acid in your body, which contribute to the development of gout, arthritis, and arteriosclerosis. They also encourage tissue anoxia, literally bringing a state of slow oxygen starvation to your cells. All three of these effects of excess fat intake are important contributors to the etiology of many degenerative illnesses as well as premature aging. They probably affect mental functioning detrimentally as well.

WHAT IS A FAT?

The term "fat" includes fats from meat, fish, poultry, and dairy products as well as vegetable oils and the nuts, seeds, and grains from which they have been extracted. There are two basic kinds of fats—saturated, occurring mostly in animal foods (although some vegetable fats such as the kind that coconut contains fall into this category too), and unsaturated, in the form of vegetable oils such as safflower, corn, and sunflower, and in seeds and nuts. Fish tends to contain more unsaturated than saturated fats, meat more saturated than unsaturated.

Whether saturated or unsaturated, all the fats you eat rapidly form a film around blood cells and platelets, creating a kind of sludge which causes them to stick together. This clumping significantly interferes with circulation by clogging blood vessels and even temporarily closing down small capillaries. As a result, your cells do not receive all the oxygen and nutrients they need to function efficiently. They only run at about 80 percent capacity. This interferes with cell metabolism as well as with the efficient elimination of cellular and tissue wastes.

The chemical structure of an unsaturated fatty acid differs from its saturated brother in that at least two of the carbon atoms in its formula are free. This means that they have no hydrogen atoms attached to them, as the molecule of a saturated fatty acid does. It was long thought that while saturated fats were bad for you, unsaturated fats were good. For unsaturated fats have been shown to reduce cholesterol levels in the blood, and therefore were believed to be helpful in preventing arteriosclerosis and coronary heart disease. That is the reason we have been encouraged in the last thirty years or so to include plenty of polyunsaturates in our diet by switching from butter to margarine and vegetable oils. The catch is that although unsaturates do this, like all fats they still raise triglyceride levels (another factor linked with coronary heart disease) and they also create the same clumping as the saturated fats do, which leads to tissue anoxia.

Women have also lately been encouraged by poorly informed writers to include lots of polyunsaturates in their diet for their beauty's sake. Unsaturated fatty acids are an important constituent of skin and muscle tissue and so it was thought, quite wrongly, that we need more of them. For what we have not been told is that the chemical structure of unsaturated fats with their free carbon atoms makes them extremely unstable compounds, and that when an unsaturated fat is exposed even to the smallest trace of a catalytic agent it begins a process of autooxidation which results in the fat molecule's breaking down to produce what are known as free radicals.

Free radicals are highly reactive particles which, if left unchecked in the presence of oxygen molecules, will form toxic peroxides. These peroxides can damage and destroy cells. They have also been implicated as a primary cause of the aging process itself. When a cell, or the genetic material of a cell, is destroyed by free radicals, the result is something known as a lipofuscin pigment granule—often referred to by biochemists as a "clinker." With age, ever more cells are damaged or destroyed as tissue degenerates, leading to increase in the number of these pigment granules. This is something you want to avoid in every way you can if you don't want to look and be old before your time.

To some extent, the presence of sufficient amounts of an antioxidant such as vitamin E in the system may prevent this from happening, because it minimizes the damage done by free radical chain reactions by breaking the chain. Vitamin E, like other antioxidants, helps block the oxidation that turns fatty acids into harmful peroxides. The more unsaturated fatty acids in your diet, the greater will be your need for the vitamin.

An interesting dietary survey that was done at the University of California at Irvine looked at over 1,000 patients and examined the degree of wrinkling and crow's-feet, frown lines, and other indications of skin degeneration such as damage to the collagen and elastin fibers and the irregular pigmentation characteristic of old skin. The subjects ranged in age from seventeen to eighty-one and 76 percent of them were women. Cadvan O. Griffiths, M.D., the professor of surgery who carried out the study, discovered that there is an undeniable link between marked clinical signs of aging and the intake of unsaturated fats in one's diet. Those who regularly and frequently included polyunsaturated fats and oils in their diet had marked signs of premature aging. Some looked as much as twenty years older than they were. Very few of those who had made no special effort to eat more polyunsaturates showed any clinical signs of premature aging. Evidence is also accumulating that links free radical reactions to the etiology of cancer, senility, atherosclerosis and hypertension—all of them disorders generally associated with aging. This is all the more reason to limit the amount of every kind of fat you eat to no more than you actually need.

HOW MUCH FAT DO YOU NEED?

Very little. Just about any food you can think of contains some fat, and when your diet is made up of at least 75 percent vegetables, fruits, and grains with a few nuts and seeds but without added oils, fats, cheese, or butter, as in the Lifestyle Diet, about 15 percent of your calories will be in the form of fat anyway. This is all you need. The body is capable of making its own fatty acids from the foods you eat with the exception of linoleic acid, and the mere three grams you need per day is more than supplied by eating a couple of tablespoons of sunflower seeds or one small dish of oatmeal. Even leafy green vegetables such as kale or spinach contain about 10 percent of their calories in fat. It is hard to be fat-deficient. Studies of people put on very low-fat diets, even when as little as .7 percent of their calories are taken in the form of fat as linoleic acid, have shown no adverse physical or psychological effects.

Even official bodies have recently begun to recognize the need to reduce dietary fats for the sake of preserving health. The U.S. Senate's Select Committee on Nutrition and Human Needs recommended in its report "Dietary Goals for the United States" a reduction of fat intake from the present 45 to 30 percent as well as a decrease in sugar consumption to 15 percent of total calories and a corresponding increase in the consumption of complex carbohydrates—the fruits, vegetables, and grains that are the foundation of the Lifestyle Diet. For long-term health and beauty, you should make an even greater reduction so that only about 15 percent of your daily calories are taken in fat.

This is in line with the Pritikin and other low-fat, low-protein diets which have recently caused great interest in both the medical profession and the general public. Pritikin recommends a diet of 80 percent complex carbohydrates, 10 percent protein and 10 percent fat. Although a radical departure from the traditional British, European, and American dietary habits, regimens like the Pritikin diet can not only substantially reduce cholesterol and triglyceride levels, high blood pressure, and high blood sugar, but can also lead to an automatic weight loss and leave people feeling and looking years younger. Such a low protein, low fat diet can also literally beautify a woman both physically and psychically.

At first such a change takes a bit of getting used to, but soon it becomes second nature and the increased vitality, slimness, and good looks it brings you in a few weeks help make it an easy way to eat permanently.

WHY NO SUGAR?

The case against sugar is a complex one. Besides the fact that refined sugar is a totally unnatural substance that has been stripped of its nutritional value—fiber, vitamins, and minerals—apart from the calories it provides, sugar in concentrated form is very hard on the pancreas. The pancreas, which is responsible for the production of insulin and therefore the regulation of blood sugar and energy levels in the body, has adapted through evolution to deal with a steady flow of glucose in small quantities such as those that result from the intake of complex carbohydrates.

When these are broken down slowly throughout the day, they provide the pancreas with a steady flow of glucose at a rate of about two calories a minute. When you eat something sweetened with refined sugar, the glucose poured into the system (say 100 calories or more all at once) suddenly soars. So does the production of pancreatic insulin in reaction to the insult. When this insult occurs repeatedly, as it does in the usual Western diet, with its average of two pounds of sugar per person per week, the blood sugar levels become depressed, then soar, then become depressed over and over again by a pancreas made trigger happy. In many people this leads to hypoglycemia or low blood sugar, with its corresponding fatigue and mental and emotional symptoms. It can also result in diabetes and in the development of allergic reactions to foods and to petrochemicals, which have recently been linked with diverse mental disorders as well as many acute and chronic forms of illness.

Repeated eating of sugar and products containing it can also result in deficiencies in the B-complex vitamins and an imbalance in certain important minerals. And just in case you are reassuring yourself that you, after all, only eat raw sugar, you should know that one sugar is just about as bad as another. Raw sugar does contain some of the natural vitamins, minerals, and fiber that are found in the sugar beets or sugarcane from which the sugar has been taken but raw, brown, and turbinado sugars are all still highly concentrated simple sugars which create the same metabolic problems as white sugar. As such, they are potential disease-makers. The Lifestyle Diet excludes every form of refined sugar—from chocolate to jams to packaged breakfast cereals with their hidden sweetness. It does allow a little honey for sweetening muesli (two tablespoonfuls a day) plus one tablespoonful of blackstrap molasses if you want it for its nutritional value.

CUT YOUR PROTEIN

One of the biggest beauty cons of all is the idea that if you eat lots of protein your muscles, skin, hair, and nails will grow strong and you will stay young. Like the old-fashioned high protein diet for building up athletic strength, it doesn't work. The human need for protein has been grossly exaggerated. At the turn of the century, respected opinion held that we need between 120 and 169 grams of protein per day. Then Chittenden showed in human experiments that far better performance and health were possible on fifty grams, a much lower amount. Another scientist named Hindhede set the figure at thirty grams. Then Oomen in Amsterdam and Hipsley in Canberra discovered a population in Australia which develop not only full health, but exceptional muscular structure and performance on a diet of merely 15 to 20 grams of protein per day.

Later in the United States, the American Research Council's Food and Nutrition Board agreed on a daily requirement of 70 grams for adults. One member of the board, named Sherman, described how this figure was arrived at. The evidence the committee examined indicated that a much lower amount was needed, somewhere around 35 grams, but there was agreement that if so low a figure had been set there would have been a public outcry, so a corresponding "margin of safety" was decided on and the 70-gram figure was published. But because the scientific basis for the figure was nonexistent, the word "recommendation" was chosen instead of "requirement." Current recommendations for protein intake hover about the 50-gram mark, although there is strong evidence now that we probably need even less.

Your body needs amino acids, the constituents of protein, for its metabolic processes, for growth and the repair and maintenance of body tissue. Proteins are made up of twenty-two different amino acids; all but eight of them your body can manufacture itself. These eight, which have to be taken in through your foods, are referred to as "essential" amino acids.

A large portion of a protein molecule is made up of nitrogen, and one of the important things about taking protein is that it helps keep a good nitrogen balance in the body, so there is as much nitrogen coming into the body as there is leaving it. This balance helps maintain body health and muscle strength, so that you don't go into what is known as a negative nitrogen balance, when you lose muscle tissue from your body. To keep your nitrogen right, 10 to 15 percent of your total calorie intake should be from protein.

But when a greater percentage than this of your calorie intake comes from protein foods, then your body goes into a negative mineral balance and you start gradually losing precious minerals and trace elements such as zinc, calcium, magnesium, iron, potassium, and chromium from your system. These nutrients, so easily lost from the body, are vital not only to physical health but also to emotional stability and well-being (more about minerals later). Wachmann and Bernstein of the Department of Nutrition at Harvard University investigated the high protein diet and came to the conclusion that the protein-rich (especially the meat-heavy) diet plays a strong role in the genesis of osteoporosis, a softening of the bones, particularly in women after menopause, caused by the loss of minerals. This is probably because of the high protein diet's tendency to leach valuable minerals (in this case calcium) from the system. And purely from the point of view of physical beauty, many of these lost minerals, such as sulfur, selenium, zinc, magnesium, and calcium, can make the difference between prematurely aging skin caused by a rapid collagen and elastin breakdown, nails that split, or hair in poor condition, and radiant looks glowing with strength and health.

Finally, the breakdown and metabolism of proteins in the body lead to the formation of a number of complex by-products such as urea, nitrogen, and ammonia, which can be toxic. These wastes need to be eliminated. This isn't always easy, and it puts great strain on the liver and kidneys. This is why, on the well-known high protein reducing diets, you are advised to drink large amounts of water in order to water down these poisons and help excrete them.

WHAT KIND OF PROTEIN IS BEST?

There is a lot of confusion about "superior" and "inferior" proteins—so-called "complete" and "incomplete" foods. At the beginning of the century, researchers doing animal experiments discovered that rats could live and grow on a single food such as eggs. Eggs, like meat, fish, and cheese, were therefore dubbed "complete" proteins. Vegetable foods such as rice, legumes, seeds, nuts, corn, and wheat were called "incomplete" since on their own they were unable to maintain life and growth. What all this meant is that the so-called "complete" proteins contain all the eight acids which humans cannot make for themselves in adequate amounts. But what they didn't take into account is that vegetable food—say, corn—together with another—say, red beans—also contains the eight essential amino acids and, provided you eat one vegetable together with another, you are getting the full complement of the eight essential amino acids in good balance. Better still, you are getting them without the fat that accompanies protein from animal foods. The idea that we need animal foods in order to be healthy is simply untrue. Populations numbering in the millions in different parts of the world have lived and developed enviable health and strength for thousands of years on a purely vegetable diet.

The best—and often the cheapest—sources of protein are the unrefined, unprocessed vegetable foods—complex carbohydrates complete with their natural fiber content, vitamins, and minerals—whole grains such as rice, wheat, oats, barley, legumes including lentils and beans; mixed seeds or mixed nuts; fruits, and vegetables from salad greens to carrots and potatoes. Eaten together in salads and casseroles, bread and soups, they provide low calorie menus without the danger of high fat from the intake of animal foods. The Lifestyle Diet provides 15 percent of your daily calories in the form of protein. It allows you to eat four ounces of meat, fish, or poultry (preferably fish) three times a

week. On the days when you choose not to eat these foods you can have
instead four ounces of mixed nuts or two eggs. It completely eliminates
all cheese except those such as cottage cheese and curd cheeses made
from low-fat milk.

If you prefer, you can take *all* your protein from vegetarian foods.
The question of a vitamin B_{12} deficiency on a vegetarian diet is always
brought up as evidence of the need to eat meat, although long ago biochemist Schweigert of the American Meat Institute researched the question and discovered that the need for B_{12} rises and falls with the amount
of protein eaten. B_{12} is available in dairy products and eggs included in
the Lifestyle Diet. In this kind of protein-economical diet it is corre-
spondingly low. Schweigert also discovered that the whole wheat grain is
a usable source of B_{12} provided it is not processed into white flour. If it
had not been, then the millions of people in different countries who have
lived almost exclusively on a vegan diet (vegetarian with no milk, dairy
products, or eggs) would have suffered B_{12} deficiencies.

THE VITAL ACID–ALKALINE BALANCE

Another important aspect of any diet for super health and beauty is one
that most nutritional systems completely overlook. It is the question of
using foods to help maintain the delicate acid–alkaline balance in your
body. For we can reach truly positive health—health beyond the simple
absence of disease—and remain permanently healthy only when the
foods we eat supply us with a surplus of alkaline-reacting foods. These
include green and root vegetables, avocados, fruits (including citrus
fruits which, though acid, have an alkalinizing effect on the body), seeds
such as sunflower, sesame, and pumpkin, and yogurt.

Your body contains mineral salts. Some of them are alkaline and some
are acid. In a healthy body the ratio between alkaline and acid is four to
one—that is, 80 percent alkaline to 20 percent acid. To maintain this natural balance, you need only to eat foods which, when digested, produce
alkaline salts in approximately these proportions. If, instead, you eat a
diet that is highly acid-forming, as the typical Western fare is, then your
body is forced to work very hard indeed to regulate the internal
acid–alkaline balance and keep your blood slightly alkaline. Without this
natural slight alkalinity, your body is unable to repair tissues and heal itself. Overacidity can lead to acidosis, chronic indigestion, irritability,
nervousness, excess appetite, rheumatic and arthritic conditions, as well as
skin problems and cellulite. Stress, too, is an acid condition. The acid-
forming foods, which should make up 20 percent of any diet but no
more, include meat, eggs, hard cheese, bread, cereals, sugar and honey,

some nuts, and some fats. Coffee, ordinary tea (not green tea or herb teas), and alcohol are also acid-forming.

To give you some idea of what it feels like when your body is too acid, think back to the last typical "good" breakfast you ate—processed cereal with sugar, perhaps an egg, bacon, white toast and jelly, and coffee. Do you remember the immediate feeling of stimulation followed in an hour or two by an unpleasant sense of jangly nerves or tiredness, so that by eleven you had to reach for another cup of coffee to keep yourself going? That is an acid state. In fact, this breakfast is made up of almost all acid-forming foods—the bacon, the white toast and the coffee, the packaged cereal, sugar and so forth. A far better breakfast would be a bowl of Birchermuesli (not the kind of muesli you find in supermarkets, which may be labeled "natural" but is chock-full of sugar) made from natural yogurt, a tablespoonful of rolled oats, a couple of teaspoonfuls of honey and a little cinnamon. On such a breakfast where the fresh fruit and yogurt, which are the alkaline-forming foods, balance the small quantities of acid-forming foods—the grains and the honey—to maintain the ideal ratio of 80 percent alkaline to 20 percent acid, you will find you can work well throughout the morning without suffering "acid rebound." Your body will also be protected against the unnecessary stress of having to work hard to rebalance the blood.

FORGET THE SALT

Recent studies indicate that the daily sodium requirement for a human being is probably not more than 200 milligrams a day, perhaps slightly higher in someone who performs great physical exertion or in nursing mothers. This small quantity is available naturally in foods alone—vegetables, meats and fish, fruits, and grains for instance—without our ever having to add salt to our foods. Where we do add it, not only when cooking but also at the table, the average sodium intake is thought to be more than twenty-five times that amount. Thanks to the research of Professor Lot Page at Harvard, salt—the ubiquitous substance which the ancient Greeks considered divine—has now been shown beyond all reasonable doubt to be at the root of hypertension, one of our most common twentieth-century illnesses.

Excess salt intake can also severely upset the body's water balance. Along with potassium, which also occurs naturally in fresh foods, the sodium in foods and in salt itself (which is sodium chloride) plays an important part in the movement of electrons through the body's water-based protoplasm. This is why sodium and potassium are known as electrolytes. Potassium tends to concentrate in the cells, sodium in the fluids outside the cells. The balance between sodium and potassium, when it is right, sets up a dynamic tension that makes it possible for the living cells to react quickly and efficiently to nerve stimuli, to exchange nutrients and wastes easily through the cell wall, and to maintain the proper interior and extracellular water balance. Too much sodium, which most of us get from eating salt, upsets this balance altogether and can cause troubles. It forces the body to hold on to extra amounts of water to make up for the extra salt one has eaten. Tissues become bloated, and this salt-caused edema can interfere with the blood's oxygen transfer to cells as well as creating extra pressure against the blood vessel walls themselves. These are some of the reasons the Lifestyle Diet eliminates salt both in cooking and at the table. It relies instead on fresh and dried herbs, garlic, and spices for seasoning.

THROW OUT THE COFFEE

Caffeine, a trimethylated xanthine, is found in coffee beans, tea leaves, cola nuts, and cacao, from which chocolate is made. Together with nicotine and alcohol, it makes up a trio of the most widely used psychoactive drugs in the world. The xanthines are stimulants to the central nervous system. They increase heartbeat rate, increase the volume and concentration of acid in the stomach, relax the smooth muscles in the body, raise blood lipids, stimulate the cerebral cortex (which means they heighten the intensity of mental processes), banishing drowsiness and feelings of fatigue. Caffeine and alcohol also have a diuretic effect on the system, causing frequent urination.

The average cup of coffee contains between 100 and 150 milligrams of caffeine per cup, instant coffee somewhat less, tea between 60 and 75 milligrams, cola drinks between 50 and 60 milligrams. This means that if you are drinking four or five cups of coffee each day you are getting a dose of 700 to 750 milligrams of caffeine. To any pharmacologist a dose over 250 milligrams is considered large, although about a third of people in the West get twice as much each day and one person in ten actually imbibes more than 1,000 milligrams of the drug caffeine every twenty-four hours. The full long-term implications of drinking coffee (and, to a lesser degree, tea and cola drinks) are still not clear. However, enough is known already to inspire any woman concerned about the preservation of her health and beauty to give them up completely. For caffeine is a stimulus you do not need on a healthful low protein, low-fat diet high in unrefined carbohydrates.

The link between caffeine intake and anxiety symptoms has been well established. Dr. John Greded, associate professor of psychiatry at the

University of Michigan, and his colleagues and others have reported that high caffeine consumers have statistically significant elevations in anxiety scores. The risk of developing peptic ulcers is also 1.4 times greater among coffee drinkers than among non-coffee drinkers. There is now evidence that coffee consumption by pregnant women can be dangerous to the unborn child. Caffeine has been shown to cross the placental barrier where its mutagenic and perhaps even teratogenic potential may cause genetic changes and, therefore, birth defects.

Finally, a daily intake of caffeine from coffee drinking is the same as continuing to supply your system with any other drug to which it has to adjust and which ultimately it has to detoxify and eliminate. One of the main principles of any long-term diet for health and beauty is, *never* add to the body anything which is not necessary and with which it has to deal. The fewer toxic substances there are, the less contribution they will make to tissue sludge, premature aging of skin, and the subclinical vitamin and mineral deficiencies which result in falling hair, breaking fingernails, chronic fatigue, and mental disorders. In the Lifestyle Diet, coffee, tea, cola drinks (even those without sugar), and cocoa are out. Instead, you can drink mineral waters, herb teas (but always in moderation since some of them in excess may not be good for you either), fresh fruit and vegetable juices, and coffee substitutes made from roots and grains.

THE QUESTION OF ALCOHOL

Alcohol, like caffeine and nicotine, is a drug. As such, it is capable of bringing about serious damage to mind and body when taken over a long period of time. Made from the fermentation of carbohydrates with yeast enzymes, alcohol is rapidly absorbed through the digestive system, affecting coordination of the muscles, nerves, and vision. It also stimulates stomach secretions, inhibits mobilization of lymphocytes so that the body's ability to fight infection is reduced, and causes sludging in the red blood cells, thereby reducing oxygen to the heart and lungs. And it affects the brain, adversely affecting the specific centers that govern self-control, judgment, and personal inhibitions.

Alcohol is a depressant. The transient feeling of well-being that goes with a couple of glasses of whisky or a dry martini—the "lift"—is followed by a series of miseries to which your body is subjected, not the least of which, for a woman, is the effect drinking alcohol has on the liver. And the insidious thing about the detrimental effects which alcohol has on health and beauty is that they occur even to the average social drinker, not just to the serious drinker and the alcoholic.

A joint study by Dr. Charles S. Leiber of the Section of Liver Disease and Nutrition at Bronx Veterans Administration and Dr. Emanuel Rubin of the Department of Pathology at Mount Sinai School of Medicine showed that too much social drinking can cause serious damage to the liver, even though the drinker may feel fine, act normally under the influence of alcohol, and not be an alcoholic. Leiber and Rubim took a group of healthy nonalcoholic volunteers and put them on a carefully controlled eight-day drinking regimen. Then they tested the subjects' livers to see what changes, if any, the alcohol had caused. The amount given to a particular group was considered equivalent to the average intake of a business executive—7 ounces of 86-proof whisky per day for the first four days, 11 ounces for the new two, and then 14 ounces for the last two. The results were surprising: there was an increase in the fat levels in the subjects' liver of from five to thirteen times, all in only eight days, and in spite of the fact that the diet of the subjects had been supplemented with vitamins.

Similar studies have turned up similar results. Researchers have also found that liver-cell damage and the increase in fat in the liver can be *reversible* if the drinker abstains from alcohol for long enough. But long-term damage to the liver resulting from daily consumption of alcohol over the years can be *irreversible*. Persistent drinking can also be a precursor not only to specific diseases of the liver such as cirrhosis, but also to other toxic conditions in the body.

Next to the skin, your liver is your body's largest organ. In many ways it is also the most important. One could, for instance, live without a stomach if necessary but never without a liver. It is the body's chemical purifier, performing more than five hundred different functions, many concerned with detoxifying the system from all the drugs, pollutants, and poisons you take in every day, including alcohol. If the liver is overworked or worn out by excess alcohol consumption, eventually and unavoidably your whole body suffers. Biochemists used to believe that excess alcohol was no more damaging to the liver than too much sugar or too much fat in the diet; that the real damage to the liver came only from malnutrition. But these theories have been disproved. Both the quantity of alcohol you drink and the duration of time over which you drink it are important factors in determining liver damage.

Because the liver is responsible either directly or indirectly for controlling levels of many hormones in a woman's body (particularly estrogen), when liver damage occurs as the result of a diet too high in fats or of drug taking or long-term alcoholic consumption, the endocrine balance can be severely upset, leading not only to disruption of the menstrual cycle but also indirectly to feelings of depression, anxiety, and chronic fatigue.

These troubles may have another cause, also related to alcohol. In order to metabolize alcohol, your body calls on its reserve of many B-complex vitamins which act as coenzymes in the process. When one eats foods containing natural concentrations of carbohydrates or sugar, such as grains and fruits, the B-complex vitamins necessary for their proper digestion and assimilation are provided by nature in the foods themselves. But the B-complex vitamins have been discarded in the processing of highly refined sugars and alcohol. So the body's own reserves can easily get depleted when you drink alcohol and eat refined sugars. Results of this depletion are many, the most common of which can be fatigue, a craving for more alcohol or sweets, or diverse emotional complaints from severe premenstrual tension to simple feelings of chronic misery.

These are just some of the reasons why the Lifestyle Diet excludes alcohol in quantities of more than a glass of wine a day. This may seem like a tremendous sacrifice to you if you are used to taking a great deal more, but once you eliminate stimulants such as coffee, tea, and alcohol from your life and begin to experience the enormous sense of well-being that comes with the low fat, low protein, complex carbohydrate diet (and all the other important things that also go with discovering and expressing your potentials mentally and physically, such as deep relaxation and exercise), you will never miss it.

WHAT PRICE CONVENIENCE?

The Lifestyle Diet also excludes all highly processed prepared foods. Convenience foods such as canned soups and vegetables, instant mashed potatoes, whole meals packaged to be easy to use, ready in a minute, are all created by a highly sophisticated food industry. These foods have been stripped of their natural fiber, denuded of most of their vitamins and minerals, and reduced to easily regulated chemical substances. They also contain a vast quantity of food additives: into them are poured some 3,000 chemicals, the long-term effects of which no one is sure. Some food additives are designed to prevent spoilage or to replace a few of the vitamins lost in the manufacturing process. But about half of them are used only for cosmetic effect. They make our foods appear smoother, more colorful, thicker, clearer or cloudier, more cohesive and so on—in other words, by artificial means they make our foods appear to be what they are not. Only 7 percent of food additives have any nutritional value whatever.

Consumption of such convenience foods is growing. Spokesmen for the food industry speak in self-congratulatory phrases about the great variety of nourishing foods they now offer us and extol the virtues of being able in twenty years to "feed the hungry masses," thanks to the inventive technology that underlies instant mashed potatoes and synthetic meat. Meanwhile eminent scientists such as Ross Hume Hall, biochemist at McMaster University in Canada, and geneticists Joshua Lederberg at Stanford and Bruce Ames at the University of California have issued sharp warnings that things are not as rosy as the industry's public relations people would have us believe. Ames and Lederberg are concerned that our pool of genes is being poisoned by the indiscriminate use of these additives.

CHOOSE YOUR POISONS

Food additives vary tremendously in character, from diethylstilbestrol (DES), a synthetic female hormone used to stimulate cattle growth by 15 percent and boost efficiency of feed by 12 percent, to butylated hydroxyanisole (BHA), an antioxidant used to retard or prevent rancidity and flavor deterioration. Then there is glycerol monostearate, an emulsifying agent derived from partial decomposition of fats, which is used in making ice cream, and a wide variety of artificial coloring compounds (there are now thirty-three permitted in Britain, only nineteen in the EEC, ten in the U.S., and four in the U.S.S.R.). Much of our animal food is laced with antibiotics, which are given to retard meat spoilage. They are also used to suppress evidence of disease in animals that are raised in adverse circumstances and are, therefore, prone to illness. They offer *no* nutritional benefits.

There are three main ways that food additives can be threats to health: they can be carcinogenic (tending to produce cancer), teratogenic (tending to harm the unborn child in the womb), and mutagenic (tending to produce changes in the gene pattern which can be passed on to future generations). One can add the danger of producing genetic changes in the cell material which promote early aging in the body—of particular concern to a woman intent on preserving her youthfulness and good looks.

Government agencies try to regulate the safety of additives in fabricated foods, but judging from the Canadian and American records of failure and the number of permitted additives that have in recent years been suddenly whisked off the market, this is an impossible task. Only 60 percent of the additives used in Britain have been tested at all and even then only for *acute* toxicity—that is, to determine whether or not they bring immediate adverse reactions to an organism ingesting them—not for teratogenicity nor for possible genetic effects. In fact, there is simply no way for them to be tested. The tests that are done are carried out on animals, not humans, and as the thalidomide tragedy showed, a substance can appear quite safe from teratogenic effects in laboratory animals, yet result in tragic consequences for a human fetus.

But even our methods of testing are outdated. According to Ross Hume Hall, this is because we have all our assumptions wrong. "Both the standards of nutrition by which these foods are judged and the methods of toxicology used to determine their safety are outmoded nineteenth-century models," he says. Nineteenth-century nutritional theory is based on the notion that all we need from food is protein, carbohydrates, fat, vitamins, and minerals regardless of their source. It is unaware of the interrelationships in natural foods, and of the implications of possible nutrients as yet undiscovered (as with fiber until fifteen years ago) which may be vital for good health. "This limited concept of what constitutes nourishment persists," says Hall, "even though it has been completely outmoded by the enormous advances in understanding of cell and molecular biology."

The nineteenth-century toxicology still practiced today assumes that each chemical tested has its own level of toxicity. As long as one's consumption of that chemical remains below that level, it says, one is safe. It gives no consideration to how different chemicals, tested separately, affect an organism when they are consumed together; nor is any thought given to the cumulative effects of taking a substance regularly over the years.

"What we are beginning to realize," says Hall, "is that not only can chemicals poison in the short term, they can also cause long-term subtle and undetected changes in personal biology. These changes can show themselves in devastating ways such as cancer and other degenerative diseases and birth defects."

Food additives are not the only problems with convenience foods either. Their simple nutritional worth is highly questionable. For in addition to their lack of fiber (natural fiber is largely removed in the manufacture of convenience foods), government surveys in Canada and the United States—where 80 percent of food eaten is now factory-produced—show that in spite of the great wealth of these countries and the availability to the public of a vast variety of foods, in general people are not getting enough vitamins and minerals in their diet. This is in large part because so many of the nutrients are lost in processing.

Researchers at Rutgers University experimented with frozen chicken pies to see what vitamin loss, if any, had taken place in the processing. They chose vitamin C levels. To their amazement, researchers found no vitamin C whatever in commercially prepared frozen pies. Then they added vitamin C to the pies and refroze them. When they were reheated two days later, three quarters of the vitamin had disappeared.

A random sampling of 6.5 million elderly people in Britain, in an investigation sponsored by the Ministry of Health, revealed that four out of five were suffering from vitamin deficiencies—a factor that is probably responsible for a large number of illnesses, including many mental disorders suffered by the elderly. According to Dr. Geoffrey Taylor, who has made a long study of the problem in Britain, "There is every reason to believe these deficiencies are present in other age groups of the population as well."

These are a few of the reasons why the Lifestyle Diet does not include convenience foods. For lasting health and beauty you need the very best complement of nutrients you can get. The McCarrison Society, an organization of doctors and dentists in Britain dedicated to the study of the relationship between nutrition and health, issued a directive that expresses it very well: "Food should be left as close as possible to its natural state. It should be grown on healthy soil. Stored, canned, packaged or precooked food should, whenever possible, be replaced by fresh food. The protective value of a wide range of fresh vegetables, fruits, and low-fat dairy produce is particularly important. Cereal carbohydrates should not be refined and sugar consumption should be at an absolute minimum." These are the basic principles of the Lifestyle Diet. Now let's see how to put it all into practice.

7

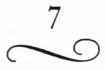

Putting Lifestyle into Practice

It is certainly important to know and understand a lot about the complex science of nutrition and how it affects health. Without this knowledge there is no way of being able to be personally responsible for what you eat. But knowledge is only half the key; practical application is the other half. How then do you put the Lifestyle principles into action?

TAKE A LOOK AT YOUR FOOD SHELVES

What do you see there that doesn't fit in with the low fat, no sugar, no refined carbohydrate principles of Lifestyle? Spaghetti made from white flour? Use it up, then next time you buy pasta, go to a health food store for the whole-wheat or buckwheat variety instead. Jams and jellies? Next trip to the health food store, look for the variety that contains no sugar and no preservatives and if they don't have it, get them to order it. It is delicious—far nicer, really, than the sickly sweet ordinary variety, and you can eat it on your bread with impunity. Or make some sugarless apple butter.

Get rid of the chocolate and cocoa, and substitute carob powder for recipes that call for chocolate. Look for the coffee substitutes made from grains or roots. They are delicious and can be drunk with powdered skimmed milk if you like. Also stock up on herb teas and keep a jar of country honey on hand to sweeten them.

THEN OPEN THE REFRIGERATOR

What in your refrigerator doesn't belong there? Let your family eat that rich cheese if they must, but you go for the nonfat cottage cheese instead, mixing it with fruit, herbs, and spices for variety. For milk, substitute nonfat dried milk—mix it with water and keep it on hand for cereals and drinks.

Eggs are OK. So are the lean cuts of meat, poultry, and fish. But when buying fish, make it fresh fish or go for the simple frozen fish steak or fillet *without* all the breading and food additives.

For ordinary yogurt complete with its undesirable butterfat, sugar, and fruit flavorings, substitute your own homemade variety (see recipe page 94). If you want it flavored, add a teaspoonful of honey or a few raisins, a little cinnamon and a grated apple or any other kind of fresh fruit. Instead of butter to spread on bread, create your own low-fat spreads with cottage cheese and fresh or frozen fruits or herbs and vegetables. A little mustard, tomato, and green pepper combined in a blender with half a cup of low-fat cottage cheese and then sprinkled with fresh chives makes a super spread you can refrigerate and use for several days.

TO SWEETEN

Instead of sugar, remember that on the Lifestyle Diet you have two tablespoons of honey to "play with" each day for sweetening. You can make another sweetener of dates puréed in a blender with a little water, of mashed bananas and other fruits, or of raisins plumped up in water overnight and then puréed in a blender. Another useful sweetener is concentrated frozen orange juice straight from the container.

Get rid of your white flour too. Recipes calling for it have to be altered to use whole-wheat varieties instead. For thickening sauces you can use whole-wheat flour or cornstarch; for thickening a vegetable stew try simply putting a cupful or so of the stew through a blender and then pouring it back into the pot. Usually no other thickener is necessary. Another way to thicken a sauce or gravy is simply to let its water slowly evaporate as it cooks.

WHEN YOU HEAD FOR THE STOVE

Forget about frying things in oil. Instead, buy yourself a good nonstick frying pan and use it without fat to cook meat, scrambled eggs, pancakes and anything else that has to be fried. When you prepare chicken, stew it or braise it, removing the skin first because it is particularly high in fat, or simply bake it and then take off the skin from your piece before you eat it.

Some of the most nourishing and inexpensive main dishes you can make are based on grains and such legumes as dried peas, beans, and lentils; chick-peas, red beans, black-eyed peas, broad beans, lima beans, and red, black, and brown lentils. The list seems endless. The only variety of bean that is excluded from the Lifestyle Diet is soybeans, as they are too high in protein and often hard to digest. You can make excellent stews or casseroles using these legumes by boiling them and then adding chopped onions, carrots, celery, or other vegetables, and herbs such as marjoram, thyme, basil, or oregano. They add such wonderful flavor to dishes—each has its own character and own personality imprint, quite different from all the others. Buy yourself a little book on herbs (there are many on the market) and experiment to find out which herbs you particularly like.

Whole grains, too, make delicious main dishes. Groats, or hulled whole wheat, soaked and then boiled for an hour or so, can be served hot as you would serve rice, perhaps with some onions or chopped vegetables added, or you can chill it after cooking to make a delicious salad. Brown rice can make an excellent main dish—a pilaf—when it is cooked together with mushrooms, carrots, green or red peppers, onions, and peas. For variety you can boil it in tomato juice or vegetable broth instead of water, or you can add curry powder to the dish. You can often spice up a dish by adding lemon juice, Worcestershire sauce, horseradish, mustard or Tabasco.

SOUPS ARE SUPER

Soups are a mainstay of the Lifestyle Diet. Easy to make, they are low in calories but very filling. In principle, you just put everything you are going to use into a pot, add water, and let it simmer until cooked. But in practice, the art of good soup-making takes a little time to master.

I always save the water in which vegetables have been cooked (when I don't steam them) for stock. I keep it in the refrigerator and then use it to give my soups a fuller, richer flavor. This makes sure you will get the nutrients that have been leached out of the vegetables into the water in which they were cooked. You can also boil up chicken and meat bones for stock, but be sure to chill the stock and then lift off the fat that congeals on the top and discard. You can make soups with simple vegetables of almost any variety and then either serve them as they are or put them through a blender to make a "creamed" soup. Or you can make a dried pea or other legume the basis of your soup to make it heartier and more of a meal in one dish.

If you are cooking not only for yourself but for a family, it is not as difficult as you might think to make use of the Lifestyle principles without causing yourself any extra work. Others too will enjoy the casseroles, soups, and whole-grain dishes made without sugar or added fats. You can still put butter and cheese on the table if they want them and they can have whole milk on their cereals instead of skimmed milk that you use. The good thing about the Lifestyle principles is that not only are they useful in terms of improving, protecting, and preserving your own health and beauty, they will also help make the rest of your family healthier too.

GRAIN—THE STAFF OF LIFE

There are all sorts of delicious breads and biscuits you can eat on Lifestyle. All of them should be whole-grain, though. This includes crispbreads made from rye or wheat flours (not the "starch reduced" varieties), Greek pita bread, whole-grain scones and rolls, whole-wheat Indian chapatis and Mexican corn tortillas, so long as they are made without oil. The breads you make yourself (see recipe on page 95) are best since they can be made without added fats, although most of the crispbreads are also fat-free.

Whole-grain cereals are an important part of the diet too. Hot cereal made from oats or cracked wheat, millet, or whole-grain semolina makes excellent breakfasts. So does homemade muesli. The packaged mueslis are out unless you can get the kind made with no sugar. But you can also make your own muesli from the mixed whole grains you can buy in health food stores to which you add raisins, chopped dates and nuts, fresh fruit, and milk. Eat your cereals with skimmed milk and add a little cinnamon if you like, or a mashed banana, grated apple, or some raisins for sweetening.

RAW POWER

Some of the most important ingredients of all in the Lifestyle Diet are the raw ones—salads made from every possible fruit and vegetable combination. Raw vegetables are a delight not only in salads but also to nibble any time between meals. I often even make raw soups; the recipes in the Raw Energy Diet (see Chapter 4) make super soups that you can vary to suit your own personal tastes and designs. The salad suggestions in the Raw Energy Diet go equally well in the Lifestyle Diet. Try to make a salad (or even two) the center dish of both lunch and dinner, and experiment with making salad dressings that are nonfat. This is one area in which I think it is sometimes useful to look for proprietary brand products; there are some excellent low calorie nonfat salad dressings on the market. Read labels carefully and only choose those that do not contain monosodium glutamate or oil. Keep them at hand for when you are too busy or too lazy to make your own.

There are so many amazing things you can do with raw vegetables—grate them, slice them, chop them, or simply cut them into beautiful pieces to serve as munchers between meals. Salads can be a symphony of color, taste, and nourishment—experiment and you will find lots of delicious possibilities. Grow your own sprouts (see page 97) and use them in sandwiches, salads, and omelets and just as snacks; you'll never find a better source of nourishment anywhere.

SPECIAL EQUIPMENT FOR THE KITCHEN

Another mainstay of the Lifestyle Diet is fresh juices made from vegetables and fruits. There is a list of them in the section on *Rohsäfte-Kur* to get you started but there are so many different combinations you can concoct. Try to drink as many as possible—get into the habit of taking a glass of carrot and apple juice before dinner instead of an apéritif, or as a snack or whenever you feel tired or on edge. They alkalinize a system that is overacid because of fatigue or stress. I find they have a way of clearing my head when I am working too hard or just feeling self-indulgently lazy. To make fresh juices (except orange and grapefruit, which you make in an ordinary juicer of course), you need a centrifuge or juice extractor. It is a handy gadget that takes in the vegetables or fruit, separates the pulp from the liquid, and produces a glass of juice within seconds. This is a piece of kitchen equipment I personally would not want to be without. You can buy juice extractors that also double as choppers or blenders or graters when you add separate attachments to them.

Whether or not you have a centrifuge juice extractor, you will certainly want a blender, to make drinks and soups, or a food processor that blends, chops, grates, or slices in a couple of seconds. They are wonderful for chopping vegetables for soups or stews, for beating eggs, for making grated salads, and any number of other tasks in the kitchen. They help make the preparation of fresh, simple foods a real delight too because they are so easy to use and clean and the foods look so good when they have been prepared.

LEARN TO SUBSTITUTE

Don't throw out all your old cookbooks and look upon the Lifestyle Diet as a horrible deprivation you have to endure bravely for the sake of your skin and hair. Keep them and experiment by substituting permissible Lifestyle ingredients for the usual old favorites. Also look around for new cookbooks that offer low fat recipes or whole food cookery and adapt their recipes to suit, leaving out such ingredients as sugar, high fat cheese, and whole milk where necessary. The process can be fun and you will discover a whole new world of tastes—hardly a deprivation. And what is even better is that after a couple of weeks on Lifestyle you will probably feel so well you won't even miss the sweets or rich foods you thought you couldn't live without.

WHAT HAPPENS WHEN YOU ARE STUCK IN A RESTAURANT?

There is no great problem, particularly if the restaurant is a good one. They can easily adapt their fare to suit your wishes. I ask restaurants to do it all the time, since I eat at least a third of all my meals in them one way or another. Vegetarian restaurants are usually very good, as are health food restaurants. They have a lot of whole-grain products (although you sometimes have to question them about the fat added) and an excellent selection of salads, casseroles, and soups. Just avoid the cheesy dishes and desserts and you're pretty safe.

Chinese restaurants are also good provided you can get them to leave out the monosodium glutamate, which they tend to add to everything as a flavor enhancer and which has a nasty habit of making you retain water. It even makes some people quite ill.

In an ordinary—American restaurant, French, Italian, or any other kind—order your main course as simply prepared as possible: grilled liver without butter or bacon, poached fish, grilled chicken (and then remove the skin before eating). The vegetables they offer are fine if you ask the waiter to leave off the butter, and of course a green salad or mixed salad is an excellent standby anywhere, provided you ask for no dressing. You can dress it with lemon juice or a little Worcestershire sauce. For dessert you can always have raspberries, pineapple, or another kind of fresh fruit.

Dinner parties are not that much of a problem either. Friends are usually quick to understand the way you eat, particularly when you explain beforehand. Certainly I have never had anyone take offense. And it doesn't mean extra work for the hostess either, provided you just eat the dishes that are acceptable and politely decline the rest. If ever you find your plate piled high with something very greasy or rich, simply take a bite or two and then rearrange the rest on the plate (a technique I discovered as a child to make my father think I was eating my dinner when I wasn't hungry).

If occasionally you have to eat something you shouldn't be eating, then don't worry about it. Lifestyle isn't a rigid regimen—it is a long-term way of eating. Just make sure, when you have to go off it, that it is not more often than *occasionally*—that's what matters.

WHAT IF YOU CHEAT?

Everybody cheats sometimes. So what? Provided you are following the principles of Lifestyle, you can eat the occasional extra piece of meat or dish of ice cream, or tablespoonful of mayonnaise with your poached salmon, without doing damage. But when you do cheat—when you go off your regimen—do it *openly* and *enjoy* it. Remember that the good effects of a long-term way of eating for health and beauty only come by eating that way *long-term*. There is no way you can continue to eat pieces of high fat cheese, slices of chocolate cake, or bars of chocolate without affecting your body and your psyche.

Don't worry too much at first about slipups; just concentrate on getting the principles right in the way you cook and eat and the kinds of food you buy. And remember that *you alone* are *responsible* for what you do—no one else. You must *choose* to cheat when you do, not pretend it is some kind of unavoidable compulsion. Chances are that the urge to take something which is not part of Lifestyle will fade pretty quickly when you are tolerant of yourself about slipups and when you get to know from experience how much better you look and feel by following this kind of diet.

HINTS AND HELPS FOR THE LIFESTYLE DIET

How to Keep Fats Out of Your Life

* Choose only the leanest meats and trim all fats from them *before* cooking.
* Make your own yogurt with nonfat dried milk.

* Chill all soups so that the oils float to the top and solidify. Then you can lift off the solid fat and discard it before you reheat the soup to serve.
* When you cook vegetables, steam or boil them in a very small amount of water which you can reserve for soup stock.
* For frying, use a nonstick skillet and no fat. (You can make delicious sautéed vegetables in a few tablespoons of quite concentrated fat-free broth which quickly boils away, browning the vegetables and giving them a super flavor.)

WHAT ABOUT NIBBLING BETWEEN MEALS?

Yes, absolutely. Do a lot of it. Don't let yourself go hungry—you can make a bag of raw vegetables such as carrot sticks, green pepper slices, tomatoes, celery, and cucumbers, and keep them in the refrigerator all scrubbed so you need just reach in and take some whenever you are hungry. You can also make up a dip from cottage cheese (be sure to deduct it from your daily protein allowance) mixed with chopped carrots and chives, or with fruit, to spread on crispbread or whole-wheat bread between meals. A plastic bag of such goodies can go with you to an office or to work or school to be on hand always.

Another good snack is a bowl of soup left over from a meal. It is particularly warming in winter. One good thing about Lifestyle is that you can keep eating all the time if you like and it will not make you fat, provided you follow its principles, get no more fat or protein than you are allowed, and take no sugar. This is a godsend to women who have spent all their lives, literally, trying not to gain weight.

Here is a quick reference chart for planning your Lifestyle meals:

Quick Reference Chart of Foods to Eat and Foods to Avoid for

THE LIFESTYLE DIET FOR HEALTH AND BEAUTY

Foods to Choose	*Amounts and Restrictions*	*Foods to Shun*
VEGETABLES	You must eat at least 2 salads a day made from all sorts of raw vegetables. You can have unrestricted amounts of vegetables at mealtimes and between meals. When cooking vegetables, it is best to either to bake them (potatoes, sweet potatoes and yams, squash, carrots, onions) or steam them. They must be served without butter or oil. You can always munch raw vegetables when you are hungry between meals (carrots, celery, radishes, cucumbers, watercress, green peppers), and you may have up to 3 glasses of fresh vegetable juice a day.	
	Wipe sugar completely off your nutrition map. You may take 1 tablespoonful of blackstrap molasses a day (rich in sulfur, vitamins, and other minerals) and you can use 2 tablespoonfuls of honey a day for sweetening if desired. Recent studies raise suspicions about long-term use of artificial sweeteners, so don't try to replace the sugar you have been used to with saccharine or other artificial sweeteners. Your palate will soon adjust to the natural sweetness of fresh	SUGAR Sugar in any form. Also reject anything made with sugar such as candy, desserts, chocolate, jams, jellies and convenience foods that contain hidden sugar. Don't eat any condiments that contain sugar.

Foods to Choose	*Amounts and Restrictions*	*Foods to Shun*
	fruits and you will get over your sweet tooth.	
FRUIT	Eat at least 1 piece of citrus fruit a day. You may have up to 6 pieces of other fruit as well. Fresh fruits are far superior to canned ones. If you have to eat canned fruits, make sure they are not the kind that have been canned in syrup. You may have as many as 2 glasses of fresh fruit juices a day and up to 1 ounce of dried fruits such as raisins, apricots, peaches, pears, dates, and figs per day in place of 2 or 3 pieces of fresh fruit.	
GRAINS	You should eat all whole grains such as brown rice, wheat, rye, barley, corn, oats, buckwheat, and millet. Have 2 or more kinds of whole grains each day as breads or cereals, whole-grain pasta, or in casseroles. You may also have 1 table-spoonful of fresh wheat germ a day if desired, and if ever you experience constipation you may add 2 tablespoonfuls of unprocessed bran to your salads, cereals, and soups.	WHITE FLOUR, WHITE RICE Avoid these and any-thing made from refined grains such as ordinary pasta and most packaged breakfast cereals (they have hidden sugar as well as refined flours in them). Avoid breads with added oils (read la-bels carefully). When you make your own, make it without oil or fat.
DAIRY PRODUCTS	You may have skimmed milk or nonfat buttermilk up to ½ pint daily; cheese made from skimmed milk, such as nonfat cottage cheese, up to 4 ounces a day; or homemade yogurt made from skimmed milk, up	WHOLE MILK Contains too much fat, as do ordinary cheeses —both soft like Camem-bert and hard like Ched-dar—cream, and sour cream.

Foods to Choose	*Amounts and Restrictions*	*Foods to Shun*
	to 4 ounces a day. If you eat both cheese and yogurt in one day, then don't have your meat or fish or poultry allowance for that day.	FATS Avoid all added fats including butter, margarine, and oils. Trim all visible fat from meat and fish before cooking. Dress your salads with dressings containing no oil.
NUTS AND LEGUMES	Two or three times a week eat legumes—all sorts of beans and peas except soybeans. You are allowed only 2 ounces of nuts, a day—raw and unsalted and preferably mixed—but no peanuts.	
FISH, MEAT, POULTRY AND EGGS	Eat no more than 4 ounces of meat, poultry, or fish three times a week or 2 eggs daily. No smoked foods, and no fatty meats. All fat must be trimmed from meat and fish before cooking. (Try to eat 4 to 6 eggs a week as they are an excellent source of the sulfur amino acids, which are esential for beautiful skin, hair, and nails.)	
CONDIMENTS	Use as many herbs and spices as you wish in cooking. Avoid all bottled condiments that contain sugar or oils or fats. Worcestershire sauce, Tabasco, and prepared mustard can be used without restriction. Mayonnaise is out, as are gravies, sandwich spreads, and monosodium glutamate. Do not add extra salt to your foods.	

Foods to Choose	*Amounts and Restrictions*	*Foods to Shun*
DRINKS	You can drink up to 3 glasses of fresh vegetable juice made with a juice extractor and 2 glasses of fresh fruit juice a day. You can have unlimited fat-free, clear vegetable or chicken broth, and up to 4 cups a day of herb teas—camomile, spearmint, and rose-hip—sweetened with some of your daily honey allowance if desired. You can take coffee substitutes made from roots and grains. You are allowed 7 glasses of wine per week and unlimited mineral water and fresh spring water.	COFFEE, TEA

RECIPES

How to Make Raw Vegetable Salads

Choose three or more of the following and mix them together: lettuce, chicory, watercress, chopped apple, white heart of cabbage, carrots, radishes, fennel, raw sliced mushrooms, red and green peppers, Italian red lettuce, romaine, endive, spring onions, cucumbers, celery, herbs.

Year-round Salad Suggestions

IN SPRING

Choose one of the following mixtures:

1. Oranges, almonds, hazelnuts, knob celery, white cabbage, raw peas, celery, and fresh mint
2. Apples and raw beets
3. Strawberries, pine nuts, watercress, and lettuce
4. Avocados, watercress, tomatoes, scallions
5. Oranges, nuts, finely chopped spinach, a dash of horseradish

IN SUMMER

1. Red currants, raspberries, nuts, and finely grated carrots mixed with fresh peas and finely chopped lettuce
2. Peaches, cherries, almonds, garnished with lettuce and finely chopped tomatoes and sprigs of mint
3. Apples, nuts, peaches, kohlrabi, parsley, and red cabbage finely chopped
4. Lettuce, watercress, grated carrots, celery, and spring onions
5. Avocado, grapefruit, watercress, surrounded by a wreath of radishes and garnished with sunflower seeds

IN AUTUMN

1. Pears, almonds, hazelnuts, chicory, beets, and apples
2. Knob celery, apples, nuts, and spring onions garnished with finely chopped spinach
3. Cucumber, dill, lettuce, chopped spring onions, and tomatoes
4. Grapes, nuts, grated raw turnip, and grated raw carrot

IN WINTER

1. Oranges, nuts, winter cabbage, carrots, and watercress
2. Tangerines, almonds, celery, watercress, and chicory
3. Apples, nuts, grapes, turnips, and lettuce
4. Fennel, spinach, chicory, and chopped tomatoes on a bed of lettuce
5. Celery, pears, nuts, and Jerusalem artichokes garnished with chopped parsley

Salad Dressings

YOGURT SWEET DRESSING

1 cup nonfat yogurt
1 large orange, peeled, with seeds removed
1 tablespoon lemon juice
4 pitted dates
Dash of cinnamon, if desired

Put into blender and mix well. Store in refrigerator.

TOMATO DRESSING

3–5 tomatoes (depending on size)
2 tablespoons lemon juice
½ teaspoon basil

Put into blender and liquefy. Store in refrigerator.

ALMOND-DATE TOPPING

1 cup raisins or dates, soaked in water for several hours to plump them
up
½ cup blanched almonds

Put into blender and liquefy. Store in refrigerator.

AVOCADO-TOMATO DRESSING

4 small tomatoes
1 avocado
2 tablespoons lemon juice
Dash of Tabasco
Crushed clove of garlic or dash of garlic powder

Mix in blender. Store in refrigerator.

YOGURT AND EGG DRESSING

1 egg yolk
1½ cups nonfat yogurt
3 tablespoons lemon juice or cider vinegar
Pinch cayenne pepper
Fresh or dried herbs to taste
2 teaspoons honey

Put ingredients into the top of a double boiler and stir over hot water
until the mixture thickens. Refrigerate to serve cold or use hot on hot
potato salad or hot rice salad.

THOUSAND ISLAND DRESSING

1 hard-boiled egg, chopped
5 teaspoons celery, finely chopped
3 tablespoons onion, finely chopped
2 tablespoons black olives, chopped
1 tablespoon green pepper, finely chopped
½ cup nonfat yogurt

Mix all ingredients and serve chilled.

NON-OIL VINAIGRETTE

3 tablespoons dried skimmed milk
½ teaspoon Dijon mustard
2 teaspoons honey
Dash of pepper
Pinch of basil
1 clove garlic, crushed
2 tablespoons vinegar

Mix ingredients, adding vinegar last. Beat well or blend until smooth. Chill and use same day.

Fresh Juice Drinks

Any combination of raw vegetable juices such as carrot, apple, celery, made in a juice extractor. Fresh fruit juices such as orange, grape, grapefruit. (See Chapter 4 on juices.) You may also have herb teas, coffee substitutes, and mineral waters.

CINNAMON-APPLE SMOOTHIE

1 large apple, cored
1 tablespoon lemon juice
½ cup water
1 tablespoon honey
½ teaspoon cinnamon

Mix in blender.

SWEET LHASSI

½ cup nonfat yogurt
¼ cup ice water
4 ice cubes
Dash of cinnamon
Dash of ground cloves
Dash of nutmeg
Dash of mace
1 tablespoon honey

Mix in blender.

GRAPE DELIGHT

Handful red or white grapes, seeded
1 tablespoon raw honey
Juice of ½ lemon or lime
½ cup Perrier or seltzer
2 ice cubes

Mix in blender.

Soups

CUCUMBER

1 cup nonfat yogurt
½ cucumber, peeled
6 leaves fresh mint
Juice of ½ lemon

Mix in blender. Serve chilled with a thin slice of cucumber on top.

CREAM OF GRAPE SOUP

½ pound of grapes, washed and seeded
½ cup fresh orange juice
1 tablespoon raw honey
12 blanched almonds

Chill all ingredients before mixing in blender. Serve immediately.

CREAM OF TOMATO SOUP

3 medium tomatoes, peeled
2 teaspoons scallions, chopped
½ teaspoon parsley and/or sweet basil
½ teaspoon prepared mustard

Blend and serve.

GAZPACHO

First chill the following ingredients, then put them into the juice extractor:

2 tomatoes
4 carrots
1 stalk celery

Add

Juice of ½ lemon
1 teaspoon scallions, chopped
Dash of Tabasco

Serve immediately.

Grain Treats

FRESH FRUIT MUESLI (for one)

1 tablespoon of natural mixed grain flakes or rolled oats
1 tablespoon water
½ banana, mashed
1 apple, grated or minced fine
1 tablespoon mixed ground nuts
Juice of ½ lemon
3 tablespoons low-fat or nonfat yogurt
¼ cup fresh orange juice or honey to taste
Raisins

Soak the grain flakes or rolled oats in the water overnight to soften. In the morning add the mashed banana and apple plus the mixed ground nuts. Mix with the lemon juice and yogurt. Add the orange juice or honey. Sprinkle with raisins and serve.

DRY MUESLI

The nutritious version of the packaged mueslis you find in supermarkets and health food stores. Unlike most of them, it contains no sugar. It is very good to mix up in bulk and then keep for when you want a fast breakfast or for traveling. It can also be cooked on a low heat for 20 minutes to make a delicious porridge.

1 cup rolled oats
1 cup barley flakes
1 cup rye flakes
1 cup wheat flakes
1 cup powdered skimmed milk
1 cup mixed dried fruits, such as raisins, apricots, peaches, apples, and bananas (sun-dried, unsulfured)
1 cup mixed ground sunflower, sesame, and pumpkin seeds

Cut up the larger dried fruits into small pieces. Mix all the ingredients together and store in a cool, dry place. Serve with fruit juice or water poured over and with a dash of cinnamon, if desired.

Homemade Nonfat Yogurt

¼ cup low-fat natural yogurt
4 pints lukewarm water
Powdered skimmed milk, the quantity to make 1½ quarts when reconstituted.

Mix ingredients well with a wooden spoon in a sterilized nonmetallic container. Cover and leave to stand in a very warm place until it has set. You can use the top of a radiator or another warm place, or you can place it in the oven at its lowest temperature for 10 minutes. Then turn it off and leave it there until set. If necessary, you can light the oven again for 2 minutes after a couple of hours to keep the temperature level. Never leave it on longer and never heat the yogurt above lukewarm or you will kill the lactobacillus and the yogurt won't set. It usually takes about 4–6 hours for a large pot of yogurt to set. Allow to cool and then refrigerate and serve cold. Save 3 or 4 tablespoons from the last pot to use as a starter for the next time you make yogurt.

Dessert Recipes

SUGARLESS JAM

For serving on whole-grain toast. Mix a selection of fruit such as strawberries, peaches, pears, apples, cherries, apricots, pineapples, blackberries, raspberries, red currants, and black currants with orange juice and blend to a purée. Add a little cornstarch and, stirring constantly, heat until thickened. Add a dash of cinnamon, nutmeg, ginger, or vanilla to taste. Store in refrigerator. Serve hot or cold.

BANANA TOPPING

Purée bananas with strawberries, blackberries, raspberries, or loganberries. Add honey. Serve immediately at room temperature.

APPLE BUTTER

Skin and core 2 pounds of sweet apples. Put into a heavy-duty saucepan with a couple of tablespoons of water (just enough to prevent burning), the juice of a lemon, a cup of raisins, and a teaspoon of cinnamon. Cook slowly and long until the volume is only a third of what it was and the mixture thickens. Remove from the heat, put through the blender, and store in the refrigerator to spread on toast, pancakes, and fresh fruit.

MOCK CREAM

1 banana
1 tablespoon powdered skimmed milk
1 egg yolk
4 drops vanilla extract

Mash banana, add other ingredients, and mix well. Serve cold on fruit salads.

MILK PUDDING

4 ounces long-grain brown rice *or* whole tapioca *or* whole-grain bread
Powdered skimmed milk (the quantity to make 1 quart when reconstituted)
2 eggs
3 cups water
4 tablespoons honey *or* blackstrap molasses
½ cup raisins
Freshly ground nutmeg

Wash and drain the grains. Mix milk, eggs, and water and add the grains or bread. Sweeten with honey or blackstrap molasses. Add raisins. Sprinkle nutmeg over surface. Bake in moderate oven (350°) for 45 minutes. Serves 4.

Whole-meal Bread

This is an excellent bread recipe originally created by Doris Grant.

The Grant Loaf method for 3 loaves:

1 ounce fresh yeast
2 tablespoons honey
Up to 1 quart lukewarm water
3 pounds stone-ground whole-wheat flour

Mix yeast and honey in small bowl with ½ cup of lukewarm water. Leave in a warm place for ten minutes or so to froth up. Pour the yeasty liquid into the flour and gradually add the rest of the water, until the right consistency is attained—dough should be firm and pliable. Mix well, preferably by hand. Divide the dough into three 1-quart bread tins that have first been greased and warmed. Put the tins in a warm place, cover with a cloth, and let dough rise for about 20 minutes, until it is within half an inch of the top of the tins. Bake in a hot oven (400°) for 35 to 40 minutes. Allow to cool for ten minutes and turn out onto wire rack.

Baked Egg Soufflé (savory or sweet)

8 egg whites
8 egg yolks
Pepper
Parsley

Fillings (Optional)

Beaten tuna fish (canned in water, not oil)
Chopped sprouted grains, green peppers, and tomatoes
Seasonal berries and currants

Beat egg whites until they form firm peaks. Whisk pepper and parsley into yolks. Beat in any filling, if desired. Fold the whites into the yolks. Turn into a nonstick container and cook for 25 minutes in a 325° oven.

SUPPLEMENTS—GET TO KNOW THE SUPER FOODS

Some of the best supplements you can take for maintaining sleek, shining hair, youthful skin, a well-shaped body, and the unmistakable energy that marks a beautiful woman no matter what her age are not pills at all but foods such as liver and blackstrap molasses that are packed full of nutritional value in beautifully balanced forms that make them easy to assimilate. They are special foods—not exactly "wonder foods," but then not far from it either. Many of them are rich sources of the "protectors"— such nutrients as the important antioxidants vitamins C and E, the B complex with all its important value to nerves, hair, and skin, selenium to improve the action of vitamin E and perhaps preserve cellular youth, and the sulfur amino acids. Get to know each of the super foods and make them an everyday part of your Lifestyle Diet, week after week, year after year. Twenty years from now, you will be glad you did.

Live Sprouts

Sprouted grains and seeds are without equal anywhere as powerhouses of *live* food nourishment. You can grow them on your windowsill or even in a warm dark cupboard. They are an excellent source of protein, minerals, complex carbohydrates, vitamins, and small quantities of essential fatty acids. Germinating seeds and grains *enormously* increases their nutritional value. Sprouted wheat, for instance, contains 30 percent more vitamin B than ordinary wheat grains, 200 percent more B_2, 90 percent more niacin, and 80 percent more pantothenic acid. The vitamin C content increases 60 percent during sprouting. Similar increases occur in the germination of all the other sprouts too—alfalfa, adzuki, mung beans, lentils, fenugreek, and beans. Nowhere will you find a food more potent and valuable for health and beauty than sprouts. Germinated soybeans are so very rich in vitamin C, for instance, that a mere 2 tablespoonfuls will supply you with the minimum daily requirement of vitamin C. (But don't stop at two—eat more.)

Sprouts are delicious on salads and in yogurt and they are easy to grow in jars. The seeds themselves can be purchased from health food stores and ordered from seed suppliers. They can be sprouted literally anywhere during summer or winter, with or without light. So potent are they that if you lived on a mixture of sprouted grains alone you would have everything you need for health and long-lasting beauty.

HERE'S HOW TO SPROUT

Put a heaped tablespoonful of seeds or grains into a jar, cover it with lukewarm water, and leave it overnight. In the morning, covering the jar with a piece of muslin or cheesecloth held in place with a rubber band, pour off the water and rinse the seeds in fresh lukewarm water (never *hot* or you will kill them). Now pour off the excess water through the cloth and put the jar on the windowsill. In the evening, rinse again and pour off excess. Repeat the rinsing twice a day, and in three to six days (depending on the kind of seeds you have used) you will have sprouts to sprinkle on your salads, fill omelets, or just eat as a snack. Grow a different kind in each jar and you will have a veritable larder of nutritional delight.

Seeds to sprout include alfalfa, wheat, mung beans (Chinese bean sprouts come from these), buckwheat, lentils, sesame seeds, chick-peas, soybeans, fenugreek. But be sure you get *untreated* seeds and grains or they will not sprout at all.

Eggs

Eggs have been much maligned in recent years because of their cholesterol content, which was assumed to raise cholesterol in the blood and therefore was thought to contribute to coronary heart disease. Thinking on the subject is changing, for the egg is a balanced combination of nutritional goodness. It offers not only cholesterol (something your body makes anyway) but also zinc, sulfur, iron, phosphorus, unsaturated fatty acids, and lecithin, all of which enable your body to build its cholesterol into valuable steroid hormones that help protect against disease.

Eggs are also the richest source of choline known, and they contain good quantities of biotin and also vitamins A, B₂, D, and E. Finally, they are a good source of the sulfur amino acids cystine and methionine, which appear to be important protective substances in warding off the aging process. Try to eat four to six eggs a week, but never eat *raw* egg white because the uncooked protein avidin it contains can block the absorption of the vitamin biotin.

Blackstrap Molasses

A tablespoonful of blackstrap molasses supplies as much calcium as a glass of milk, as much iron as nine eggs, more potassium than any other food, and the B-complex vitamins in good balance. It is an extraordinarily valuable food for women who tend to be anemic. The by-product of sugar refining, blackstrap molasses contains all the minerals, vitamins, and trace elements lost in the refining process that makes sugar such an empty food. Blackstrap molasses is also rich in magnesium, vitamin E, and copper. It is a great natural sweetener for yogurt, muesli, or drinks. A lot of skin troubles and hair problems respond to supplementing your diet with a tablespoonful of molasses a day. The taste varies greatly from one brand to another, so try them all until you find one that suits you. A cup of hot water into which you have squeezed the juice of half a lemon and added a tablespoon of molasses is an excellent way to start the day or a great pickup when you have been working long hours and need extra nutritional support.

Garlic

A powerful detoxicant, garlic, like onions, helps to clear fat accumulations from the blood vessels, lower cholesterol, and protect against bacterial and viral infections. This evil-smelling little bulb has been used throughout history for a variety of medicinal purposes. Recently research has established that many folk uses of garlic are much more than old wives' tales. Garlic plays two important roles in the prevention of aging. The first is to clear out wastes from the system and to render harmless toxic substances that can cause cell damage. (Garlic can even help clear dangerous heavy metals from the body.) The second is to lower serum cholesterol and therefore help protect against arteriosclerosis, one of the worst manifestations of aging. If you are offended by the taste of the stuff, you can buy tiny capsules of garlic oil from health food stores to swallow. They leave no aftertaste and don't affect your breath.

Kelp and Seaweed

Sea plants grow in mineral-rich seawater, which means that they contain a beautifully balanced combination of all minerals essential for life and health in an easily assimilable form. Kelp, or seaweed, is a superb source of iodine, which helps protect the body against the radioactivity in the atmosphere that contributes to early aging. It also strengthens hair and nails. Kelp is also rich in B-complex vitamins, vitamins D, E, and K, as well as magnesium and calcium. You can use it dried in soups, fresh in salads, or in the form of kelp tablets to supplement your diet (useful in dealing with many skin complaints). But be sure you take enough of them. The tablets are not concentrated; they are simply dehydrated seaweed, so you need to take six to eight of them after each meal for good results.

Wheat Germ

The heart of the wheat kernel, wheat germ is the richest known source of vitamin E. It is also rich in magnesium, copper, manganese, calcium, and phosphorus. And it is a superb source of protein to sprinkle on muesli or yogurt. But be sure to keep it refrigerated in a tightly closed container and if possible buy it in vacuum-packed tins, because the oil in it oxidizes rapidly and it can go rancid. And don't eat too much, for wheat germ is rich in fat: a tablespoonful a day is ideal.

Lecithin

High in phosphorus, lecithin joins with iodine, iron, and calcium in the body to give energy to the brain, and helps in the digestion and absorption of fat, apparently breaking up cholesterol so that it can pass through artery walls. It has also been shown to increase immunity to virus infections and help prevent gallstones. This natural constituent of every cell of the body is available in some foods such as egg yolk, soybeans, and corn. Supplementary lecithin comes in capsule, liquid, and granule forms. It is a good source of essential fatty acids and choline. Lecithin has some rather remarkable benefits for beauty and health when taken daily—say, sprinkled into yogurt or on a salad or simply taken from a spoon. It encourages the even distribution of body weight and helps to cleanse the liver and purify the kidneys. As a result, and also because of its choline and unsaturated fatty acid content, it is wonderful for skin. Lecithin is important in maintaining a healthy nervous system and vital to the resistance of stress-caused damage in the body. I would never let a day pass without taking a couple of tablespoons of the granular form.

Liver

A powerhouse of anti-stress vitamins and protein, liver also contains good amounts of trace elements and minerals such as potassium, sodium, and magnesium. It is a good source of phosphorus and sulfur amino acids —free-radical scavengers thought to help protect against radiation. They may also play a part in the repair of damaged cells. The B-complex content of liver recommends it to any woman suffering from fatigue, working under stress, or suffering from an illness. It can also improve the health of your hair. When these B-complex vitamins are undersupplied, emotional and physical troubles can develop as well as some of the most annoying beauty problems—falling hair, prematurely graying hair, and poor nails. Liver is also one of the richest sources of vitamin A, which is used successfully with zinc and the B vitamins in the treatment of many skin troubles including acne.

Yogurt

A fermented milk product that is a mixture of lactobacillus acidophilus and other bacteria, yogurt furnishes the helpful bacteria that keep the human intestine clean. The bacteria in yogurt are antagonistic to the putrefying bacteria that can cause toxicity in the body. This is one of the reasons yogurt is often useful in the treatment of skin disorders. It provides the B-complex vitamins, and it is richer in vitamins A and D than the milk from which it comes. Eating yogurt daily—as well as raw vegetables in salads or whole-grain foods—prevents hidden constipation, which is so detrimental not only to health but to beauty. It is a source of protein that is alkaline-forming in the body, so it is excellent for avoiding hyperacidity. It is best to make your own yogurt with powdered skimmed milk (see page 94), for the yogurt you buy commercially often has preservatives and flavorings added to it that interfere with its benefits. Fruit yogurts commercially made also contain a lot of sugar and many are too high in fat.

Brewer's Yeast

One of the best sources of B vitamins you can find, brewer's yeast contains seventeen vitamins, fourteen minerals, and sixteen amino acids. An excellent source of enzyme-producing agents, it is a nonlevening powder that you can add to juice, soups, and breads. It has a slightly bitter taste (some brands are more bitter than others), but you get used to this if you start off with only small quantities of the stuff stirred into a glass of juice (tomato and pineapple mix with it particularly well) and then gradually increase the amount. You can also get brewer's yeast in tablets but in this form it is much more expensive and you have to take quite a few tablets to get even a teaspoon of it. Although there are other foods that are higher in chromium, the chromium is more nutritionally available to your body in brewer's yeast than in any other food. Chromium is essential for the maintenance of good blood sugar levels. There is also evidence that brewer's yeast may contain a factor vital to the body's immune response and, therefore, to your ability to resist infections and diseases; also, brewer's yeast and wheat germ taken daily may aid the prevention of heart trouble. Because the ratio between calcium and phosphorus in brewer's yeast is high on the side of phosphorus, it is a good idea to mix the brewer's yeast with nonfat skimmed milk in a ratio of 4 tablespoons of dried milk to 1 tablespoon of brewer's yeast or to take a supplement containing calcium and magnesium with it.

Mixed Three Seeds

Pumpkin, sesame, and sunflower seeds ground in a blender or coffee grinder in equal proportions make a wonderful complete protein to sprinkle on yogurt, salads, or fruits. They are exceptionally rich in vitamins and have other qualities that make them excellent for hair and skin as well as overall health. They are all available in health food stores. You can grind a good quantity and then store them in the refrigerator. Pumpkin seeds are rich in B vitamins, phosphorus, iron, and zinc. They are known to have a strong antiparasitic ability, and some European nature-cure specialists believe that they contain plant hormones which directly improve the hormonal functions of human sex glands. Sesame seeds, which the Romans first used along with honey as emergency supplies for their soldiers, are rich in magnesium and potassium and have been used for generations to treat chronic fatigue, insomnia, and sexual dysfunctions. They are also very rich in calcium. In fact, they contain more calcium than either milk, cheese, or nuts. They are also a good source of vitamin E. Sunflower seeds are also high in vitamin E, containing an amazing 31 milligrams of the vitamin in each 3½-ounce serving. They have twice the iron of raisins, three times as much as cooked eggs. This makes them particularly useful for women. They too are rich in the B-complex vitamins and are especially high in magnesium and zinc. The pectin in sunflower seeds is said to help eliminate radioactive strontium. Mixed together, the three seeds are a wonderful source of the essential fatty acids.

CAN HEALTH AND BEAUTY SURVIVE
IN THE MODERN WORLD?

Of all the nutritional questions, "Do we need vitamin supplements?" is probably the most difficult to answer. Recently attention has been particularly drawn to it as reports come in from all over the world linking large doses of vitamins with the prevention and treatment of many serious illnesses such as schizophrenia, cancer, heart disease, diabetes, infectious diseases, and even premature aging. There is evidence that supplementary vitamins *can* help protect the human body from external environmental pollutants such as pesticides, harmful gases, smog, and cigarette smoke. Studies also show that extra vitamins and minerals may be helpful in guarding the body from the possible carcinogenic effects of food additives. Finally, and of great interest to a woman concerned about lasting fitness and good health, there is some evidence that vitamins may help retard the aging process.

YOU ARE BIOCHEMICALLY
AN INDIVIDUAL

But the main reason the question is hard to answer is simply how, short of obvious clinical symptoms of a particular vitamin deficiency, are you to know just *how much* of each vitamin is enough for you? There is no way to test adequately if a woman who feels generally well is getting enough of each vitamin she needs. Too, as biochemist Roger J. Williams has pointed out, each woman is an individual, not only in her physical and emotional makeup but also in her requirements for different nutrients. What is plenty of one vitamin—say, B_6—for one woman will be far too little for another whose endocrine system, digestive system, and stress level are very different.

Of course, there are always government tables. But minimum daily requirement tables are rather arbitrarily set and tend to vary greatly from one country to another. And although they are a fairly good indication of the amount of a specific vitamin you will need in order to avoid suffering the obvious clinical symptoms of deficiency disease associated with it—say, scurvy in the case of vitamin C or beri-beri from too little B_1—in no way do they give any indication of *optimum* levels of a vitamin needed to help keep you fit, well, and full of vitality, let alone to ensure that your skin does not age rapidly and your hair keeps its shine.

Certainly the most important factor in ensuring that you have adequate vitamins and minerals is your diet, day to day, year after year. The

Lifestyle Diet is excellent for this because it supplies the full complement of nutrients as they occur naturally in foods which are as unadulterated as possible; because it is both low in protein to help preserve the mineral balance in the body instead of promoting mineral loss; and because its low fat content reduces the body's need for certain nutrients such as vitamin E, which is important in the prevention of aging.

HOW MANY VITAMINS ARE ENOUGH?

But is the Lifestyle Diet all you need? It is a question that can only be answered individually. For some women yes, for others *probably* not—in which case vitamin supplements are necessary. The answer for you personally will depend on your age, your previous dietary habits, your general state of health, where you live in the world (in a polluted atmosphere or on top of a mountain), whether or not you take the Pill, and finally on your individual genetic makeup. Rigid recommendations from nutritionists or rules from government tables can only act as guidelines. And unless you are one of the fortunate few with a physician who understands the vital role nutrition plays in health and the prevention of aging, this is ultimately something you will have to decide for yourself. But it has to be a decision based on knowledge—knowledge of the functions and actions of the different nutrients, knowledge about which nutrients work together and which are antagonistic, knowledge about what role pollution, alcohol, drugs, and cigarettes play in using up your body's stores of nutrients, knowledge about how supplements may be useful in preventing the damage these cause, and finally an awareness of the specific effects on beauty that different vitamins, minerals, and combinations of both can have in alleviating a problem, whether it be skin eruptions or falling hair. Then you can decide for yourself.

My own personal answer to the vitamin supplement question is simple: "How do I look and feel?" There are periods in which all is well and the Lifestyle Diet itself appears to be all I need. During other periods—from, say, a couple of weeks to up to six months at a time—I will take different vitamin supplements for just as long as I feel I need them. I have always had a great respect for the French idea of a "cure," where you take something only for a limited period of time so that it acts as a stimulus to the organism but your body does not become dependent on it. I find this works well when it comes to vitamin supplements. Another thing I have found (and so has everyone else who has tried the Lifestyle Diet) is that the longer you remain on the low-fat, low-protein regimen with its high fiber and large quantities of fresh vegetables, the less you feel the need for supplements. It appears that your system gradually rebalances itself so that they are no longer necessary. But of course they are always there when I want them—for instance, under periods of particular stress or when I'm traveling in an area where the air pollution is bad or the food available to me is poor, or when my hair suddenly begins to lose its luster. In fact, there is quite a science to the use of food supplements and it is important to know very well what is good for what, how to mix—and *not* to mix—vitamin and mineral supplements, and how to avoid mistakes. We will be looking at all this, but first let's examine an aspect of modern life that poses a serious threat to any woman's health and beauty: environmental pollution. Then let's take a look at the process of aging itself. Both are intimately connected with vitamin and mineral balances in the body. And in both areas the use of food supplements can be useful in helping to maintain that balance.

POLLUTION BRINGS PROBLEMS

Our air is polluted by an enormous number of toxic substances. They include poisonous gases such as sulfur dioxide, nitrogen dioxide, carbon monoxide, and ozone, as well as smoke and particles of solid matter such as lead dust and other heavy metals. Our drinking water contains detergents, chemical salts, pesticides, fertilizers, and radioactive wastes from power plants. They also have residues of heavy metals and human wastes. Our agricultural lands have been sprayed with thousands of pesticides and fungicides, weed destroyers and other toxic agents, some of which we eat directly, others of which are taken into the bodies of the animals that we then consume. Of course, the fact that our air and water are polluted and becoming more so all the time is no news to anyone. But the important questions now are:
1. How exactly does pollution affect health and the aging process in the long run? and
2. What, if anything, can we do to help protect ourselves from it? That's where extra vitamins and minerals may come in.
Researchers studying the effects of various pollutants on animals and humans have little doubt that they contribute greatly to the development of some diseases, particularly respiratory ailments (such as asthma, bronchitis, and even chest colds), cardiovascular diseases, and eye troubles. Pollution from gasoline fumes alone has a significantly detrimental effect on health. For three months during the fuel shortage a few years ago, researchers in the United States counted the number of deaths from heart and lung diseases and compared them with figures for the same three months the preceding year. Even though only 10 percent less gasoline

had been available for cars during the period, deaths from cardiovascular disease had fallen by 17 percent.

Another pollutant that is causing concern is ozone. Nowadays, in many areas, ozone levels are even used as a measure of general pollution in the atmosphere. Relatively new to public attention, ozone is a kind of oxygen with three atoms to a molecule instead of the usual two. It is a strange substance which in terms of animal life seems to be both hero and villain. In its helpful aspect it forms an invisible protective layer fifteen to twenty miles above the earth which shields us from the otherwise lethal amounts of ultraviolet radiation from the sun, and which environmentalists are, therefore, anxious to preserve and protect.

The villainous face of ozone, which is probably the most toxic constituent of city smog, is that of an unstable gas which poisons the air, hinders the activity of some important enzymes in the body, and can produce chest pains, headaches, coughing, and eye and heart problems. It also causes harm to plant life, damages tires and buildings, makes fabrics disintegrate and, like most of the other pollutants, damages skin by altering its electrical charge, interfering with its respiration, and changing the qualities of its protective acid mantle, thereby making it more susceptible to external aggression.

SMOG MAKES YOU LOOK OLDER

Some researchers, such as Dr. Daniel Menzel at Duke University, also believe that ozone, like many other and wider-known pollutants, encourages aging, since it is an oxidizing agent that promotes breakdown on a cellular level. Like soot, coal dust, cigarette smoke, and noxious chemicals, it is probably high on the list of causes of premature wrinkles and loss of skin tone, quite apart from its known detrimental effects on the lungs and the body as a whole. To petrochemicals and ozone one could add dozens of other classifications of pollutants to which our bodies are being dangerously exposed day after day as they have never been before throughout the history of the world. The specific long-term effects of these substances cannot be known, for we have no way of studying them in isolation. What is known is that breathing polluted air and drinking polluted water taxes your body's supply of vitamins A, C, and E as well as some of the B-complex vitamins, and also tends to upset its mineral balance while also making it prone to collect poisonous heavy metals, such as lead, aluminum, and mercury, in the tissues. And what is also becoming increasingly apparent is that supplementing the diet with some of these nutrients which become used up in the process of dealing with day-to-day pollution appears to have protective capabilities. Menzel, for instance, has found that vitamin E, which is a natural antioxidant, is helpful in counteracting the effect of both ozone and nitrogen dioxide (another constituent of smog). He believes that most people need supplements of 100 international units of the vitamin a day. In experiments where animals were exposed to lethal doses of ozone, those animals receiving vitamin E survived 50 percent longer than the unprotected group. Other studies have shown vitamin E to be good insurance against the ravages of X-ray radiation.

Among their other actions, air pollutants such as ozone directly oxidize lung tissues. This results in a decrease of the body's ability to extract oxygen from the air, and can eventually lead to disease. The antioxidant vitamin E helps protect against this oxidization. Another thing pollutants do is destroy the vitamin A in lung tissue that is required for the health of a mucous membrane. When your lungs are deficient in vitamin A their first line of defense against carcinogens is threatened. Supplementary vitamin E can help keep this from happening by protecting the stores of vitamin A in lung tissue.

Two other researchers, Dr. Fred R. Klenner in the United States and Dr. Walter Blumer in Switzerland, have found that another antioxidant, vitamin C, used either on its own or together with calcium supplements, will go a long way toward detoxifying poisons that have entered into the body either from drug taking or environmental pollution of one kind or another. This may be because vitamin C is capable of increasing the activity of enzymes that are responsible for detoxifying the liver. It seems to attack chemical pollutants in the body similarly to the way our own antibodies fight off infections. Vitamin C also helps detoxify heavy metals such as lead, cadmium, and mercury and appears to offer useful protection against the potentially cancer-causing nitrates that have infiltrated our drinking water as a result of a long-term use of chemical fertilizers on our farmlands.

FIBER PROTECTS

Natural fiber or roughage appears to have a protective factor too that goes far beyond its recognized ability to ensure that wastes from digestion are quickly and efficiently eliminated. Researchers have reported that dietary fiber appears to remove radioactive strontium from the body and to help flush out several heavy pollutants such as lead and cadmium. A high fiber diet has been shown to protect animals from developing tumors after being bombarded by radiation and greatly to moderate the harmful effects of large doses of sodium cyclamate (the chemical sweetener) as well as to render harmless large doses of the artificial food coloring Red Dye No. 2. Finally, two of the B-complex vitamins, riboflavin and nicotinic acid, and the trace element selenium (which occurs naturally in eggs, brewer's yeast, bran, wheat germ, cabbage, tomatoes, and tuna fish) are also believed to be helpful in guarding the body against the harmful effects of pollution.

THE QUESTION OF AGING

Sleek, shining hair, youthful skin, a well-shaped body, and the unmistakable energy that marks a beautiful woman no matter what her age are not accidents of nature. They depend on care. They also depend on protection. For aging is no longer considered an inevitable consequence of the passage of time. How quickly and how badly you age depend not only on your genetic makeup but also on how you live and what kind of attack you are exposed to in terms of stress, environmental pollution, and wrong nutrition, all of which help bring about aging on a cellular level.

The aging process itself is not completely understood. But scientists are in agreement that the foundation of the aging process lies in the individual cells themselves, which in turn make up the tissues, organs, and systems of the body. At cell level two important things happen as you get older. First, there is a disruption of the DNA and RNA—the systems in your cells which are responsible for preserving and reconstructing genetic information for growth, synthesis of new proteins, and reproduction. Second, there is a progressive tendency for more cells to die than your body is able to replace.

Radiation is one cause of these things (and one of the reasons lying in the sun causes the skin to age rapidly). The genetic material, the DNA with its chromosomes, needs to remain intact in order for cells to reproduce themselves accurately. Radiant energy penetrating the cell membrane can result in the formation of "free radicals." These are highly reactive molecular groups that combine with the DNA enzymes or cell membranes and cause damage, particularly to the chromosomes so that the whole genetic record of the cell becomes distorted.

But free radicals are not only the result of radiant energy, they are also produced by the interaction of oxygen with polyunsaturated fats, which results in formation of semistable peroxides that are in turn destructive to body proteins. When chromosomes are damaged either by free radicals or chemical reactions, some of the genetic information carried by the DNA is lost so that either the life of the cell itself is endangered or vital cell functions are impaired. This in turn leads to a further mis-synthesis of protein in the making of new cells and creates "clinkers" that interfere with the normal immunological reactions and use up important nutrients needed for other things in the body, as well as strangling the life in cells with waste material.

The whole process is not yet completely understood, but what is known is that protection from radiation and from other factors which bring about alterations in the genetic material is an important part of any program for preserving youth and beauty. Experimentally, one of the most successful ways to slow down the aging process has been to destroy the free radicals before they can produce their multiplicity of harmful reactions.

Another phenomenon in aging is the formation of "cross-linkage" of molecules, where neighboring molecules are chemically joined by a bridge or bond between an atom of one and an atom of the other. Well-known age researcher Johan Bjorksten has studied this cross-linkage phenomenon and pointed out that "Many of these cross-linked molecules lead to agglomerates which cannot be broken down by any body enzyme, but will increase in the cell and gradually crowd out other constituents, thereby causing a continual decline in the cell's activity and ability to cope with stress."

Certainly, cross-linking is an important phenomenon in the aging of the skin. Collagen, a protein that makes up 30 percent of the body's total protein and that is largely responsible for giving young skin its resilience and muscles their firmness, is particularly vulnerable to cross-linking. When collagen fibers start to cross-link and to bind together, wrinkles form and the body loses its firm curves and perfect shape. Whatever can be done to neutralize the effect of free radicals and thereby protect the genetic material of cells, or to inhibit the process of cross-linking, will also help to preserve skin and body shape and hold back the rate of aging.

RADIATION PROTECTORS AND ANTIOXIDANTS

In animal experiments many things have been tried. Researchers have found, for instance, that a combination of radiation absorbers and antioxidants such as vitamins E and C, which are scavengers for free radicals and deactivate them, can significantly prolong lives. Several researchers, including Denham Harman, Alex Comfort, and Richard Passwater, have significantly increased the lifespan of mice by feeding them antioxidants. Passwater believes that collagen, which is highly subject to cross-linking as a result of free radical attack, can to some degree be protected from the destructive aging process by supplements of vitamin E to neutralize the effect of the free radicals and vitamin C to promote the health and growth of collagen. Another leading gerontologist, Bernard Strehler, also believes that antioxidants can play an important role. As far back as ten years ago he was saying, "Autooxidation appears to play a key role in aging; experiments have shown a striking increase in the longevity of laboratory animals whose diet was supplemented with antioxidants such as BHT [a preservative used in food]. The natural antioxidant vitamin E also seems to be important in the maintenance of cellular function. There appears to be little reason to doubt that the judicious use and development of dietary supplements and restriction of calorie intake to optimum levels will add significantly to healthy life expectancy."

Other researchers have found that vitamin E will prolong the lifespan of cells by reducing damage to them. And although by no means all researchers accept that vitamin E has a role to play in slowing down the aging process in humans, there is already enough evidence to make any woman concerned with the problem of aging sit up and take notice.

Where the antioxidant vitamin E appears to work particularly on the fat-based membranes of the body, vitamin C works on its water-based fluids. It enhances vitamin E's protective abilities and helps protect the body from damage due to environmental poisons. Smoking robs the system of vitamin C at an estimated rate of 25 milligrams of the vitamin per cigarette and is consequently one of the skin's worst agers. A group of researchers studying longevity recently found that the women studied who ate diets rich in vitamin C lived longer. There is considerable evidence that supplements of vitamin C plus a diet high in raw fruits and vegetables are of help in preserving skin from premature aging. (More about this in the section on skin.)

The second challenge in retarding aging, and one which as yet has had little experimental success, is that of not only *inhibiting* mis-synthesis of protein and damage to the cells' material as may be possible with antioxidants, but also of finding a way of *repairing* proteins already mis-synthesized. Passwater believes that these nutrients spur the breakdown of wrongly made proteins into their component parts, which then become nourishment for the cells' undamaged DNA. He also believes that selenium and vitamin E together act as a stimulus to the body's immune system which may help destroy the aged cells that interfere with the body's proper functioning.

Passwater singles out five nutrients he thinks are particularly important in retarding the aging process and helping to protect the genetic material of cells and perhaps correcting damage: vitamin E, vitamin C, the B complex, selenium, and the sulfur amino acids, which are found in eggs, cabbage, muscle meats, and onions. But in its own way each nutrient, each vitamin and mineral, has a contribution to make. Let's look at them in detail and see what they do.

VITAMINS

Vitamins are organic substances that occur only in living things. There are about twenty of them so far known to be essential for human growth and the maintenance of health. Each is present to varying degrees in specific foods. With a few exceptions, vitamins are substances your body cannot make for itself. They have to be taken in through the foods you eat. Although they have no energy value, they are essential constituents of enzymes, the catalysts on which almost all metabolic processes in the body depend. They also help form bones and tissues, convert fat and carbohydrate into energy, and regulate metabolism. And they can play a vital—and often underestimated—role in keeping a woman well, youthful-looking, and emotionally balanced.

There are two different types of vitamins: water-soluble and fat-soluble. The water-soluble vitamins are usually measured in milligrams. They include the B-complex vitamins, vitamin C, and the bioflavonoids. They are not stored in the body, so they need to be taken daily in your food. Any excess you take in of these water-soluble vitamins—any extra that your body doesn't need—is simply eliminated as waste.

The fat-soluble vitamins, which include A, D, E, and K, are usually measured in international units, each unit representing the amount of the substance necessary to bring about a specific change in the state of health of a laboratory animal. Because they are oil-soluble, they are stored in the body. Excessive amounts of some of these vitamins in the body—particularly vitamin A—may result in toxicity.

Many studies have been done to try to establish vitamin requirements according to sex, age, and physical condition such as pregnancy or illness. Most governments have published recommended daily amounts which are believed to be adequate to meet the nutritional needs of healthy individuals living in temperate climates. But recommended amounts of many vitamins vary considerably from one table to another and even from one decade to the next. The human requirements of other nutrients has not even been established yet. And the amount of a particular nutrient *you* need, not only to keep you in optimum health but even to keep you free of obvious clinical symptoms, is difficult to determine.

Specific vitamin needs vary tremendously from one woman to the next because of biochemical individuality as well as age, changes in climate, your sex, your general state of health, and the environment in which you live. And although science has been able to establish approximate amounts of some of the specific nutrients that will keep a human being from suffering the obvious symptoms of deficiency disease (vitamin C for scurvy, thiamine for beri-beri, or vitamin D for rickets), this amount does not necessarily represent the ideal necessary to keep one in optimum health, to protect against premature aging, and to ensure mental balance.

Also, the amount of any specific vitamin you take in through your foods or in the form of nutritional supplements will not necessarily be the amount of vitamin available for your body's use. Often absorption problems in the digestive system or an insufficiency of another nutrient on which the use of one vitamin or mineral is dependent will result in a vitamin's being wasted.

The subject of vitamin and megavitamin therapy is an extremely complex one which, for the sake of lasting health and beauty, is worthwhile investigating in depth. For a vitamin or mineral supplement or two can often make the difference between smooth, unlined skin and a face that is aging rapidly, between high reserves of energy and chronic fatigue, or between thick, glossy hair and constantly splitting tresses. To get the maximum benefits from vitamins and minerals, it is important to familiarize yourself with them, their health and beauty benefits, how they are absorbed, stored, and how they interact with other nutrients, signs and symptoms of deficiency, and what dosages have been found useful. That is why I've included information about specific vitamins in some detail— so one can get to know them and will have a source of quick reference when it is needed.

The quantities given are, of course, not prescriptive. They have merely been reported in studies as being useful. Individual demands and tolerances vary tremendously from person to person and from time to time. A few of the dosages of some of the vitamins which have shown themselves to be beneficial can be very high. If ever you take large quantities of any specific nutrient, you should first consult a doctor who has been trained and who understands the principles of nutritional therapy.

Vitamin A

An important anti-stress vitamin, vitamin A is intimately involved in all the body's repair and growth processes. A susceptibility to infection can result from insufficient vitamin A. So can a thickening of the cornea of the eye. Called xerophthalmia, this condition can result in an inability to see at night, styes in the eyes, burning, itching, inflamed eyes, poor night vision, and even ulceration and blindness, as well as frequent fatigue, loss of smell, skin blemishes, and softening of bones and teeth. When there is a deficiency of vitamin A, vitamin C depletion will also result. Rough, dry skin and prematurely aging skin are all signs of a vitamin A deficiency. Therapeutic doses of A have been used to correct and prevent acne, maintain smooth, young-looking skin, and protect from infection. Also to correct excessively oily hair and skin. Sufficient vitamin E and D and adequate zinc are necessary for proper absorption and use of A, which plays a large part in the health of eyes and bones.

RECOMMENDED DAILY ALLOWANCE (RDA): 5,000 iu.
THERAPEUTIC DOSE: 50,000 iu. Up to 200,000 for short periods under supervision.
SOURCES: Green and yellow vegetables (spinach, cabbage, carrots), eggs, fish-liver oils, liver.

B-complex Vitamins

Occurring in whole grains, liver, brewer's yeast, wheat germ, the three seeds, and blackstrap molasses, the B complex is essential for brain and nervous system health. The B vitamins also help keep skin healthy and hair lustrous, and ensure proper metabolism of carbohydrates and fats. Drugs, pollution, estrogen, alcohol, nicotine, stress, physical and mental fatigue, and sugar all use up the B vitamins and increase one's need for them. A deficiency in the B group often leads to chronic fatigue, irritability, indigestion, depression and insomnia as well as falling hair, skin troubles, anemia, constipation, acne, and prematurely graying hair. In nature the B-complex vitamins always occur together. If you take any single B vitamin, you need to take it together with the complete group either by eating foods rich in them or by taking a natural full B supplement. The B complex is more effective when taken with vitamins C and E, calcium and phosphorus. Let's take a look at each B vitamin separately.

SOURCES: Made in the body. Also from raw fruits and vegetables, whole grains, liver, and brewer's yeast.

VITAMIN B₁ (THIAMINE)

Called the "morale vitamin," B₁ aids digestion, supports good muscle tone in the heart, alleviates fatigue, and has been useful in the treatment of stress and alcoholism. It is important for stamina and mental alertness. Helps prevent premature aging.

RDA: 1.4 mg for men; 1 mg for women.
THERAPEUTIC DOSE: 75–500 mg.
SOURCES: Whole-grain cereals, blackstrap molasses, liver, pork, fresh green vegetables, potatoes, brewer's yeast, beans.

VITAMIN B₂ (RIBOFLAVIN)

Essential to the breakdown and use of carbohydrates, fats, and proteins, this vitamin is also important for cell respiration and tissue maintenance. It is also essential for healthy hair, skin, and nails, and to protect adrenal glands from stress damage. A B_2 deficiency is probably the most common vitamin deficiency in the industrialized world. Too little B_2 can result in scaling around nose and forehead, hair loss, vaginal itching, oily skin, cracks and sores around mouth corners, and itchy eyes that are oversensitive to light. Acne rosacea has cleared up by taking B_2 with each meal. Oily skin, whiteheads, and blackheads have also been cured with it. Because of its role in cellular oxidation, B_2 helps prevent premature aging.

RDA: 1.6 for adults.
THERAPEUTIC DOSE: 50–200 mg.
SOURCES: Milk, brewer's yeast, organ meats (liver and kidney), fish, nuts, green leafy vegetables and legumes. Wheat germ.

NIACIN

A coenzyme, niacin breaks down proteins, fats, and carbohydrates for use. It improves circulation, is essential to brain metabolism, and has been used in high doses to treat schizophrenia and other mental disorders. Deficiencies can result in digestive problems, bad breath, fatigue, skin problems, and abnormal skin pigmentation. Niacin has been used to clear up acne and other skin problems, to relieve arthritis pain, and to treat circulatory problems. The niacin form of the vitamin causes temporary flushing or itching of the skin when taken in large doses. The nicotinamide form does not. The flushing is of no medical importance.

RDA: 1.8 for men; 13 mg for women.
THERAPEUTIC DOSE: 100–3,000 mg. Large doses of niacin are usually given with equal doses of vitamin C—usually 2,000 mg of each.
SOURCES: Nuts, fish, poultry, whole-grain cereal, soybeans, brewer's yeast, organ meats (liver, kidney).

PANTOTHENIC ACID

An adrenal stimulant, pantothenic acid increases the body's ability to withstand stress and decreases toxicity of many drugs, as well as protecting against radiation damage to cells. It is important for health and the maintenance of strong nerves and good skin. It acts as a coenzyme in utilization of other nutrients and in energy production from food. It has been shown to improve mental processes when given in therapeutic doses, to correct enzymic disturbances present in allergic reactions and digestive problems, and to help prevent premature aging and wrinkles. More pantothenic acid is needed during illness, stress, and prolonged fatigue.

RDA: 0.5–10 mg.
THERAPEUTIC DOSE: 50–1,000 mg.
SOURCES: Whole-grain cereals, legumes, organ meat (liver and kidneys), eggs, brewer's yeast.

VITAMIN B$_6$ (PYRIDOXINE)

Important to the formation of collagen and elastin, as well as DNA and RNA in the cells, truly adequate quantities of B$_6$ may also help prevent premature aging. Stretch marks are often a sign of a B$_6$ and zinc deficiency. Therapeutic doses of B$_6$ improve many beauty problems such as eczema, acne, dandruff, thinning hair, tiny wrinkles around the mouth (although these are slow to improve), and water retention. B$_6$ is also useful for premenstrual tension. If you are on the Pill you should always take B$_6$ supplements as well as B$_2$, zinc, B$_{12}$, folic acid, and vitamin C.

RDA: 1.8 mg for men; 1.5 mg for women.
THERAPEUTIC DOSE: 50–1,000 mg. It is useful to balance B$_6$ with the same quantity of B$_2$ because B$_2$ is necessary for the use of B$_6$ in the body. B$_6$ and zinc often work together.
SOURCES: Liver, fish, lean muscle meats, whole grains, bananas, peas, brown rice, brewer's yeast, sunflower seeds, milk, peanuts, hazelnuts.

VITAMIN B$_{12}$ (CYANOCOBALAMIN)

B$_{12}$ plays a primary role in the synthesis of nucleic acid—the DNA and RNA in the cells—and therefore is probably related to the prevention of premature aging. As it is involved in the production of red blood cells, it is called the antianemia vitamin. It also helps metabolize proteins, fats, and carbohydrates. Deficiencies produce fatigue, poor concentration, and mental depression. The vitamin is useful in treatment of osteoarthritis, osteoporosis, and pernicious anemia, particularly when used with iron, vitamin C, and folic acid. It also relieves poor memory, depression, and insomnia.

RDA: 3 mcg for adults.
THERAPEUTIC DOSE: 75 mcg–1,000 mcg.
SOURCES: Yeast, wheat germ, organ meat (liver and kidneys), meat, milk, sardines, oysters, egg yolks, cheese, salmon, herring, clams.

THE FORGOTTEN FIVE: BIOTIN, CHOLINE, INOSITOL, FOLIC ACID, AND PABA

These five B-complex vitamins are often neglected and even left out of inexpensive commercial vitamin supplements, probably because inositol and biotin are commercially scarce and expensive. But all five are as important for health and beauty as the rest, and some of them have particularly vital roles to play.

BIOTIN

A coenzyme involved in nutrient and food metabolism, biotin is sometimes called vitamin H. It is needed in all the cells of the body for healthy skin, hair, sebaceous glands, sex glands, bone marrow, and nerves. Antibiotics and sulfa drugs can seriously disrupt manufacture of biotin in the intestines, as can eating raw egg whites. Grayish skin, depression, anemia, muscular pains, and disturbances in fat metabolism can be biotin deficiency signs.

Seborrheic dermatitis has been cleared up by giving biotin. It has also been used to clear up pale ashen skin and various kinds of dermatitis, and is useful in the treatment of balding.

RDA: 300 mcg usually meets needs; no RDA.
THERAPEUTIC DOSE: 100–300 mcg. When choosing a multiple B-complex supplementary formula, the amount of biotin in a tablet is often a good indication of its value. It should range somewhere between 20 and 60 mcg per tablet in a high potency formula.
SOURCES: Liver, brown rice, nuts, eggs, fish, whole grains, brewer's yeast, beans, peanuts.

CHOLINE

Important in the use of fats in the body, in the health of the nerves' myelin sheaths, and to protect the liver from fat accumulations and prevent gallstones, choline also plays a large part in the development of the immune system and therefore, along with folic acid and B_{12}, aids lifelong protection against disease. Choline has successfully been used to reduce high blood pressure, improve a fatty liver, and restore natural coloring to prematurely gray hair. It is used by the adrenals to make adrenalin, cortisone, and sex hormones.

RDA: None.
Average diet yields 500–900 mcg per day.
THERAPEUTIC DOSE: 500–1,000 mg.
SOURCES: Lecithin, brewer's yeast, liver.

INOSITOL

Eczema, hair loss, high serum cholesterol levels, and constipation may all be signs of inositol deficiency. The vitamin is important in fat metabolism, in preventing fatty buildup in arteries, and for brain cells as well as the health of the eye. Therapeutically, it has been used in the treatment of nerve damage in some kinds of muscular dystrophy, in eliminating fatty deposits in the liver, stopping hair loss, and lowering blood cholesterol.

RDA: None.
THERAPEUTIC DOSE: 500–1,000 mg. Supplements of inositol should be balanced with equal choline. A good B-complex multiple vitamin should contain between 10 and 500 mg per tablet.

SOURCES: Lecithin, blackstrap molasses, brewer's yeast, brown rice, legumes, liver, whole grains, beef heart.

FOLIC ACID

Folic acid works together with B_{12} and C as a coenzyme to metabolize proteins. It helps prevent mental illness and some forms of anemia and, because it is directly concerned with synthesis of nucleic acids such as DNA, is probably important in prevention of premature aging. Stress, surgery, and shock all increase your need for the vitamin. So does taking the Pill. Therapeutic doses have been used, together with pantothenic acid and PABA, to prevent hair turning gray, and to treat various nail problems, menstrual problems, some forms of anemia, and gastric ulcers.

RDA: 400 mcg for adults.
THERAPEUTIC DOSE: 0.5–5 mg.
SOURCES: Brewer's yeast, liver, leafy green vegetables, kale, asparagus, endive, turnips, spinach, bran.

PABA

Another coenzyme in protein metabolism and in the making of red blood cells, Para-aminobenzoic acid (PABA) also plays a large role in maintaining the health of the skin and the condition and color of hair. With folic acid and pantothenic acid, it has reversed the graying of hair. It is also used to treat some skin disorders such as vitiligo and, when used externally, to protect skin from sunburn and premature wrinkling. Sulfa drugs can cause deficiency. (Deficiency signs can be nervousness, headache, digestive problems, fatigue, and constipation.) PABA also helps prevent skin aging.

RDA: None.
THERAPEUTIC DOSE: 50–1,000 mg.
SOURCES: Liver, eggs, brown rice, wheat germ, brewer's yeast, blackstrap molasses.

OTHER B VITAMINS

Research turns up other B vitamins that may also have specific effects on health and beauty. The three most recent are B_{13} (orotic acid), used in Europe in the treatment of multiple sclerosis, B_{15} (pangamic acid), and B_{17} (laetrile). B_{15} is able to eliminate hypoxia, or insufficient oxygen supply to human cells, which is associated with degenerative illness and aging, and with alcoholism. Many athletes claim it has helped them perform better. B_{17} is used as an anticancer treatment. It is said to single out and attack and destroy the cancer cells. Toxicity levels of the vitamin have not been established, but it is generally accepted that 1,000 mg doses are all that should be given at any one time.

RDA B_{15}: None.
THERAPEUTIC DOSE B_{15}: 100 mg.
SOURCES B_{15}: Whole grains, pumpkin seeds, sesame seeds, brewer's yeast.

RDA B_{17}: None.
THERAPEUTIC DOSE B_{17}: 50 mg–1,000 mg.
SOURCES B_{17}: Apples, cherries, peaches, apricots, seeds.

Vitamin C

Probably the most important nutrient of all when it comes to protecting and preserving health and beauty, vitamin C is a natural antioxidant. It plays an important role in maintaining healthy collagen, preventing aging and skin wrinkling, easy bruising, and broken veins under the skin. It also protects the body against damaging effects of pollution, helps prevent colds, coronary heart disease, and swollen and painful joints, and counteracts the toxic effects of drugs. It is an important anti-stress vitamin. It also detoxifies heavy metals in the body such as lead, and even helps remove poisons such as DDT. Therapeutic doses of the vitamin have been used to treat many skin complaints such as eczema, burns, psoriasis, shingles, herpes simplex, acne, boils, and impetigo, as well as to retard the aging process.

RDA: 45 mg for adults.
THERAPEUTIC DOSE: 1,000 to 15,000 mg.
SOURCES: Citrus fruits, tomatoes, raw green vegetables, rose hips, strawberries, potatoes, broccoli, spinach.

BIOFLAVONOIDS

Brightly colored substances including citrin, rutin, flavones, hesperidin, and flavonals, the bioflavonoids occur naturally in foods containing vitamin C and enhance its actions. Strengthening blood vessel walls, preventing and healing capillary breakage in skin, protecting the body from infections, varicose veins, bleeding gums, and severe bruising, and increasing vitamin C's ability to preserve collagen. The bioflavonoids are useful in the treatment of eczema, radiation sickness, and hypertension.

RDA: None.
THERAPEUTIC DOSE: 100 mg upward.
SOURCES: With vitamin C in fruits and vegetables.

Vitamin D

Essential for health and growth of bones and in the metabolic functions directly related to the heart, nervous system, and eyes, vitamin D is important in the absorption of calcium from foods and in the assimilation of phosphorus. It is useful in repairing osteomalacia, preventing tooth decay, and, along with vitamin A, in reducing the incidence of colds. It prevents rickets in children.

RDA: 400 iu for adults.
THERAPEUTIC DOSE: 400 iu–1,500 iu.
SOURCES: Fish liver oils, tuna, salmon, egg yolks.

Vitamin E

Like vitamin C, vitamin E is a natural antioxidant. This is why, with vitamin C and zinc, it forms what is probably the most effective nutritional trio for preserving youth and beauty you will find anywhere. Its antioxidant properties help protect the cells from damage and genetic mutation caused by the formation of peroxides in the breakdown of polyunsaturated fats. E also helps protect the B-complex vitamins and vitamin C from oxidation and destruction in the body. It plays an important part in cell respiration, is needed for the formation of new cells, the production of pituitary, adrenal, and sex hormones, and the reconstruction of damaged tissue inside and outside the body. A deficiency of the vitamin can result in fragile red blood cells which easily rupture, in shrinkage of collagen in the skin which leads to wrinkling and muscle wasting, and to abnormal deposits of fat. E encourages the use of iron. Underactivity of the adrenal glands and the pituitary can be another sign of an E deficiency. Its health and beauty benefits are long: prevention and counteraction of premature aging (when used both internally and applied on the skin), stimulation of skin cell metabolism, healing of burns and cuts to prevent scarring, calming itchy dry skin, treating varicose veins (it can dissolve fresh clots and prevent new ones from forming), and treatment of female complaints from alleviating hot flashes to regulating menstrual flow. The vitamin also appears to protect against virus-caused illnesses and is useful in the treatment of damaged liver.

RDA: 15 iu for men; 12 iu for women.
THERAPEUTIC DOSE: 200 to 5,000 iu. Precautions: high doses are not given to sufferers from high blood pressure, rheumatic heart disease, or overactive thyroid. Then small amounts are given (approximately 30 mg a day for a month) and then increased gradually.
SOURCES: Wheat germ, seeds, cold pressed vegetable oils, green leafy vegetables, whole grains.

Vitamin F

This is the name given to a group of unsaturated fatty acids. The body cannot manufacture the essential unsaturated fatty acids: linoleic, linolenic, and arachidonic, so they must be obtained from food. They help reduce excessive cholesterol and prevent heart disease and arteriosclerosis. Needed for the health of skin and mucous membranes, they are essential for healthy gland function, and are particularly important for adrenals and thyroid. A deficiency can cause brittle and lusterless hair, nail problems, dandruff, and allergies as well as acne, eczema, and dry skin.

RDA: None; 10 percent of daily calories: men need five times more than women.
THERAPEUTIC DOSE: Obtained from foods.
SOURCES: Wheat germ, seeds, safflower, sunflower, and corn oil. Cod liver oil and lecithin are the best sources of vitamin F.

Vitamin K

Important for liver functions, needed for blood clotting, gives energy to cells. Importance for longevity. If you eat yogurt, acidophilus culture, and kefir, your body is probably able to make all you need.

RDA: None.
THERAPEUTIC DOSE: 300–500 mcg is considered adequate.
SOURCES: Yogurt, eggs, blackstrap molasses, fish liver oil, milk.

MINERALS CAN BE BEAUTIFUL

As well as protein, complex carbohydrates, essential fatty acids, and fiber, your body needs minerals and trace minerals—crystalline chemical elements and compounds such as zinc, chromium, manganese, magnesium, calcium, selenium, and sulfur. Although only 4 or 5 percent of the weight of your body is mineral matter, minerals are essential to your mental and physical well-being. They are important in the formation and maintenance of soft tissues, muscle, blood, and nerve cells. They also act to maintain the life processes, to preserve the vitality of the heart and brain, muscles and nerves, and to keep the skeletal system strong. Like some of the vitamins, they act as catalysts for many biochemical reactions including nerve transmission, the utilization of other nutrients from foods, digestion, and the production of important hormones. They also help to maintain the delicate water balance and the proper relationship between acidity and alkalinity on which the health of the body depends.

Most minerals have no established minimum dose or recommended

daily requirement. Some, such as calcium, phosphorus, potassium, magnesium, and sodium, are called macrominerals because they are needed in
fairly high amounts. Others, such as zinc, cadmium, manganese, selenium,
iron, iodine, and sulfur, are known as the micronutrients or trace elements. They are found in the body only in the most minute amounts,
measured in micrograms. Although minerals, like vitamins, are needed
for life, these micronutrients or trace elements are particularly important
to health and beauty—far more than you might imagine.

The minerals are generally less well known than the vitamins, although
the roles they play in health and beauty are equally important. Mineral
deficiencies are often the hidden causes of hair and skin troubles such as
stretch marks (zinc and B_6 deficiencies), acne, and early wrinkling, as
well as mood changes and a variety of other common miseries, from
premenstrual tension to diabetes and serious illness. Recent studies show
that even so-called well-fed people in the West often suffer serious mineral imbalances and deficiencies. Among women, the most common are
deficiencies of zinc, chromium, and manganese. Also, the presence of
heavy metals and toxic minerals in the atmosphere, water, and food tends
to deplete our bodies of the minerals we need, and our soil is also becoming progressively depleted in many of the vital minerals. This makes it
more imperative than ever to familiarize yourself with the major minerals, with what they do and how they have shown themselves to be useful in treating health and beauty problems.

Calcium

The body's most abundant mineral, calcium is needed every day for all
the vital functions of the body: for growth and the formation and health
of bones and teeth, as well as to protect the health of the heart and muscles. It is a very calming mineral that speeds healing and helps protect
against pollution. It helps the body use iron and helps regulate the passage of nutrients through cell walls. Calcium acts as a natural tranquilizer, helps prevent premenstrual problems, and, with vitamin A, helps
keep skin healthy. A high intake of calcium may protect against harmful
effects of radiation in the atmosphere and offset premature aging.

RDA: 800–1,400 mg depending on age.
THERAPEUTIC DOSE: 1,000–1,500 mg.
SOURCES: Milk, yogurt, cheese, whole grains, green leafy vegetables, kelp,
watercress, sardines, nuts, sprouted grains and seeds.

Copper

Needed for the synthesis of RNA and for the formation of elastin, an
important component of muscle and skin fiber, copper is also important

in healing and in preserving the natural color of hair. Because of the widespread use of copper water pipes and the relatively low levels of zinc in our foods (copper and zinc are antagonists), a deficiency of copper seldom exists. When choosing a multimineral supplement it is best to look for one without copper, because too much copper and too little zinc can lead to allergic problems and mental symptoms.

RDA: 2 mg for adults.
THERAPEUTIC DOSE: Seldom needed.
SOURCES: Liver, seafood, yeast, kelp, heart, brains, whole grains.

Chromium

Plays an important part in the regulation of blood sugar and therefore the avoidance of fatigue in the body. This is why it is often called the glucose tolerance factor. Deficiencies of chromium are widespread in the West. It also appears to inhibit the formation of aortic plaque. A deficiency may contribute to arteriosclerosis.

RDA: None.
THERAPEUTIC DOSE: 3 mg.
SOURCES: Brewer's yeast, clams, whole-grain cereals, meats, fruits, vegetables.

Iodine

Vital to the proper functioning of the thyroid gland and therefore concerned with the total metabolism in the body and with energy output. Protects against wrinkled and rough skin and helps keep hair strong and healthy.

RDA: 100 mcg for women; 130 mcg for men.
THERAPEUTIC DOSE: Best taken in seaweed or kelp form.
SOURCES: Kelp, onions, legumes, fish liver oils, seafood.

Iron

Needed for hemoglobin and myoglobin formation, iron assists protein metabolism, strengthens hair and nails and prevents anemia. It also helps prevent breathlessness and fatigue. Vitamin C aids iron absorption and use.

RDA: 10 mg for men; 18 mg for women.
THERAPEUTIC DOSE: 25–50 mg.
SOURCES: Egg yolk, leafy green vegetables, blackstrap molasses, sun-dried raisins, desiccated liver, whole grains, potatoes, seafood.

Magnesium

A catalyst for digestion and use of food, magnesium helps absorption and metabolism of other minerals such as calcium and phosphorus. It helps regulate body temperature. It is needed for healthy muscle tone, bones, and heart and helps prevent arteriosclerosis. A natural tranquilizer, it is used in treatment of psoriasis.

RDA: 350 mg for men; 300 mg for women.
THERAPEUTIC DOSE: 350 to 700 mg.
SOURCES: Yellow corn, nuts, rice, apples, celery, lemons, seafood, bran, figs, grapefruit.

Manganese

Manganese activates enzymes needed for normal skeletal development, plays an important role in fat and carbohydrate metabolism, helps maintain sex hormone production, and helps nourish the central nervous system and make blood cells. Manganese also plays an important role in childbearing, in maintaining the health of the circulatory system, and in resistance to infection. It is often used to treat mental illness, heart disease, and diabetes.

RDA: None.
Average diet supplies 3–9 mg.
THERAPEUTIC DOSE: 50 mg.
SOURCES: Leafy green vegetables, legumes, beets, egg yolk, nuts, whole grains, spinach.

Phosphorus

Phosphorus helps maintain healthy acid-alkaline balance in blood and tissues. It works together with calcium to maintain strong bones and teeth, to facilitate the metabolism of food, and to promote good kidney functioning. Phosphorus is important for good complexion, mental alertness and health, energy and growth.

RDA: 800 mg for adults.
THERAPEUTIC DOSE: 800 to 1,000 mg.
SOURCES: Dairy products, meat, fish, egg yolk, red cabbage, cranberries.

Potassium

Potassium is an important alkalinizer for acid-alkaline balance. It aids glucose metabolism, cell metabolism, and muscle protein synthesis. It balances sodium in the body, helps control heartbeat and prevent dry skin, acne, and dermatitis. Important in energy production, it eases premenstrual tension and protects from stress. It helps the body dispose of wastes, promotes secretion of hormones, and helps prevent female disorders.

RDA: None.
Average daily intake is 2,000–2,500 mg.
THERAPEUTIC DOSE: 100 mg depending on sodium intake. More sodium in diet demands more potassium.
SOURCES: Citrus fruits, watercress, figs, bananas, green peppers, meat, fish, whole grains, molasses.

Selenium

An important antioxidant, selenium works together with vitamin E to retard the aging process and preserve tissue elasticity. It relieves high blood pressure and protects against toxic effects of heavy metals such as cadmium and mercury. It is important for the health of the digestive system and as a protective factor against malignancies, and useful for treatment of dandruff.

RDA: None.
THERAPEUTIC DOSE: 50 mcg.
SOURCES: Varied diet of unrefined foods, broccoli, eggs, onions, tomatoes, tuna fish, garlic, brewer's yeast, liver.

Sodium

Sodium helps maintain health of the nervous, muscular, lymph, and blood systems. But too much sodium causes water retention.

RDA: 3 g–7 g but recent research indicates it should be much less: 200 mg–300 mg.
THERAPEUTIC DOSE: None—we get plenty of sodium in our diet.
SOURCES: Seafoods, poultry, cheese, bacon, bread, most prepared foods.

Sulfur

Called the "beauty mineral," sulfur keeps hair, nails, and skin healthy and beautiful. Essential for the formation of red blood cells, it is also important for tissue respiration. It helps the body resist bacterial infection and is needed for collagen synthesis. Linked with the functions of B-complex vitamins, it is important for nerve health and clear thinking. Sulfur amino acids are used with zinc for nail and hair and skin complaints.

RDA: Normal protein intake usually provides sufficient sulfur.
THERAPEUTIC DOSE: 10 to 20 mg.
SOURCES: Fish, eggs, cabbage, lean beef, dried beans, legumes, sprouts, onions.

Zinc

Essential for the formation of RNA and DNA, for collagen synthesis, and for rebuilding cells, zinc is involved in many hormone and enzyme reactions in the body such as food digestion, tissue respiration, normal gland functions. It is needed for growth and healing and is used to redress the side effects of some drugs. Zinc is essential for normal sexual development and fertility in men. It has been used to improve skin health and hair health, to help cure alcoholism and restore mental and emotional balance. White marks on nails are often a sign of zinc deficiency, as are stretch marks, which can be prevented with zinc. Zinc deficiency is widespread in the West, and is particularly pronounced in women who are on the Pill.

RDA: 15 mg for adults.
THERAPEUTIC DOSE: 15 to 500 mg.
SOURCES: Seafood, meat, nuts, whole grains, legumes, oysters. But foods must be raised or animals fed on zinc-rich soils.

PUTTING IT ALL TOGETHER

OK, so once you begin to familiarize yourself with the different nutrients, how they can be used and what they are necessary for, the next question is, "How do I know whether I should take vitamin and mineral supplements?" "And if I do, how much of each do I need?" There is no easy answer to the question. The Lifestyle Diet will give you the best all-round nutritional support for health and beauty. In addition, according to an expert in mineral metabolism, Carl Pfeiffer of the Brain Bio Centre, and others working in the field of minerals, most women need zinc and manganese as well as chromium, which you should get from taking brewer's yeast daily because the supply in our diet of these nutrients is restricted due to soil depletion and other factors. If you are on the Pill you should make sure you get adequate vitamin B_6, B_{12}, B_2, folic acid, and C and the minerals zinc and iron. Both human and animal studies have shown that estrogen in the Pill and hormone replacement therapy for menopausal women cause an increase in the level of copper in a woman's body and a decrease in the level of zinc. When you are on the Pill you both absorb more copper from foods in your digestive system and make more of an important copper-binding protein called ceruloplasmin in the liver to which 95 percent of the copper in the blood is bound. Many of the unpleasant side effects of the Pill that affect health and beauty in a woman—brittle nails, migraine, weight gain, chronic fatigue, depression—appear to be related to this high serum copper and low zinc.

Studies have also shown that the Pill changes carbohydrate and fat metabolism as well as altering the need for the nutrients zinc, copper, iron, and the vitamins B_2, B_6, folic acid, and B_{12}. When women on the Pill are given supplements of these nutrients, most of these Pill-associated problems disappear.

Apart from the question of the Pill, supplements of various vitamins and minerals have been shown to be an advantage in a rebuilding program. They supply many of the essential materials needed for speed and efficient restoration of the parts of the body and its systems that become damaged by wear and tear, as well as for correction of imbalances caused by long-term stress, poor nutrition in the past, or illness. When supplements are used in this way it is important that they be carefully chosen and regularly taken—each and every day. Your body responds to a constant steady supply of nutrients in carrying out its restorative and rebuilding tasks, such as eliminating stored wastes and deposits around joints, clearing the circulatory system, and rebalancing the hormonal system. It is also important that you buy the very best supplements you can find, checking labels carefully for quantities and balance. Some vitamins such as vitamin C are equally good in synthetic form as in natural form (that is, where they have been extracted from foods) provided that you accompany them with the other nutrients that occur naturally with them in foods. (In the case of vitamin C, the bioflavonoids.) Others, such as some of the B-complex vitamins, should never be taken in synthetic form.

It is a good general rule to do your vitamin shopping in a health food store rather than a drug store or supermarket, because they are more likely to carry the natural varieties. Minerals are best taken in the form of a good multimineral formula (one without copper) unless a specific mineral has been recommended for you by your doctor or nutritionist. Remember that in any nutritional rebuilding program for general health or for skin and hair or anything else, all of the important nutrients have to be supplied in the form of foods or supplements for them to work properly, because balance is everything and every nutrient is dependent on others for absorption and proper use in the body.

Here is an example of what a rebuilding program for health and beauty might look like. *It is given here for educational purposes only and in no way is it intended to be prescriptive.* Individual needs vary greatly from one woman to another depending on your age and condition and on whatever personal imbalances you may have.

Vitamin A and D: 25,000–50,000 iu of A together with 1,000–2,000 iu of D for skin and hair, repair and growth processes, and strengthening resistance to illness.

High Potency Natural B Complex: This should contain about 75 mg of B_1, B_2, B_6, pantothenic acid, PABA, niacin, choline, and inositol, and 75 mcg of B_{12} and biotin as well as 400 mcg of folic acid. For healthy hair and skin, to combat fatigue and strengthen resistance to stress, and encourage mental and emotional clarity.

Niacin: 100–250 mg. For improving circulation and skin condition, combating fatigue, and helping to clear up any toxic waste deposits in tissues.

Vitamin B_6 (Pyridoxine): 100–500 mg. For good collagen and elastin formation in muscles and skin, for DNA and RNA synthesis, and for help in preventing premature aging. Good for tiny wrinkles, hair and skin problems, cellulite and water retention problems, as well as stabilizing nerves.

Vitamin C with Bioflavonoids: 1–8 g for detoxifying the body, as a natural antioxidant to help prevent premature aging, skin wrinkling, and broken veins, to strengthen resistance to stress and increase resistance to illness.

Vitamin E: 200–1,600 iu. A natural antioxidant, vitamin E helps retard the aging process and protects cells from genetic damage, rebuild tissue and skin, combat shrinkage of collagen fibers and therefore counteract wrinkling, stimulate cell metabolism, and keep the circulatory system clear. (Anyone with high blood pressure or an overactive thyroid would have to start with a small dose of vitamin E and then work up gradually.)

Multimineral formula of chelated (that is, protein-bound) minerals for better absorption: 1 or 2 tablets containing, say, 1,000 mg calcium, 25 mg iron, 5 mg zinc, 100 mg potassium, 10 mg manganese, 500 magnesium, 200 mcg iodine, and 200 mg phosphorus. For healing and maintaining mineral balance.

Lecithin: 2–4 tablespoons of granular lecithin for strengthening stress resistance and balancing hormonal system.

A program such as this for rebuilding and restoring might last from six weeks to a couple of years depending on your present state; then you would reduce the quantities of supplements as your body restores itself, using them from then on only to offset the effects of pollution and stress.

My Own Regimen

I am often asked what supplements I take. It varies depending on the season and the situation in which I find myself. I often take none at all (except extra vitamin C and lecithin) when I am at home in the country where most of my foods are organically grown and I am under no particular stress. At other times, I take:

Vitamin C, 3–10 g a day in the form of a sustained-release tablet
A bioflavonoid tablet
A high-potency B complex that also contains A, D, and a few chelated minerals
A multimineral tablet
Vitamin E, 800 iu just before bed
Brewer's yeast, a heaped tablespoonful stirred into a glass of juice three times a day
Lecithin, four tablespoonfuls a day with water or stirred into yogurt
Kelp, six tablets morning and night

The Third Dimension
Movement

∽

Introduction

There is a new elite appearing in the West. It has nothing to do with social position, education, or money. It is concerned with the condition of
one's body and one's psyche. The new elite is made up of men and
women who have discovered the power of the third dimension of health
and beauty: *movement.* They have learned for themselves the fact that
each of us lives at a level far below that of our potential energy, and they
know from experience that regular vigorous exercise is the way to tap
these resources. Members of the new elite come from all ages and all
backgrounds. You'll see them out on the roads bicycling or running, on
the courts playing, almost anywhere these days, dressed in a wide range
of clothing. They come in all shapes and sizes. But in spite of their
differences they all have a few things in common—shining eyes, enormous vitality, and a childlike enthusiasm for *play.*

This section deals with their discoveries. It is all about movement and
what it can do for you. It will tell you about the different sorts of exercise you can take and what each is good for, about the importance of
aerobics and stretching, about what good posture has to do with health

and beauty and how permanently to protect your back from anguish, and it will tell you how you can profit from going Outward Bound.

But more than anything else, I hope that it will encourage you to put on an old shirt and a pair of shorts and *do* something. For that's where the rewards come from.

8

The Joy of Exercise

The idea that you should exercise because it is good for you is all wrong. Not that exercise is *not* good for you—it is indeed. It is probably the single most important thing you can do to stay well and beautiful. It will help you live longer, get slimmer, have more energy, look younger, and stay healthier. But any woman who still faces a thirty-minute run, swim, or cycle as a chore hasn't yet discovered the secret of what exercise is all about. For movement—exercise—whether it be in the form of running, dancing, swimming, yoga, bicycling, or other sports, is far more than something you do to keep fit and trim down a spreading waistline. It is also a key to extraordinarily high energy levels and to a sense of tremendous physical and psychic freedom, which are fundamental to true beauty.

Taken regularly over weeks and months, strenuous exercise can also help you discover the truth that all things are possible. It is a discovery that can literally change your life. And if this sounds exaggerated or if this is not what some complex and tedious exercise program has brought you in the past, then you have a whole new world of enjoyment and experience just waiting to be discovered.

YOUR BODY THRIVES ON MOTION

The human body, which we often treat like a machine, is in reality nothing of the sort. For unlike a machine, which wears out with use, the more your body is used, the stronger, healthier, and more expressive it becomes. Most women tend to ignore their body and its needs. Or they treat it in a narcissistic way—more like an object to be pushed and pummeled and pampered than a living thing. Many of the exercise programs one finds in books and magazines have been geared to this attitude—calisthenics designed for the self-obsessed woman who literally spends hours doing some boring movement in the hope that it will whittle away yet another inch from her right thigh (something which seems of prime importance to her although probably nobody else will ever notice). This kind of attitude really misses the point.

In part, it comes as a result of our culture. Woman's body has traditionally been regarded as a passive sex symbol, beautiful in its quiescence. Seldom is it recognized as the simple physical expression of the woman herself—an inseparable part of her and, as such, a vehicle for her to communicate and respond to life, to experience pleasure and pain—a means of relating intimately with her environment. If a woman's feelings about her body and her relationship with it are not as intimate and as at ease as this, it probably means that she is not experiencing her life fully. Neither is she using her mental and creative abilities as successfully as she could. Regular exercise can change all this. For in addition to all the well-known physical benefits, such as firm muscles and increased strength and stamina, it will also bring you a feeling of being intensely alive, along with greater self-confidence and a lively sense of play that comes from knowing you are able to meet each new challenge in your life spontaneously with openness and enthusiasm. For to be beautiful, your body needs to move—it needs to be put through its paces, pushed near the limits of its heart and lungs, freed from the habitual day-to-day restrictions on muscles and joints that result from living the modern life, which is strongly mentally oriented.

Once you discover this for yourself, then far from being something you do quickly to get it over with—a chore you virtuously suffer through because you know it is doing you good—exercise will become one of the most enjoyable parts of your life. American cardiologist Dr. George Sheehan has done much to make people aware of the essential nature of exercise and has said, "Exercise that is not play accentuates rather than closes the split between body and spirit. Exercise that is drudgery, labor, something done only for the final result is a waste of time." Moving freely down a country road at dawn, gliding through water, speeding down mountains covered with fine snow are things that you will do for their own sake, for the pleasure of it. The fact that these activities are good for you will become incidental to the lovely unexpected pleasure. Then you will have discovered for yourself what exercise is really all about. But let's begin at the beginning. What happens when you exercise regularly?

KEY TO A STRONG HEART

A number of recent inquiries into the relationship between levels of physical activity and the incidence of coronary heart disease confirm what experts in sports medicine have been saying for years, that regular exercise significantly reduces the risk of heart attack. A recent ten-year study of 17,000 men between thirty-five and seventy-four, for instance, showed that those who spent less than 2,000 calories a week in exercise were 64 percent more likely to suffer a heart attack than those who spent more (2,000 calories are burned off in two and a half hours of running a week, four hours of swimming, or three hours of squash or bicycling).

In fact, there is a lot of evidence now to indicate that the benefits of regular exercise far outweigh those of dietary management in the prevention of heart diseases. A joint research project between Harvard University and Trinity Medical School in Dublin looked at 600 Irishmen between thirty and sixty who had lived in Boston for ten years or more and compared them to their brothers who still lived in Ireland. The Irishmen ate 500 more calories per day than the Americans, and they consumed double the eggs (Ah! the poor maligned egg). In fact, they average fourteen to eighteen eggs plus a pound of butter a week. Yet for all that, the Irish weighed on average 15 percent less than the Americans, had lower cholesterol levels and only half the incidence of high blood pressure. The reason? They got far more exercise.

Your heart is fed by coronary arteries on its outside surface. When fats are deposited inside these arteries, a kind of plaque forms on them which can impede the flow of blood. If the plaque builds up so much that the blood supply is cut off, then the area of the heart muscle that is nourished by that blood vessel dies. You suffer a heart attack. When this happens to a large portion of the heart muscle, it is no longer able to pump blood throughout the body and the body dies.

Strenuous physical activity, taken regularly, can help prevent this in several ways:

1. Your heart is a muscle and, like any muscle, when it is put to work as it is during physical exertion and made to beat harder and faster it becomes stronger, larger, and more efficient. It is able to process more blood with each beat and doesn't have to work as hard as it did before it was strengthened.

2. Exercise lowers the concentration of blood fats such as triglycerides so they do not form the heavy plaque in the coronary arteries which results in heart attacks.

3. Exercise enlarges the coronary arteries which nourish your heart and increases the number of auxiliary capillaries that feed an area so that if

the blood does become blocked in one coronary artery, blood from another can supply the area.

4. Exercise lowers blood pressure.

5. Finally, exercise trains the heart to draw oxygen from the blood with greater efficiency; it simply works better.

Other organs in your body, such as the liver and the lungs, are also pushed to greater efficiency with physical exertion so that the whole organism is able to maintain itself in more optimum condition. When you exercise regularly and strenuously, your lungs become stronger. You also learn to breathe more deeply and soon are able to draw more oxygen from each breath you take. (While you are running, for instance, the oxygen the lungs process increases twelvefold over the resting state.) Your nerve reflexes become brisker too. This has the effect of making your body muscles able to respond to commands more promptly and to resist stresses and strains.

STAYING SLIM

The old injunction to eat less and exercise more is good not just for overall fitness but for weight loss itself—but probably not in the way you imagine. For burning calories is not the only way exercise helps you lose weight and stay thin—probably not even the most important way.

Many women neglect exercise because of the mistaken idea that physical activity increases the appetite. This is not true. On the contrary, studies show that people don't react to physical activity with a blossoming appetite. Regular exercise, unless it is excessively strenuous, will *decrease* your appetite. There appear to be several reasons for this:

1. You get hungry when your blood sugar level drops drastically. Regular exercise keeps blood sugar levels from fluctuating dramatically, because when muscles are regularly exercised the amount of fat they oxidize is increased and the amount of carbohydrate burned is reduced. Since your muscles are using more fat, they don't take as much sugar from the bloodstream.

2. When you exercise, peristaltic movement in the intestines increases. The transit time for foods to pass through the body and wastes to be excreted is diminished. As a result, your body actually absorbs fewer calories.

3. Exercise also raises your metabolic rate so that your cells burn oxygen more efficiently, make better use of nutrients from your diet, and more

thoroughly eliminate waste products. This also probably contributes to the appetite-decreasing ability of exercise—because you are getting better nourishment value from your foods, you are inclined to eat less.

4. When you exercise, your temperature is raised. The elevation of body temperature brought about by physical activity also helps inhibit the feelings of hunger. Fat mobilized in the process supplies enough energy to inhibit the desire for food for up to forty-eight hours after strenuous physical activity, probably because your body is producing enough blood lactate to affect the metabolism of glucose in the satiety center. And this beneficial exercise-caused elevation of temperature, or "thermogenesis," is not short-lived either. Your resting basal metabolic rate remains raised by as much as 10 percent for up to forty-eight hours after strenuous activity.

Exercise can also make you lose inches because it helps turn fat into energy while at the same time building muscle. Muscle tissue weighs more than fat which is why, when you begin to exercise, you find you are losing inches more rapidly than pounds. In fact, to lose weight successfully and keep it off you *have* to exercise. Researchers have shown that about a quarter of the weight lost by restricting calories alone is lost in muscle tissue. If you go on a slenderizing regimen without exercising, you will lose this muscle tissue and then later, if you regain any of the weight lost, you will regain it in fat, not in muscle. This means you will be even more flabby than you were to begin with.

And just in case you have fears of exercising because you think you will develop big bulky muscles, forget it. This won't happen with any kind of rhythmic exercise such as running, swimming, bicycling, or dancing. These activities tend to form long muscles and beautiful bodies. Only resistance exercises, such as certain kinds of weight lifting, will bring that kind of bulk, and even that is unlikely for a woman as big muscles occur only in the presence of sufficient male hormones, and most women have far too few in their bodies to make it possible.

STAYING YOUNG

Premature aging is one of the worst threats to your good looks, and one of the best ways of avoiding it is by getting plenty of exercise. This is not only because exercise stops your body from losing its youthful shape, firms muscles that could go flabby, and helps keep you slim. Physical activity is also essential in maintaining the strength and form of your whole muscle-skeletal system. When bones are not used they lose calcium, become weak and brittle, break easily and are slow to repair. They also actually shrink in mass. What is worse, physical decay is progressive; a lack of physical activity results in an almost inevitable further lack of activity and further shrinkage.

When muscle mass shrinks, so does the production of steroid hormones from the adrenal and sex glands—in direct proportion to the loss of muscle tissue. (This occurs as a natural process in the passing of years as well, but more slowly.) These hormones are essential for the maintenance of young-looking, wrinkle-free skin and healthy hair. They also fulfill numerous other roles in the maintenance of internal health. Your level of physical activity is an important factor in the maintenance of optimal functioning in your endocrine system, helping to make possible the continued flow of sufficient hormones for youth and vitality.

RESHAPE YOUR BODY FROM WITHIN

Each body has its own potential perfect shape. It is how your body was meant to be, regardless of how much until now it has been distorted by neglect, overweight, or habitual poor posture. I know women who have spent enormous amounts of money and undergone expensive medical treatments in an attempt to restore their bodies to their normal form. Exercise can do it better, more cheaply, and more rapidly than anything else. And this is something that occurs naturally as part of the process of the body's getting back into shape—the line of a thigh changes, an obscured waistline begins to reappear, a breast becomes firm and rounded again and loses its sag.

One of the things that worries women most is cellulite—the lumps and bumps that simply won't go away and are the result of toxic wastes, fat, and water stored in the body. In a sedentary person these by-products of metabolism are not fully oxidized. Instead, they get deposited in the tissues and there they stay as a kind of tissue sludge to make thighs pucker and bottoms sag. Later the flesh hardens and becomes lumpy like suet under the skin to mar the line of even the slimmest body. Exercise helps prevent this because it increases oxidation and stimulates metabolism and the elimination of wastes, both from the individual cells and the body as a whole.

MOVEMENT GIVES YOU ENERGY

Many women don't function at anywhere near peak. They tire easily. They feel under strain and look for any escape from fatigue. When the body is under stress it produces large quantities of adrenalin, a powerful substance that is a chemical product of the sympathetic nervous system. Adrenalin is the emergency hormone that mobilizes the body for fight or flight, giving extra power when it is needed most. It increases your heartbeat, calls forth sugar reserves, and causes your muscles to contract.

In modern life the adrenalin produced through emotional and physical stress is not all used up as often as it should be in physical movement. Instead, it is stored in your heart and brain, a phenomenon known as the adrenalin buildup. When this buildup is great, as it often is in city dwellers, the efficiency of your heart decreases while excess adrenalin in your brain adversely affects your moods and emotions, making you feel tired, irritable, and at the end of your tether.

Exercise will call forth these stores of adrenalin, dispersing them into the system, burning the adrenalin up and so clearing away the buildup and resulting in a renewed feeling of vigor and freshness. This is why after a hard day when you feel completely exhausted or very irritable, if you can resist the temptation to collapse on the sofa and instead take exercise, you will be amazed to find that in about thirty minutes your energy returns.

But there are other reasons for the increase in energy that sedentary people experience when they take up regular exercise. When you exercise regularly, changes occur in the cells of your body. There is an increase in the number of mitochondria, the microscopic factories in each cell where energy is produced. This creates more sites for the production of an energy-rich compound called adenosine triphosphate (ATP) so the quantities of this mitochondrial enzyme increase and it is produced more rapidly than before. Recently, two researchers showed that as a result of the increase in this enzyme and others in the cells after an eight-week training program, the cells' energy content had increased dramatically.

EXERCISE IMPROVES YOUR MOOD

The positive effect exercise has on your mental and emotional state is well known to anyone who exercises regularly. Ask anyone who in the past couple of years has taken up running or other vigorous activity and he will tell you that it has brought him enhanced mental energy and concentration plus a feeling of heightened mental acuity. Some claim too that, as a result of taking up regular exercise, they discover a sense of willpower they didn't know they had. It seems to pervade their whole life, making it possible for them to carry through arduous tasks or bear with difficult situations without becoming discouraged even when they are fatigued.

A number of studies have also shown that vigorous exercise taken regularly every day or so alters one's mood for the better and is capable of
bringing about a long-term sense of well-being. Professor Tom Curetin
at the University of Illinois studied 2,500 sedentary people who took up
exercise. He discovered that they quickly developed significantly greater
energy and less tension than they had when the study began. Herbert de
Vries at the University of Southern California looked at stress levels and
muscle tension in subjects who had either been given tranquilizers or
who engaged in physical exercise every day. He found that even as little
activity as a fifteen-minute walk is more relaxing and efficient in dealing
with stress than a course of tranquilizers. At the University of Arizona
Medical School, psychologist William P. Morgan discovered that exercise significantly lowers anxiety levels.

In an interesting study, psychiatrist John Greist experimented with depressed university students, treating some with conventional psychotherapy and others by asking them to run for a few minutes each day.
After ten weeks he found that the runners felt significantly better, studied better, and did better on their exams than the conventionally treated
group. Another psychiatrist, Dr. Thaddeus Kostrubala, has been treating
a variety of emotional disorders successfully by getting his patients to
run. He has even found it useful in severe cases of paranoid schizophrenia
as well as in helping drug addicts and alcoholics to kick the habit.

Scientists are not yet able to explain fully why these positive mental
effects come about from simply exercising regularly, but many believe
that they are at least in part related to increased levels of norepinephrine
in the brain. This is a hormone essential for the brain's messages to be
transmitted along certain nerves in the body. People with high levels of
norepinephrine in their blood tend to be cheerful and happy, while those
who suffer from moodiness and depression show low levels. Taking up
regular exercise can turn the moody into the calm. Another possible contributor to the sense of well-being and positive mental attitudes exercise
brings may be its ability to increase the blood supply to the brain so that
brain and nerve tissue receive more oxygen, enabling the cells to function
better.

Finally, exercise improves your ability to sleep deeply. Recent studies
have shown that people relatively free of emotional conflicts and depression sleep deeply, while at least 85 percent of those with psychological
disturbances have long-term insomnia in one form or another.

IS EXERCISE A POSITIVE ADDICTION?

Many researchers into sports have commented on the ability regular
strenuous exercise has of developing qualities of courage and character as

well as greater physical stamina. Some even believe that this is because regular strenuous movement is a natural *need* of human beings, one for which we have been genetically programmed and one which, if denied over a period of time, leads to feelings of timidity, negativity, lack of creativity, and chronic fatigue as well as physical illness. Psychiatrist William Glasser, author of *Positive Addiction,* and others have noticed that once people become regularly involved in an exercise program for several weeks and months, they develop a kind of addiction to it that replaces many of the negative habits they had before they started, whether it be the excessive use of alcohol, smoking, or self-deprecating thoughts and unproductive behavior in relationships.

It is certainly true that once you discover the joy of exercise, and the feelings of well-being and mental and physical freedom that come with it and carry over into the rest of your life, you don't want to give up. Meanwhile the negative addictions tend gradually to disappear, almost automatically. For instance, you almost never meet a swimmer or runner who smokes, although many did before they took up the sport. The whole process of eliminating negative addictions appears to be quite simple and to require no great effort of will. It is just that the pleasurable feedback you get from the habit of overeating or smoking in no way approaches the sense of exuberance and satisfaction that exercise brings. And since cigarettes interfere with running by making it harder for you to breathe, and overeating interferes by making you feel sluggish and creating more weight to carry about, you find (even unconsciously) that you no longer want to sustain your negative habits. They are just not as satisfying as the positive ones. This is something that large numbers of people have experienced, and something that I know firsthand because it happened to me.

EXERCISE IS A FINE TOOL FOR PERSONAL GROWTH

We live in a culture that puts increasing emphasis on the use of human potential and individual growth. Exercise can contribute a great deal to both. In *The Complete Book of Exercise* by James Fixx, the author (himself a runner) comments on this when he says, "Zen Buddhism, transcendental meditation, assertiveness training and similar movements are all directed at making us fulfilled human beings. Sometimes, however, they do not, and I suspect the reason in many cases is that they fail to mesh with the inescapable peculiarities and idiosyncrasies of individual character. In contrast, while running often alters a person profoundly, the changes all come from *within* and are, therefore, tightly integrated with the total personality." To some extent, of course, this is true of all athletics since they alter the mind by altering the body. Dr. E. J. Kane of the University of London, who is well known for his investigations of the psychology of sport, has written, "The way an individual characteristically perceives his body has long been held as an important factor in forming his image of himself and his general integration."

I believe this aspect of exercise is particularly important to women. The cultural roles imposed on women too often limit a woman's habitual assumptions about her body, its strengths and weaknesses, what she is capable of and what is impossible for her. She finds herself having to fulfill others' expectations or having to rely heavily on other people because she feels she has not yet found her own strength and a sense of her own identity apart from the roles she fulfills. Her sense of her body is often distorted or restricted, and so her sense of her life and its possibilities becomes limited. Exercise can alter this dramatically. I have seen it happen to women of all ages who took up daily running, swimming, or bicycling.

When it comes to the specific relationship between exercise and beauty, a change in body image can also play another important role. As anyone with an interest in observing female beauty will tell you, there is a certain charisma that surrounds some women. It is not altogether connected with the form of a woman's body or the shape of her face (the conventional criteria for judging someone beautiful) nor with the perfection of her skin and bone structure. It is a kind of vibrance of personality that is reflected in her physical appearance. It is this difficult-to-describe quality that makes one woman a great beauty regardless of her age and another, with what would seem to be equal physical endowments, simply plain. Charisma has a great deal to do with body image, self-image, and overall energy level—all significantly improved by strenuous exercise.

TRANSCENDENTAL MOVEMENT

In many ways the most interesting results of exercise lie in its ability to induce a state of stillness of mind and inner peace which meditation aims at and which was, until recently, considered the exclusive province of religion and mysticism. In *The Psychic Side of Sports*, Michael Murphy and Rhea A. White record numerous phenomena that have been experienced by people during the self-imposed physical stress of exercise. Murphy and White draw strong parallels between the experiences of mystics and the descriptions athletes have given of altered states of consciousness that happened on the road or playing field. They say:

> The many reports collected show us that sport has enormous powers to sweep us beyond the ordinary sense of self, to evoke capacities that have generally been regarded as mystical, occult, or religious. This is not to say that athletes are yogis or mystics. Very few of us approach games with a lifelong dedication and conscious aspiration for enlightenment that the mystical path requires. It is simply to recognise the similarities that exist between the two fields of activity, both in their methods and in the states of mind they both evoke.

Murphy and White, commenting on the fact that until now we have been but little aware of the parallels because athletes tend not to talk about this kind of experience, say:

> There are probably several good reasons for this, among them a wisdom about talking the spiritual side of athletics to death and a refusal to build up false expectations about it. The athletes' silence about these matters is not unlike the old Zen Buddhist attitude: if you experience illumination while chopping wood, keep chopping wood. If there is something in the act that invites ecstasy, it doesn't need an extra hype or solemn benediction. And there is a wisdom in letting people discover these experiences in their own way, for too many expectations can dampen the spontaneity and sense of release that are part of sport's glory. They can take the fun out of sports in the name of religion.

This sums up well my own feeling about exercise. It really is something you need to find out about for yourself by doing it, for in the last analysis words are dead—only symbols used to describe what can never be conveyed by description. The reality behind them can only be experienced.

9

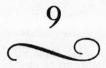

What Kind of Exercise Do You Need?

There are several different kinds of exercise: aerobic, anaerobic, isometric, and isotonic. Each can be useful but by far the most beneficial for overall health and vitality are the aerobics. The name "aerobic" was popularized by Kenneth and Mildred Cooper in their books *Aerobics* and *Aerobics for Women*. It means "living, acting or occurring in the presence of oxygen." What makes aerobic activities different from all other kinds of exercise is that they demand your body's efficient use of oxygen throughout the whole time you are doing them.

AEROBICS

Oxygen is the ignition factor in the burning of energy from the foods you eat. A good supply is always necessary for your body's metabolic processes to take place efficiently. When your cells (particularly the cells of your brain) have an adequate supply, you feel well, have stamina, and don't tire easily. If you tend to feel tired often, get depressed easily, or have trouble thinking clearly, it is likely that your body is not getting all the oxygen you need. In short, you are physically *unfit*.

Unfit people find themselves breathless after climbing stairs, lack concentration when they get involved in a demanding mental task, and are often too weary in the evenings to do anything but plunk themselves in front of a television set. They also tend to rely on stimulants or depressants such as alcohol to relax or to keep going.

Taking aerobic exercise changes all that. Any sustained-rhythm movement that puts constant demand on your heart, raising your pulse rate to between 120 and 160 beats a minute, and continues to develop your lung capacity will bring about a number of important changes in your body. It will:

1. tone your muscles and improve your circulation.

2. increase the number and the size of the blood vessels that carry blood from your heart all over the body so you will have better transport of oxygen.

3. strengthen your chest wall, making you breathe more easily, as air will come in and out of your lungs with less effort. Soon your body will become capable of taking in far more oxygen than it could before. This oxygen will generate energy for sustaining mental and physical effort.

4. make your bones, joints, and ligaments stronger so they have a natural resistance to injury.

5. increase the level of enzymes and energy-rich compounds in your body. You will be better able to assimilate and make use of nutrients from your foods.

6. make your body more efficient. And as the efficiency of your heart increases and you pump more blood with each beat, your basic pulse rate will decline.

Aerobic activities include long-distance running, steady swimming, bicycling, rowing, cross-country skiing, and even long, *brisk* walks.

ANAEROBICS

Anaerobic exercise, such as running a hundred-yard dash or gymnastics, involves a high level of effort sustained over only a short period of time. The effort is such that during the activity you run into "oxygen debt" which means that you use up more oxygen than you take in. This is the opposite of an aerobic activity where, once you are relatively fit, you are able to process oxygen efficiently enough to continue running or bicycling for hours without incurring any oxygen debt. Anaerobic activities can be useful for developing muscle tone and power and for training your body to produce great bursts of strength and movement, but an anaerobic activity cannot be sustained long enough to be of real value to your lungs and heart and so to overall fitness.

ISOMETRICS

Isometric exercises are those you do without any actual movement in your joints. They are muscle-tensing exercises. For instance, try putting your palm against the wall and pushing hard. Nothing happens in terms of body movement, although the muscles of your arm become very tense. All isometric exercises are based on the idea that you push or pull against objects that are immovable. Tensing muscles in this way brings about an increase in their size in the same way that weight lifting does, for whenever a muscle is put under strain it gradually increases in endurance and bulk. Isometric exercises are often "sold" to women on the grounds that they are effortless—the lazy way to exercise. In fact, they do require some energy to perform but nowhere near enough to be useful in building overall fitness. They have another disadvantage, for contracting muscles in this static way causes blood pressure to rise. In anyone with a tendency to heart disease this can be dangerous.

ISOTONICS

Isotonic exercises such as calisthenics, yoga, weight lifting, ballet bar work, and many sports are more dynamic. They demand real movement in muscles and joints and the rhythmic lengthening and shortening of your muscles. For instance, with weight lifting, when you bend your elbow to raise the weight to shoulder level, your biceps contracts as the triceps at the back of your upper arm lengthens. Then when you straighten out your arm again, lowering the weight, your triceps is contracted and the biceps is lengthened. This kind of repeated lengthening and shortening of antagonistic muscles helps you develop muscle strength and tone and freedom of movement in your joints. It is also useful in correcting a muscle area, such as the abdomen or the upper leg, that has become flaccid and flabby. Some isotonics, such as yoga or stretching exercises, are important for developing flexibility and suppleness.

The best total exercise program you can devise for yourself involves some form of isotonics, such as the stretching exercises in the next chapter, done for at least fifteen minutes three times a week, and thirty minutes of aerobic activity, also done at least three times a week. You can alternate doing aerobics one day and isotonics the next if you like. Unless you are determined to become an athlete and the particular sport you have chosen demands work in isometrics or anaerobics, you need not worry about them. Your aerobic activity will build overall fitness, improve your mental and emotional state, and give you energy. The isotonic stretching will give you grace and suppleness and will fill in any muscle-toning gaps your aerobic activity leaves, as well as improving the extensibility of your muscles and tendons. For you are after freedom of movement and endurance, not building big muscles, which is decidedly *not* what health and fitness are all about.

WHAT SPORTS ARE BEST?

There have been several studies of the physiology of exercise, and now it is generally agreed that the best sorts for overall fitness are aerobic activities—running, swimming, rowing, and bicycling. You can add to that list cross-country skiing, disco dancing (providing you do enough of it and really get your heart beating and lungs working). Walking is acceptable too if you walk *fast* and *far* enough and if you go over hilly ground as well as over flat terrain. For only these activities offer the kind of steady, sustained movement that builds muscle strength, increases the flexibility of joints, and also fortifies the heart and lungs. You may be able to exert yourself by playing tennis or squash or golf, but how well depends on how you play the game and whom you play with. You can win sets of tennis without moving more than a few feet from one place or you can be all over the court and totally exhaust yourself. A recent study of men from thirty-five to seventy-four at Stanford University concluded that these games do not give as effective protection as swimming or running or cross-country skiing. So play them and enjoy them, but take up something else too. Let's take a look at aerobic exercises first.

TAKE TO THE WATER

Swimming is one of the best of all the aerobic activities to start with, particularly if you are very much overweight. The support the water gives your body makes you able to put all your effort into participating in the movement, instead of having to direct some at just keeping yourself erect as you do in running. Swimming is also a wonderful way to build beautiful muscles if you are very thin, or to pare down and firm up muscles if you are flabby. This is because swimming develops long muscles in the legs and back, gradually reshaping and reforming any body that has lost its shape, no matter what its age.

If you are going to take up swimming, arrange things so you can do it *regularly* and without fail at least three times a week. The fitness that comes with aerobic exercise is built gradually and depends on consistency. No amount of weekend heroics will accomplish it.

You will need to set yourself a goal—say, at first fifteen minutes of constant swimming from one end of a pool to the other without stopping —and stick to it. If you are troubled by chlorine in public pools, then buy yourself a small pair of racer's goggles. They will keep your eyes protected. Begin slowly. Swim a couple of laps and then stop and, using a watch with a second hand (which a friend can keep for you or which you can leave at the side of the pool), take your pulse.

Here's how: put the tips of the first three fingers of your right hand against the artery of the inside edge of your wrist, count the number of beats you get in six seconds, and then multiply by ten. This will give you your heartbeat rate for one minute. If it is 120 then you are doing well. If it is less than that make yourself swim a little harder, and if it goes above 160 then you are exercising too hard for your present level of fitness so draw back a little. After a few weeks you will find you are able to exert yourself much more and still your pulse will remain within the safe range. Besides being sure the level of exertion you are making is safe for you, the main reason for taking your pulse is to discover how much effort you need to make to continue to improve your level of fitness.

It is important to understand the difference between *work* and *effort*. Two people may swim a mile in sixteen minutes and do equal *work*, but if one raises his heartbeat by 60 percent over what it was in a resting state and the other only by 30 percent, then their *effort* has been different. *Effort* in this sense indicates the effort your heart is making in response to the work your body is doing. In order to increase your level of fitness, you have to keep up a certain level of *effort* for a specific period of time. The amount of work you will have to do to achieve this, the distance you will have to cover, and the speed at which you will have to swim (or run, walk, dance, or whatever) will constantly alter as you get fitter.

There has recently been a lot of medical research done to find the ideal range of effort. This is measured by the heartbeat rate during exercise. As usual, opinions vary, but there is a pretty good consensus that you need to exercise within a pulse range where your heartbeat rate is between 75 and 80 percent higher than in its resting state and then to sustain this pulse rate for thirty minutes three times a week.

Taking your pulse can seem a nuisance at first, but it is worthwhile until you get used to exercise and get to know by the feel of things how much effort you are making. After a few weeks you will never need to consult the second hand of a watch again. You will simply know.

Begin slowly. Swim for fifteen minutes the first three or four times. Then you can gradually add a couple of minutes each week until you work up to thirty minutes, three times a week. At this level, provided you monitor your effort by taking your pulse occasionally, you can be assured of gradually and steadily building fitness. Then if you want to do more for fun, that is up to you. However much you do, watch your breathing while you swim. It is important to breathe regularly, for oxygen is what gives you the power to sustain the physical effort you are making. This is what aerobic fitness is all about.

BUY A BICYCLE

The same basic principles apply to bicycling. It too is an excellent endurance sport that promotes coordination and muscle strength, particularly in the lower half of your body. The other good thing about bicycling is that it gives you a feeling of getting good return on energy expended, as a bicycle will carry you a lot farther than a run or swim with the same effort, preferably in the early morning or on country lanes. Then you will be able to keep up a steady pace without having to stop for signals, cars, or pedestrians, and the air is free from dust and gasoline fumes. You can take your pulse in the same way—after, say, five minutes of bicycling—to ensure that you are making the right effort. And you can start off with fifteen minutes' bicycling and then work up to half an hour or more three times a week. Make sure that the seat and the handlebars on your bicycle are the right height for you or you can end up with back strain. And be sure to look after your bicycle well so it offers little resistance, for although working against unnecessary resistance from a machine may be physically beneficial when you are using an indoor bicycle exerciser, it can be an awful bore and very discouraging. Bicycling is a particularly good sport to take up if you have a family, as children delight in going on bicycle outings. An ideal Sunday afternoon activity is to make a fifteen- or even twenty-mile bike ride together, especially if there is a delicious picnic in the middle.

WALK TO FITNESS

Probably the most neglected of all activities that can build health and fitness, walking can be tremendously enjoyable no matter what your physical condition. The rewards are many, varied, and immediate. There are the delights of feeling fresh pure air entering your body, the tingle of a cold morning, the wind and rain on your face. You can become absorbed in the sights you see—wild honeysuckle on a summer evening, the antics of birds, the fascinating patterns made by water, the power of the wind, the delightfully absurd goings-on of other people, the sounds and smells. Such things, if you have the eyes to see, can engage your mind and dissolve your sense of time and thoughts about stressful aspects of your life.

As with most physical activities, the rewards of walking are directly related to the effort you make doing it and to the spirit in which you do it. A gentle stroll without purpose or a grudging constitutional with the dog will do little for you. But taking a brisk walk with good will and a sense of purpose while breathing deeply will put a glow on your skin and help improve your posture, the condition of your muscles all over, and your circulation.

If you choose walking as an aerobic activity, make a date with yourself to spend thirty minutes a day at it. It doesn't matter what you wear as long as it is comfortable and unrestricting. But you do need a good pair of sturdy shoes. They should be stout so that they give you a feeling of security and reliability over even the roughest and wettest ground; thick rubber soles are particularly good because they both grip and act as shock absorbers. Natural fiber socks are better than the synthetics because they are more absorbent. You needn't be deterred by wind or weather either; walking in the rain, provided you are well dressed for it, can be a delight. A lightweight wind- and water-proof jacket is a great help.

Start off walking briskly—fast enough that you will be a little out of breath. Feel the rhythmic movement of your body and the way your legs swing freely from your hips. Get into the swing of it all, then after the first week or two increase the time you spend to forty-five minutes and vary your pace. Try not to walk over flat ground all the time—the hills and valleys, the ups and downs are what bring real physical rewards.

Walking regularly can bring fitness slowly but surely without ever taking a pulse or timing anything. A walker can measure her progress by self-observation alone. Ask yourself how you feel and compare your performance walking with that of six weeks or a few months earlier. You will notice that very soon you are walking faster and farther. More important, you are getting ever greater pleasure from the time you spend on the roads and pathways so that before long you won't want to let anything interfere with your daily exercise. You will also probably notice that work has become less of a burden for you, perhaps that you sleep better, think more clearly, and feel more emotionally balanced.

Another good thing about walking is that no matter where you are living or visiting, there is always somewhere interesting to go. In town there are always parks and recreation areas, and even industrial areas can be fascinating in the early mornings or late evenings when the air is relatively free of pollution.

HIT THE ROAD

My favorite aerobic sport is running. One of the main reasons I was determined to try it was that running was the one sports activity I did at school at which I was no good at all. Running my first mile was the hardest thing I have ever done in my life, but now that I have been running for a year, covering as much as eight miles at a time, I have quite literally developed a passion for it.

I decided to run because I had read all about the psychological benefits of running and because, after several years of being somewhat a lounge lizard (apart from mountaineering, swimming, and sailing), I felt I needed to get fit somehow. I began one cold November morning at five. It was the only time, apart from the middle of the night, when I could be relatively sure that there would be practically nobody on the roads. I did *not* want to be seen. Mustering all the courage I could, I made a dash through the front door, up the drive, and along the street. I went about fifty yards before I felt that I would die from the exertion and had to stop and walk.

It wasn't my legs, it was my lungs—I just couldn't get enough air. I walked panting for another fifty yards or so and then resumed my jog. I found I could sustain the running for just about the distance between one set of lampposts, then I would walk between the next. In this way I finally completed my circuit—the mile distance (I had measured it by driving it in my car) around a large cemetery near my house and then home again. I arrived home exhausted, dispirited and depressed.

The next day I found a hundred reasons why (no matter what all those books said about running) I should *not* repeat my performance. But something, I'm not quite sure what, had got hold of me. And when 5 A.M. came around again there I was, with aching hips and ankles, ready to submit myself to the same torture. I did just as badly.

PAINFUL PROGRESS

Three or four days later, to my amazement, I found I could run between *two* sets of lampposts before having to walk the next set. Ten days later, somehow—with tears streaming down my cheeks and curses at my own stupidity for taking up such an absurd activity—I actually ran a mile. I couldn't believe that it had happened. I had the same desire to stop and walk several times but for some reason I didn't. I kept saying to myself, "Just a little farther and then I'll stop"—but when a "little farther" came I pushed on again and again.

When I finally arrived home, instead of being pleased with my triumph I had the feeling that I had not really done it. That I had made it all up the way a child does a story about what he has done at school today. Or that my having run a mile was an accident of fate which I would never be able to repeat.

But fate was with me, and I did repeat it the next day and the day after. Soon I was running two miles a day and then, one wintry morning about six weeks after my first painful attempt, to my amazement I found I actually *enjoyed* it. I don't mean just the feeling afterward when you have pushed yourself hard, your face is flushed, and you feel alive and good. I mean the actual running itself. There was something about it that was wonderful to me. In a fit of exuberance I came home and scribbled down my experience:

> This morning I ran along a road where I had run before;
> Yet I saw things which I had never seen.
> Legs heavy, breathing hard, my heart was light.
> My body was full of life.
> Then it began to rain.
> Such joy.

I had caught the running bug, which everyone I have ever read on running warns will happen sooner or later, and I wasn't going to give it up. Oh, there have been days here and there when I lay in bed and convinced myself that running was a bore and that I was too tired, too busy, or too something else to go out that day. Some days I've indulged my laziness, but never for long because to my amazement my love of the bed (which has always been very great indeed) doesn't seem to come up to my love of being on the road. So next day I put on my running shoes and I'm off again.

I've found out a lot about myself and a lot about living from my hours on the road. I have learned that I am capable of succeeding at things I never thought I could accomplish. I have gained a better sense of my own strengths and my own limitations. I have grown thinner, firmer, fitter, and happier. I've rediscovered the fun of play, the idea of doing something for its own sake—an art that I had long ago forgotten. Running has also given me more physical and mental perseverance. Where before I was always inclined to give up when things got difficult, now, although I'm just as *inclined* to give up, I do it far less often because I have found out that if you concentrate on putting one foot in front of the other you can get there—wherever "there" happens to be at that moment. Perhaps most important of all, I have learned that you have to go through discipline to get freedom.

Dr. George Sheehan took up running in his forties, and has since gone on to become one of the world's experts on the psychology and physiology of exercise. In *Sheehan on Running*, he describes with great charm the feeling of your life "opening out" and the kind of rewards that can come from the challenge of running (although they can certainly come from other aerobic activities too). He says:

It may be common sense of the common man to consent to be ordinary, but now, everything instinctive, everything intuitive, everything beyond logic tells me otherwise. It tells me that compared to what I *ought* to be, I am only half awake. It tells me, as William James did, that I am using only a small part of my mental and physical resources. Running gave me these insights. It made me an athlete, albeit an aging one, and started my ascent toward a new goal. . . .

OBJECTIVE VALUES

My enthusiasm for running is not all the result of a personal bias, either. There are several objective reasons why running appears to be the best form of aerobic activity for most people. For instance, it is something everybody knows how to do already, so no special training is needed for it. Secondly, it is something you can do anywhere so long as you have a good pair of shoes and a street or a field or a beach to run on. You can run if you live in the city. You can run when you travel—it is simply a matter of tucking your running clothes and shoes into your suitcase wherever you go. Running is also something you can do at any time— during a lunch hour or in the early morning while your husband is still in bed if you have children who can't be left alone. You can even run in the middle of the night provided you wear white (and preferably reflectors) and run toward the oncoming traffic.

GETTING STARTED

Before beginning any program of running you need to check up on how fit you are *now*. If you are over thirty-five or you suffer from high blood pressure, have a family history of heart disease or are recovering from an illness, you should have a checkup with your doctor to be sure that what you are planning to do is safe for you.

In the past few years a number of complicated tests for cardiac and pulmonary strength have been devised by our ever more high technology medicine. Most of them are expensive and unnecessary—that is, unless you happen to be recovering from a heart attack. Do you need an EKG stress test first? Probably not. They are not only overpracticed and overpriced, they are also by no means the perfect indicator of heart trouble that we have been led to believe. For instance, in one study of people with heart disease given an electrocardiographic stress test, as many as 62 percent of them showed up normal while in another study 47 percent of those who showed up abnormal in the testing did *not* have heart disease.

Although the EKG is far from foolproof it is certainly useful in determining a person's state of health. If you have any of these warning signs, then it is a good idea to see your doctor and get his approval for any exercise program you are planning:

• Are you short of breath at even the mildest exertion?

• Do you ever have pain in your legs when you walk which goes away when you rest?

• Do you often have swelling in the ankles?

• Have you ever been told you have heart disease?

• Do you get chest pain when you perform any strenuous activity?

If you have none of these warning signs, there is a simple way to check yourself out for fitness. Walk a brisk two miles in thirty minutes. How do you feel afterward? Do you have any nausea or dizziness? No? Then, so long as you have no medical condition that indicates caution, you are certainly fit enough to start at the bottom of a slow, graded program for joggers. If, however, you have any difficulties on the walk, then keep up this two-mile walk every day until such time as you can do it easily in the half hour before you start running (you will be surprised at how rapidly your condition improves even from daily walking). Don't get discouraged, just keep things up and you will soon be running.

THE GRADED PROGRAM

There are a number of good graded programs you can follow in some of the good books on exercise: Mildred and Kenneth Cooper's *Aerobics for Women;* James Fixx's *The Complete Book of Running,* or Dr. Joan Ullyot's *Women's Running* for instance, or you can try the program outlined below, which a friend who is a physical training expert and another friend—a sports medical man—helped me put together:

FIRST WEEK

Take a brisk walk of one mile, breaking into 50- or 100-yard jogs when you feel like it. Walk at a steady pace in between the jogs but never force yourself. Fitness is gained by steady work. You only end up with injuries and anguish when you push too hard. Take a look around you and enjoy your surroundings. Explore the feeling of your body in motion and discover what it feels like to be *you*.

SECOND WEEK

Walk/jog a mile, alternating about 100 strides of each at a time.

THIRD WEEK

Walk/jog 1½ miles, increasing your jogging intervals to 150 strides with 100 strides of walking in between.

FOURTH WEEK

Jog for a mile at any speed that is comfortable for you. If you find you can't make it all the way without stopping to walk, don't worry. However, by now you should be able safely to tolerate a little discomfort. It soon passes.

FIFTH WEEK

Run one mile in less than nine minutes.

SIXTH WEEK

Jog/run 1½ miles or more. By now you will be over the hump and beginning to feel all the benefits of your perseverance. You will have started to be aware of your body and to be able to listen to what it is telling you. You will no longer need to monitor your pulse. Now you can even begin to move differently, varying your pace, for your stamina and willpower have increased. You can start to push yourself a little bit further some days and to let yourself go more slowly than normal if you are feeling a little low. You can trust your sense of things.

ON TO THE FIFTEENTH WEEK

Play about with your speed and distance, increasing your distance when you want. Try to alternate a long run—say five miles—with a short run of one or two the next day. By the end of six months of running you will be able to run easily and steadily for from half an hour to an hour, covering between three and nine miles.

LISTEN TO YOURSELF

The best way to use a graded program like this is with flexibility, always adapting it to your own individual needs and level of fitness. If in the early stages you find weeks one, two, and three are very easy for you, then you can try a higher level instead. Someone else might decide to work through only the first four levels of the program and then not go further.

So long as your pulse rate when you are running lies somewhere between the 120 and 160 beats per minute range, what you are doing is right for you. And although there are rules to follow, you should never let yourself get bogged down with rigid training schedules or obsessed by standards. They will only detract from the real purpose and pleasure of your running. Aim to spend thirty minutes at least three times a week on the road. By all means do more if you want, but to build fitness you need short periods of exercise, half an hour at a time, done often instead of one long period of 1½ hours a week. If, like me, you find you want to run every day, try leaving off Sundays each week. This gives your muscles a chance to restore themselves and to build up their store of glucose again. You will probably find, as many runners do, that your running will be better for your day of rest.

GETTING INTO GEAR

It doesn't matter what you wear to run, provided it gives you freedom of movement and doesn't inhibit the elimination of perspiration. Clothes made from natural fibers such as cotton and wool, which "breathe," are much better than those made of nylon. In summer you probably won't need more than a pair of shorts and a cotton vest or T-shirt. Bare legs give you a sense of freedom when you run and help keep you cool. In winter (Oh yes, runners tend to run all year round in all kinds of weather including rain and snow) you will need something warmer—a fleecy lined cotton sweat suit or warm-ups, shirt and light sweater are fine. You can add a light waterproof jacket or parka when it rains. If you are large-breasted you will probably want to wear a bra for comfort. When the weather is particularly cold you may need a wool cap or a scarf tied around your head to protect your ears. For night running, wear white or light colors, preferably with reflectors, so you can easily be spotted by cars.

RUNNING SHOES

While the clothes you run in can come from anywhere and look like anything so long as they are comfortable, choosing your running shoes is a different matter. They need to be specially designed to absorb the powerful impact of your feet hitting the road 1,600 times with every mile you cover. The first few times you run, you can wear an old pair of tennis shoes, especially if you run on dirt roads or grass. But as soon as possible you should purchase a pair of proper running shoes. They are not cheap but they are an excellent investment, probably the best you've ever made for fitness—provided, of course, you continue to *use* them. They should not be too flexible. They should be without studs and they need to have a high-density sole. Some of the best soles are made in microcellular rubber. Some soles on running shoes extend up the toe and heel in order to take the rocking motion from heel to toe that running brings. A good pair of running shoes enables you to run on roads without risking shin splints or the injuries to your knees or Achilles tendons that are easy to come by when you wear just an old pair of tennis shoes. The padded instep in your shoes is also useful in absorbing the shock of each step on hard pavement.

When choosing a pair of running shoes, take your time and be sure they fit properly. There should be enough room inside for your toes to move about. Your heel should be slightly raised as this will help protect you from injuring your Achilles tendon, which can be very painful if you overstretch it. The shoe should lace up with five or six pairs of holes so that when it is tied it will hug your foot comfortably. Ideally, your training shoes should fit so well—they should be comfortable but firm— that they begin to feel as though they are a part of your feet while you are on the road.

Training shoes come in all different materials. Some older styles are light leather, which can be very good indeed. The newer designs are in nylon, which dries faster and is easier to care for. Plastic and artificial leathers are not very good because they make your feet sweat.

The question of socks is a moot point among runners. Some wouldn't dream of wearing them and others wouldn't ever go without them. I find socks are useful because they keep your feet and your shoes dry inside and protect your shoes from odor. I like the bobble socks that don't even come up to the ankle, the kind women tennis players often wear because (here my vanity is showing) they make your legs look longer in shorts. Socks also help to absorb shock. You can keep your shoes, shorts, shirt, and socks in a little bag that you can easily carry with you to work if you want to run during your lunch hour. Most runners like to have their kit with them so whenever there is a chance of getting in a couple of miles they are prepared.

THE WARM-UP

Before you start running you need your muscles warmed up, your blood flowing in your veins, and your metabolic rate up. It is not a good idea to get straight out of bed and run. When you have been inactive and your muscles are stiff or cold you are far more apt to pull a muscle or injure a joint. A few exercises or simply moving about the house briskly for five or ten minutes will get your body ready for your run. If you have time, you can do a few exercises to limber the back of your legs, tighten your tummy muscles, and strengthen your ankles—all things that fill in the few muscle gaps that running leaves. Dr. Sheehan recommends six different stretching and firming exercises that have become regular practice for many runners. They take five minutes or so to do:

1. For your calf muscles and Achilles tendons: stand about a yard from a tree or wall. Then with your feet flat on the ground, lean into it until the backs of your legs hurt a little. Hold the position for ten seconds and then relax. Do this five or six times.

2. For tight hamstrings at the back of your legs: keeping your legs straight, put one heel up onto a table or windowsill at waist height (lower, if you cannot reach that high). Now lower your head down to your knee until you feel the strain. Stay in this position for ten seconds, holding on to your leg or foot to steady yourself if you need to. Repeat the exercise five or six times.

3. For lower back and hamstrings: lying on your back, arms at your sides, keeping your legs straight bring them up over your head. Now lower them as far as possible above your head, touching the floor if you can. Hold for ten seconds, relax, and then repeat five or six times.

4. For your shin muscles: sitting on the edge of a table, hold a 5-pound weight on the front part of your foot just back of the toes. (You can use an empty paint tin full of stones.) Now raise your toes slowly. Keep them there for a few seconds and lower. Repeat several times with each foot until you get tired.

5. For your quadriceps: sit on the table and hang the same weight over the toes of one foot so the tin rests on the floor and you don't stretch the knee ligaments. Now straighten your knee, raising the weight. Hold for a few seconds and then lower. Repeat five or six times with each leg.

6. For tummy muscles: do twenty or more sit-ups with your knees bent and your feet tucked under a heavy piece of furniture to keep your balance if necessary. You can either clasp your hands behind your head or stretch out your arms over your head, but do each sit-up by keeping your chin in and curling your body up from the floor to give the muscles of your abdomen as much work as possible.

If you don't have time to go through the whole exercise routine before a run (or, like me, you get impatient sometimes and would rather be on the road), then start your run very slowly and for the first five minutes or so keep it at a slow, steady jog until your heart and lungs get going and your muscles start to warm up. This warm-up is terribly important if you are to protect yourself against injury. And the older you are the more important it becomes. In a few people a condition known as myocardial ischemia, where not enough blood gets to the heart, can occur if they plunge into vigorous exercise without sufficient warm-up. Finally, never jog after a meal, a hot bath, or if you are really cold.

THE COOL-DOWN

Just as important as beginning slowly is how you end your run. When muscles have been very active they need help to cool off gradually. This you can accomplish by walking for five or ten minutes after each run. This keeps extra blood flowing through the muscles and helps your body to eliminate the waste products of exercise such as lactic acid, which can otherwise make you stiff or sore.

During the cool-down you can shake your legs occasionally, do some stretching exercises if you like, such as bending over from the hips, or simply shuffle along at a slow walk for a while. You will probably find, when you first start running, that you have a few aches and pains in your legs, hip joints, or ankles because your muscles are not yet in condition. This will soon change, and provided you are not in great discomfort you can ignore them. Muscle ache passes far more quickly than you would think. In a few days you should not have to deal with it anymore.

TROUBLESHOOTING

If you get a stitch in your side or your shoulder while you are running, don't worry about this either. Stitches are common and don't mean anything. You can stop and walk if you like, or just jog through it until it passes by slowing your pace a little and breathing deeply. The fitter you get, the less likely you will be to suffer one.

Sometimes you get a little chafing under the arms or between the thighs as a result of skin rubbing against skin while you move. You can remedy this or prevent it altogether by applying a little petroleum jelly to the area where it occurs before you begin. (Put some on your lips too if they chap easily.)

Most aches and twinges here and there are of little consequence and soon disappear. But if you ever have a *sharp* pain in a muscle, stop. You may have torn some fibers. This means that, although you cannot see it, the muscle is bleeding inside which will make it harden and swell slightly. Put an ice bag or cold compress on the area and get advice from a medical authority on sports injuries if the pain doesn't disappear in a couple of days. If you ever get a sharp pain in your chest, you must stop and seek medical advice immediately.

A RUN CAN MAKE BEAUTIFUL SKIN

I am always looking for ways of doing more than one thing at a time when I can get away with it. I have discovered that a run is an excellent opportunity to indulge in some first-rate skin treatments. Because aerobic exercises raise your skin temperature, opens your pores, and increases circulation to skin and muscles, it makes your skin far more receptive than it is at any other time to whatever you put on it. So before you go out, cover your face with an aromatherapy oil, treatment cream, or one of the French ampoule treatments (see Chapter 27). Your skin will take in as much as it can in twenty minutes. When you return you can simply wash it and you will have had one of the best beauty treatments you can get without taking any extra time out for it.

IN THE BEGINNING

At first it is hard. Even during the first minute or so of your jog your heartbeat rate will climb and you'll find yourself breathing deeper and faster because your body needs more oxygen to meet the demands being made on it. Once your muscles start warming up, your skin will flush as your circulation increases and you may find a little stiffness in your chest as your muscles expand to enable you to breathe more deeply and fully. These sensations may seem strange to you if you are used to being inactive, but they are simply an indication that your body is responding the way it should to this new experience and are nothing to worry about. After a couple of minutes of jogging you will probably experience an "oxygen debt"—your body is demanding more oxygen than it is yet able to process efficiently. You may feel as if you can't go on. If it is too tough, then walk slowly for a while or simply stop and wait until you recover.

After you have run for a few minutes, your joints may start to feel a bit stiff or sore and your legs may feel heavy like lead—two more unusual sensations. They are also perfectly normal since you are probably using some muscle fibers and joints in a way they are not used to being used. It is to be expected that you should creak a bit here and there.

When you are able to run for from six to ten minutes without having to stop and walk, you will experience your "second wind." Your running will suddenly get easier and your breathing freer, and you will find you are covering ground more smoothly. Sometimes this second-wind stage takes time to get to if you are a new runner. But eventually it will come each time you run.

After you have been running for several weeks and are able to run for half an hour or so without stopping, you may experience what runners call the "third wind." What happens is this: you keep running until you find your muscles beginning to feel sluggish, your breathing very hard, and your legs a bit heavy. You think you should stop because these sensations seem quite strong. Then suddenly you find all this changes. Your body becomes lighter. The running itself becomes almost automatic and you feel as if you could go on and on. You get a kind of euphoria, or "runner's high." It is with the arrival of this third-wind state that many runners experience the meditative aspects of their sport. Your mind becomes calm and clear, your perceptions heightened, your movements fluid and more effortless than ever before. It is a very exciting experience and one which, although it does not happen to every runner, is quite common.

CHANGE COMES QUICKLY

The more you run, the more in touch with your body you will feel. You will begin to notice that once flabby thighs are remolding themselves automatically. Your posture will get better, your skin will be clearer, your elimination more efficient. Your eating habits will also probably change for the better—slowly and imperceptibly, so you may not even notice until you look back a couple of months and find that you have no trouble resisting those not very nutritious goodies that looked so delicious a few weeks back. You will also find it easier to trust your body to *ask* for what it wants. Everything seems to work for you more harmoniously and better than before.

AGE IS NO BARRIER

How old you are, how overweight you are, how out of condition you may be now matters little when you take up running, so long as you follow the step-by-step program and have your doctor's OK. Where you are *now* and where you will be *then* (in three, six, or twelve months' time) are completely different. Running makes things happen from the *inside*. I know a young woman, fifty pounds overweight, who was so embarrassed about it all when she first started running that she would go out with a hat and sunglasses on as well as a heavy sweat suit that covered her from top to toe even though it was midsummer. After six months of running five times a week she had lost thirty-five pounds. At the end of a year she was truly lithe. She bought herself a beautiful pair of satin running shorts. And she has never looked back.

Another friend, a sixty-two-year-old Russian painter who lives in Paris, took up running because, as she said, "I was in so much pain from arthritis that I figured if I didn't *move*, all my joints would solidify and I would die. They all laughed at me," she said, "at the idea of an old lady running around the streets of Paris early in the morning. But I didn't care. I found it very hard, very painful to start with. Then I began to learn something about my pain. That if you are not *afraid* of it, if you just notice it and let it *be*, continuing on with what you are doing, it begins to let you alone."

DEALING WITH SCOFFERS

Another worry many women have about starting to run is that they will be made fun of by strangers on the roads and by their families. It can happen, but there is usually far less ribbing than you ever expect there to be. Most people you meet on the road respect runners—admire them, even—for their courage and perseverance. It isn't everyone, after all, who will head out into the rain at 6 A.M. to run. Friends and family will only tease you as long as they think they can get away with it. You are doing something that they would like to be able to do, but they just haven't yet come around to getting it all together.

When I started running, I got a bit of ribbing from my friends who insisted that I'd "gone weird." I think really it made them uneasy to think that the "lounge lizard" they were accustomed to was involved in something that seemed so far out. My running seemed a kind of threat to them, but they soon learned that I was the same old lounge lizard in my new skin. In fact, very soon four of my closest friends took up running themselves when they saw how much it did for me. Or maybe it was more in self-defense, since for the first six months of my running I could speak of little else to anyone and must have been a terrible bore. Perhaps they just decided to take an "if you can't lick them, join them" attitude.

If you are very self-conscious about being on the road (and most people are at first, although this soon changes), then get up early to run even if you come back to bed afterward. You certainly won't meet many hecklers at 5 A.M. no matter where you live.

IS RUNNING DANGEROUS?

In recent years, with greater numbers of people running, there has been an increasing number of scare stories in the press about how dangerous jogging is. You know the kind of thing, about all the people who supposedly suffer heart attacks from running. The latest scare is that running on roads will damage your back because of the jolt that travels upward from repeated impact of your feet against the hard surface. It is true that running can be dangerous if you are very out of condition and you go about it foolishly—that is, without your doctor's OK, without the right shoes on hard roads, and without starting gradually on a graded program. Otherwise there is no reason to fear that it will harm you. Those who speak out loudest against running are those, even in medical circles, who know the least about it. It would be very hard to kill yourself running no matter how hard you may try.

There is a true case on file with the President's Council on Fitness and Sports that provides an interesting comment: a middle-aged executive who suffered from constant fatigue and was discouraged about his life to the point of suicide had read the fitness advice that has been published widely in recent years. He knew, for instance, that it was supposed to be dangerous for someone as overweight and out of condition as he was to take up strenuous exercise at his age for fear of suffering a heart attack. Being of an unusual turn of mind he saw this as a convenient way of committing suicide without causing embarrassment to his family, since it would look like an accident. So he borrowed a sweat suit and went for a run. He pushed himself as hard as he could—way past the safety limit—and waited for the "inevitable" to happen. To his surprise, in spite of terrible pains in his chest and the conviction that he would die at any moment, no heart attack came. The next day he tried again. But though he drove his body as hard as he could, he still did not collapse. After a week or so of this, he suddenly realized that he felt quite differently about his life; all thoughts of suicide had vanished and he had more energy than he ever remembered having before. He decided he wanted to live.

CREATING ENERGY

The experience of gaining energy from running or any other aerobic activity is a common one. You will have it too. And there are things you can do to enhance it. For instance, each day before you begin your activity, try to be aware of your body as an energy factory by focusing your attention at a point a couple of inches below your navel. This is known as the "hara" center. If you are able to think of your *self* as emanating from it—not just when you are exercising but whenever you need energy—you will find this releases a great deal of vitality.

This technique is traditionally used for creating powerful yet controlled movements for the Oriental disciplines such as aikido, tai chi, and even Japanese and Chinese calligraphy. The hara, located in the abdomen, has always been considered a center of power—like a smoldering furnace in which the fire is forever waiting to burst into flame. As you begin your movements, keep focusing on this area and make every movement as though it comes from there.

When you are running or swimming, bicycling or rowing, focus on the hara center, gradually increasing the speed and force of your movements until you find your own pace. It should be one that makes enough physical demand on you (you can check that by your pulse), but not so much that you are left gasping for breath. Then you are ready to get into the second energy game, that of being *here* and *now*.

THE HERE AND NOW

Almost everyone has experienced the ability to summon up energy, almost magically, to cope with particularly demanding situations—getting a second wind when you have been up all night nursing a sick child and thought you couldn't possibly drag even one more ounce of strength from yourself . . . having an all-encompassing fatigue somehow disappear into thin air with the unexpected arrival of a much-loved friend you haven't seen for years . . . discovering the extra strength that an athlete gets at the end of a long race when he feels he has already given all he had. What, more than anything else, determines how much energy you have in any of these situations is not your physical strength, not what you ate for lunch, nor even how much sleep you had the night before. It is simply whether or not you are *totally involved* in what you are doing —physically, mentally, and emotionally. This is the theory of biologists, sports experts, and psychologists who have looked seriously at the phenomenon of energy or vitality and tried to distinguish between the traits of those people with high energy levels and the rest of us. They find that athletes, executives, artists, or whoever, all high-energy people have one thing in common: *total involvement*.

For most of us this kind of complete involvement doesn't come naturally. It probably did when we were children, but it is an ability we have since lost. While you are exercising is an excellent time to relearn it. Here's how.

While you are moving, pay attention to your surroundings—the sights, the smells, the feel of the air—and to your own inner sensations. Visualize something in graceful motion such as a horse or antelope, a dolphin or an eagle soaring in the sky, and focus on yourself as a thing in motion. It will give you feelings of strength and grace that will help you keep going. The whole experience should be demanding but satisfying, not felt to be an awful chore. When you feel you want to stop, do. But be aware of *why* you have stopped. Are you short of breath? Anxious? Did you lose the image in motion? Your reasons will probably be different each time it happens.

Practice this for three weeks or so, allowing your pace and your images of motion to change according to how you feel each day. Sometimes you will go faster. Sometimes you will hold back. That is all part of the process. Simply be aware of what is happening and let it happen. Gradually you will find your body gaining strength, your breathing becoming easier and your movement more graceful. You will find that you are also developing the art of being *here and now* in other areas of your life too. It gets easier and easier with practice. At the end of three weeks you will be bouncing with vitality and radiating a healthy glow. And your energy level—no matter what kind of energy you need, mental or physical—will have soared. That, after all, is what aerobics is all about.

10

The Fully Alive Body

There is more health and beauty through natural movement than you will get from vigorous aerobic exercise alone. For no matter how far you run, no matter how fine an athlete or dancer you are, unless your muscles and joints move freely through the *full* range of motions possible for them you quite simply won't feel fully *alive*. Neither will you have full freedom of locomotion nor will you get the complete enjoyment of your sensations.

The body is the medium of experience. Everything you do—walking, writing, playing, working, making love—you do through its movements. In fact, all life is made up of the action of living flesh and muscle on moving joints and bones. These movements are composed of finely controlled positions and motions. When your joints and muscles are supple and mobile your body remains free, glowing, alive and highly resistant to stress. To get it that way, unless you are a child or unless you happen to be gifted with exceptional flexibility, you need to teach your muscles to stretch to their limits and encourage your joints to move fully.

This calls for some slow, sustained isotonic movement such as yoga or stretching. Practicing for a few minutes three or four times a week will not only increase your vitality and your capacity for experiencing joy and pleasure, it will also eliminate the chronic tension that results in headaches and menstrual complaints and the other long-term problems some women believe they either have to suffer in silence or treat with tranquilizers and pain-killers. You don't!

A "LIVING DEATH"

Most important of all, because your body is the physical expression of your experiences and your relationship to life, when chronic muscle tension and flaccidness are widespread enough, you become pervaded with a feeling of numbness which many women experience more emotionally than physically.

The world is full of people walking around feeling indifferent to themselves and their lives. They seek highs through artificial means such as alcohol and drugs. This numbness usually develops gradually, unnoticeably, until in time the victim loses much of her sensitivity and her capacity for experiencing pleasure from everyday things. In a sense her body, which has gone unused, dies.

Many women remain unaware that the sense of ennui they have is a physical problem and not some basic disillusionment with their lives. In fact, many people come to think of it as being normal—that is, until serious depression develops or severe back pain or a chronic illness. Then they wonder what went wrong. Long-term chronic tension in shoulders, around hip joints, in the back of the legs, in the neck and head and elsewhere does something else too. It robs you of vitality simply because much of the energy you could be using for living has to go into maintaining the rigidity of the muscles.

GET TO KNOW YOUR MUSCLES

The cause of all excess tension lies in restricted muscles. It is impossible to be emotionally tense or anxious if your muscles are completely relaxed. Learning to release tension through slow, sustained stretching makes true freedom of movement possible. Muscles are elastic things, able both to contract and to stretch up to one and a half times their relaxed length. A healthy muscle can be in one of three different states:

1. It can be *contracted*, which means it is in the act of causing movement in the skeleton.

2. It can be *in tone*, which is in the normal state of an awake muscle where its power is latent but the muscle is ready instantly to contract or stretch as soon as a nerve impulse to do so reaches it.

3. It can be *relaxed*, which should only happen when you are asleep.

In a truly fit and alive body the muscles are capable of moving from any one of these states to either of the others quickly and without strain. In most of us they are not, simply because we do not use them fully so they have become neglected.

When a muscle goes unused or is only partially used it either becomes chronically tense (in which case it feels rigid to the touch) or it goes flaccid.

Muscles work in antagonistic pairs and groups. As one set of muscle fibers contracts, its opposite set relaxes and stretches. Not a single muscle in your body works alone. The ratio of strength between opposing muscles and groups is finely balanced. But inactivity and stress destroy the balance. Then as one muscle becomes chronically tense its opposite becomes overstretched or flaccid and vice versa.

When you have imbalances in groups of opposing muscles your body is more liable to damage, particularly in the flaccid areas where fibers and tendons are weaker. This can also affect the strength and health of your internal organs which, like your bones, are held in place by the body's musculature. A combination of tension and flaccidness in opposing muscle groups is why, in an unconditioned or out of shape body, you find simultaneously a state of flabbiness in some areas (thighs, stomach, and bottom, for instance) and rigidity in others (shoulder blades, calves, and sacrum, for example) which leads to the distortions in body shape that women find so disheartening and so difficult to change—the expanding midriff, the bulging thighs, the "dowager's hump" at the base of the neck.

In the areas where muscles are weak, fat forms around them for they do no work to help disperse fatty deposits. The muscles sag and the skin covering sags with them. At the same time their opposing muscles, which are chronically tense or contracted, remain in a near static state. They are hard and bulging and their movement is restricted. This stasis impedes natural circulation of lymph and blood to the area, which means that vital nutrients and oxygen are in short supply to the cells. It also interferes with your body's ability to carry out tissue repair when needed and restricts the elimination of cellular wastes.

There is also a possible fourth state for muscles. It is one that does not usually occur in everyday life. It is called the state of *full stretch*. You experience it through slow isotonic movements that will reshape your body to its natural form from the inside out.

Dance teacher Sidi Hessel describes rather well what can happen from slow, deliberate stretching in his book *The Articulate Body*. "Tense or slack muscles are like ill-fitting clothes," he says, "either too tight or too loose. This accounts for the rigid, even brittle, appearance and angular movements of tense bodies, and the blurred pendulous contours of bodies that lack good muscle tone. With tensions released and natural resilience restored, muscles *fit* the body properly. Tense muscles become pliable and slack muscles shorten and wrap more closely round their supporting frame. Like a well-fitting girdle, they take up slack flesh and redistribute it in firmer and smoother contours."

The elasticity of a muscle is the real measure of good muscle tone, not the size as many people think. Many overtense muscles in thighs and calves, for instance, appear to be overdeveloped. A woman who had them might hesitate to do any form of exercise lest they get even bigger. But excessive size is not a sign of good muscle development at all. It is, instead, a sign of chronic muscle tension. Just as stretching exercises will build up soft flabby areas, they can also reduce areas that are too big because slow isotonic stretching has the ability to normalize—to help restore true form to each area of your body.

WHAT HAPPENS WHEN YOU STRETCH?

When you stretch a particular muscle you squeeze the blood (especially the veinous blood) out of it. This blood does not depend on the beat of the heart for its circulation. It depends on the contraction and relaxation of muscles that, when they move, compress the veins and capillaries, pushing the blood back in the direction of the heart. Only by this periodic contraction and expansion will any muscle be properly cleansed of the cellular wastes that accumulate in it and only then will it get the circulation of blood needed to bring nutrients and oxygen in optimum quantities to the cells. For as soon as the stretch is finished and your muscle springs back to its normal size, it becomes automatically bathed in fresh blood which cleanses and nourishes it. This is one of the reasons stretching brings with it a wonderful sense of renewal to the whole body.

While dynamic, aerobic exercise brings great benefit to your heart and lungs, tones many of the muscles in your body, and brings you greater vitality, the slow, deliberate stretching of specific muscle groups will give you extraordinary grace, improve the flexibility of your joints, and eliminate muscle tension, which is so limiting not only to your physical well-being but also to your personal sense of being free.

TRUE GRACE

Once you start to untense your muscles by stretching, you become physically and mentally lighter as the energy that was once wasted in maintaining muscle tension is freed. Your movements become more economical and your natural grace begins to emerge. The interesting things about this natural grace is that it will differ from one woman to another because it is an expression of her individuality. It bears little resemblance to the stereotyped, controlled balletic movements or the supposedly graceful movements that have traditionally been imposed on women by teachers of one kind or another. It is, instead, a grace that speaks for itself and seems to say, "Set the body free and it will find its own way."

I first became aware of what this kind of stretching could do for me when I met two young British teachers, John Stirk and David Stebbing. Both men had discovered the value of this kind of movement and both believed that the secret to releasing chronic muscle tension and at the same time tightening and toning flaccidness lay in learning to make "effortless effort"—in other words, in putting oneself in specific postures that work *against* the tension and then learning to let it go by allowing the body to move naturally the way it falls. This is where gravity comes in. There is no need, John and David taught me, to go through complicated and exhausting movements stretching and straining one part of the body against the other as women do in the traditional calisthenic movements designed to trim a thigh or arrest a spreading waistline.

GOING WITH GRAVITY

The force of gravity imposes a natural pull on every human body. Since muscle tension is ultimately the result of strain (although usually unconscious) against the natural full movement of a muscle, why, asked Stirk and Stebbing, could one not eliminate it by putting the body in certain positions where gravity will gently urge muscles to give up their stiffness while toning their opposite flaccid muscles? Why not indeed?

They taught me a series of exercises. I tried them and they worked, beautifully. Not only did these exercises realign the body and bring areas deadened by chronic tension back to life, they also helped women find their own natural grace in movement while restoring normality to the musculature all over the body, from the top of the neck to the bottom of the foot.

In the process, these postures also whittle away excess flab far better, I have found, than the unpleasant and compulsive repetition of calisthenics designed to work on specific areas. They also restore good circulation all over the body, particularly in cellulite-prone areas where it is needed most, and they restore good tone where before there was excess tension or unsightly flab.

SENSUOUS STRETCHING

Stretching needs to be done slowly and gently. You simply sink into a posture and then gradually let go, allowing gravity to pull as it will.

There is a wonderful sensuous feeling about doing this in the different positions, which will leave you feeling not only physically more alive and mentally clearer but also emotionally calm and still, much as meditation techniques do.

It is important to breathe normally while you do the postures and to let yourself relax as completely as you can in each one. The more you practice the postures the easier this becomes. If at first you are not fully relaxed, you may be inclined to hold your breath and to breathe spasmodically. Don't. Neither should you impose any artificial way of breathing on yourself.

When you first begin the postures you may find you feel stiffness or soreness in your muscles as they start to let go their stored tension. This is a good sign that they are giving up tension. To release stiffness you first need to be aware of it, and it is normal for the awakening process to bring with it mild sensations of pain. But the pain is not the pain of doing something *wrong*. It is a good ache that comes from letting go. It is also something you are completely in control of in each posture. You can go only as far as is comfortable for you. Then, as your muscles let go a little more, you will find that you can go a little farther each time. But never strain—strain or effort to force anything will only work against the effectiveness of the postures.

HOW TO BEGIN

Choose three postures at a time, spending fifteen to twenty minutes a day doing them three to five times a week. You can do them any time, but not immediately before bed or you may feel so invigorated by them that you won't want to sleep. Doing three postures one day and another three the next and so on, you will soon learn them and may find the results and sense of enjoyment they bring give you a desire to spend more time on them. But you should never exceed thirty minutes a day. You don't need more than that and it is far better to do less and have them be something you look forward to the next time than to glut yourself on them one day and skip them when the following session rolls around. There is never any rush, so go easy and learn to let gravity work for you. The postures are particularly useful when you are tired from work, in the early evening, and are most enjoyable when done with another person or with children. But there is never any sense of competition about how far you can go compared to someone else. Everyone is different and you are only working against yourself. What matters is the continuous releasing of tightness.

Hip Bends for Grace

The Rewards: This posture eases tension in your hamstring muscles at the backs of your legs and lengthens the back. Because it reverses the blood flow to the head, it is also good for your skin, face muscles, and overall circulation as well as bringing a feeling of being revitalized all over.

Here's how: Standing straight, facing a wall, feet a few inches apart and parallel, bend your knees and bend at the hips, dropping your head and back down against the wall, letting your face go limp and your hands and arms hang free in front of you. Now straighten your legs, slowly coming back up with your back against the wall. Rest in this position for one minute (you can gradually work up to four as you get used to it). As a variation, bend one leg for thirty seconds to one minute to give added stretch to the hamstrings of the other leg. With practice, your trunk will gradually go lower and lower with your legs straight. This promotes a free movement at the hip joints for a more beautiful walk and also lengthens the spine.

Wall Splits for Awareness

The Rewards: This passive exercise will make you aware of tensions you never dreamed existed. Practicing it regularly can improve your stride, release tensions in your pelvis that interfere with sexual response, and give inner thighs the workout they need to keep them smooth and sleek. It is also excellent for learning how to let gravity work for you instead of expending energy working against it.

Here's how: Sit parallel to a wall, legs extending out in front of you, one hip right up against the wall. Now lie down, swinging both legs up in an arc along the wall as you turn your body around so that you end up at right angles to the wall with your legs in a "V" shape. Let your legs fall gently open with the force of gravity to their maximum width. They should be flush against the wall at all times with your ankles flexed so your feet form almost a right angle with your legs. Relax and let go. You'll feel an ache at the inside of your thigh caused by excess habitual tension. Just be *aware* of it. You'll find the ache will change in character until it becomes not unpleasant as your muscles start to let go. Gradually your legs will open more and more. Don't force anything—just let it happen. Stay in this position for three minutes with your eyes closed, being quietly aware of the feelings in your body.

Lean-tos for Freedom

The Rewards: This movement opens up the chest cavity, improving your breathing. It can even widen the breadth of your emotional response, bringing you a new sense of freedom all over. It also relieves lower back tension, which can result in menstrual pains, and increases the flexibility of your arms at the shoulders.

Here's how: Standing three to four feet from a wall, arms at shoulder width, place your hands against the wall two feet above your head. Lean on your hands, letting your head and neck drop forward with the pull of gravity and allowing your chest to sink downward so that your back is bowed. Spend no more than half a minute in this position. Repeat three times.

Stretch Back for Length

The Rewards: This posture eliminates excess tension in shoulders, throat, and pectorals, and is excellent for combating a double chin as well. It brings with it a remarkable sensation of loosening and freedom in the upper half of your body.

Here's how: Using a low table over which you have placed a folded blanket, push the table near a wall and then lie down on your back on it so that your shoulders come just to the edge and your legs are in a relaxed position with your feet flat against the wall. Your head needs to hang loosely over the edge (you will find that you continually have to remind yourself to let go of your head instead of trying to support it). Now interlock your fingers or loosely hold a small stick and try to keep your arms straight as they are extended over your head and allowed to drop with the force of gravity. On coming up out of this position, come up slowly and roll over to one side before lifting yourself. Begin by doing the posture for two minutes and then gradually increase your time to four.

The Neck Stretch for Beautiful Carriage

The Rewards: This challenging exercise releases the tension in your neck and promotes a fresh flow of blood to your head. It also lengthens the whole back, relaxes the muscles in your eyes, relieving eye strain, and can also help headache and migraine sufferers by eliminating tension in the neck and shoulders that spurs the pain. It is also great for relaxing if you ordinarily have trouble sleeping.

Here's how: Lying flat on your back, legs stretched out in front, hands by your sides and palms on the floor, bend your knees and lift your legs *slowly* over your body and head, pushing down with your palms until you are as far onto your neck as possible, keeping your chin well in and head straight. (If your feet don't easily touch the floor, you should use a cushion or low chair to rest them on.) Go easy. Relax and let go as much as you can being aware of where you are stretching. This exercise contains the whole secret of the effort of making no effort. At first you might feel a bit nervous about the unusual sensations it brings with it but after one or two tries you will be able to let go. Time: one minute, then *gradually* increase to five.

Twist-overs for Waist and Spine

The Rewards: This movement lengthens the chest and front shoulder muscles, restoring flexibility at the shoulder joints. It also helps trim down a spreading waistline and midriff. The twisting motion gives elasticity to the spine, making it stronger and more supple and helping to protect it from backache.

Here's how: Lying on your back, draw up your feet and cross your legs, left over right, then tuck your left foot under your right calf. Lock your legs in this position and then slowly take your knees over and down to one side to touch the floor, stretching your left arm above the head and gently working your shoulder down to the floor (it may not go all the way to begin with, but it will in time). Now, in a wide and gentle arc, move the same arm around in a half circle until it reaches your side, working your shoulder down to the floor in tiny stops along the arc. Repeat this three times, taking about half a minute for your arm to travel through the arc each time. Change legs and repeat.

Lie-backs for Beautiful Legs

The Rewards: This exercise loosens tension in the muscles all along the front of the legs and slims and strengthens the thighs. It also strengthens the middle and upper back, and used with other back exercises it can help protect you from chronic backache.

Here's how: Sit on your heels with your legs folded under you, back straight, feet far enough apart for your buttocks to rest on the floor. Place your hands behind you, palms on the floor (or, if you are supple enough, bend arms and rest elbows and arms on the floor) and keeping knees together, lean back, stretching out the muscles on the front of the legs while you look down over the front of your body. Go easy. Never strain. As you do this you will find it easier and easier and you can get closer and closer to the floor. If you find it very hard, then place a chair covered with a blanket or a pillow behind you and lean against that until you are flexible enough to go clear to the floor. Be careful—if you get any pain in your *lower* back this means you have gone beyond your present limit. Ease forward again until the pain is gone.

Hip Looseners

The Rewards: This posture helps develop full movement in the hip joint and also stretches the powerful muscles at the inside of the thighs. It leads to more graceful movement and eliminates tensions that interfere with sexual pleasure.

Here's how: Sitting on the floor with your legs straight out in front of you (use a wall for support to keep your back straight if you need to), open your legs as far as they will comfortably go and still let you keep your back straight. Now lean forward from the hips (if you find it difficult to keep your back straight in this position then you are bending at the waist). The movement should only be a slight one but you will feel a pull down the inside of your legs when you are doing it right. If you need to at first, sit on a small cushion instead of directly on the floor so you can gently lever your trunk forward from your hips. Just be sure you don't bend from the waist, for however small the bend from the hips it is doing you good. Start with three minutes and build up to five.

Side Stretches for a Slim Waist

The Rewards: This exercise stretches the side of the body and whittles away excess fat; it also stretches the tendons at the knee joint for better flexibility when you walk.

Here's how: Sitting with your feet straight out in front of you on the floor, draw one leg up and in so that your heel touches the pubic bone, and the sole of your foot rests on the inner thigh. Then draw the other foot in so that the heel touches the ankle of the first foot. Now turn and face the sides of the foot touching the pubic bone. Making your spine as erect as possible, stretch out over one knee and let gravity work for you, the center of the chest just above the knee. (In time the tummy and chest will both rest along the length of the thigh.) Reverse the feet and do the same thing for the other side. Time: three minutes each side.

Stretch Out for Slim Thighs

The Rewards: Not only does this exercise trim away excess flab on the thighs and release restricted movements in the knee joints, in time it can also help eliminate the tension in the lower back that can result in sciatica, and it will strengthen and trim ankles.

Here's how: Sit on the floor Japanese style, with your calves alongside your thighs so that you are sitting between your feet. Open your knees to their maximum width and place your hands on the floor in front of you. Gently slide your hands forward until you can rest your head on the floor. (In the beginning your bottom will lift off the floor with the movement but gradually it will stay stationary as you stretch.) Relax in this position for three minutes, breathing normally and letting gravity do its work. With practice, eventually the whole front of your chest and tummy will rest on the floor.

Lower-body Stretches

The Rewards: This posture will bring with it firmer buttocks, shapelier calves and longer, more supple hamstrings, which improves the whole shape of a leg.

Here's how: Standing with one heel back firmly against the wall to help keep your balance, and the other foot eighteen inches in front, keeping both legs straight, clasp one wrist behind your back and slowly lever your trunk forward by bending from the hips—*not* from the waist. Do the other side by swapping your leg positions. Begin with one minute each side and build up to two on each side.

11

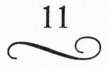

At the Back of Beauty

Posture is another important part of movement. But for most women posture is an ugly word, reminiscent of agonizing school periods in which one was urged to "Pull your stomach in, for heaven's sake, and stand up straight." No matter how hard you try or how long you hold your breath you can never seem to get it right. That is because this kind of posture is something imposed on the body from *outside*. It should be nothing of the sort. Good posture is quite simply the most efficient use of the skeleton to keep the body erect and give it freedom of movement. It is a way of standing, moving, and sitting that doesn't put excessive strain on the muscles or joints anywhere in the body. It comes from *within* and is most natural.

BETWEEN HEAVEN AND EARTH

Begin by standing as though you were suspended between heaven and earth by a fine string from the top of your head so your spine stretches out down to its very tip in a soft "S" curve. Feel your legs reach with strength to the ground and let your arms and shoulders hang loose. In this place you have a sense of balance and strength that seems to radiate from the abdomen (the energy center of the body) and that gives unbroken impetus to all your movements so that they are direct, purposeful, and an expression of what *you* at any particular moment are all about. This is truly good posture, for it is *real* and the movements that flow from it are real too—not some artificially learned form of gracefulness which may be charming or sweet but is empty of meaning.

Good posture like this also creates the correct relationship between the head and the spine, which is important in determining how you feel emotionally as well as physically. Long-term negative emotions such as sadness or resentment can lead to a distorted spine. So can a distorted spine lead to negative feelings (you have only to walk around with your head hanging over and your shoulders slumped for half an hour one day to discover this for yourself).

When you are depressed or bored or frustrated, your spine bends, your shoulders stoop, and muscles around the neck and upper back get tight and hard. This can result in headache and in restricted breathing with all the feelings of anxiety that go with it. When depression or fatigue turns into a chronic state, even a mild one, this curved configuration becomes gradually a permanent part of one's anatomy. But it all happens so insidiously and slowly that you can hardly notice it until one day you take a look at yourself in the mirror and are horrified to find you have an unattractive sway back or a dowager's hump. All of this can be avoided by a few simple exercises before your bath every day, by developing good habits of sitting and standing, by becoming more aware of your own body in how it feels and moves, and learning to move *with* it instead of imposing harsh mechanical gestures on it.

THE PERFECT SPINE

No spine should be straight. A spine is made up of a series of curves that form an "S" shape and give the back strength and resilience. But the curves need to be just right. Too great a hollow in the center of the back goes with chronic tightness in the sacral muscles, which interferes with sexual sensation and is one of the main causes of menstrual agonies. Too little a curve there leads to stiffness, poor balance on your feet, and a lack of freedom in movement. It can also result in chronic backache.

The vertebrae that make up this curve are held in place by a complex system of flexible muscles that are tremendously powerful. And in between each two vertebrae is a cushion of cartilage known as the vertebral disk. It has a soft center that makes it behave like a shock absorber to protect bones from damage and to withstand the tremendous impact every time you put your foot down to take a step. If, through injury or sudden strain, one of the soft cores starts to protrude from the edges of the vertebrae it lies between, then one ends up with what is commonly known as a "slipped disk." This, like most other back troubles, occurs when the muscles are shortened and weakened or when they are limited in their movements through lack of use or misuse. Then your back becomes vulnerable to spasm—powerful contractions of the muscles that don't let go—pain, and damage.

THE CAUSES OF BACKACHE

Backache is one of women's most common complaints, but it is not as mysterious in its origins as everyone seems to believe. Eighty percent of all back troubles can be prevented if muscles are kept resilient and strong through exercise. And although all back trouble when it strikes needs to be diagnosed by a physician before any self-treatment program, most of it can also be cured by exercise. The idea that because you have had back trouble already you will have to suffer with it on and off for the rest of your life is simply not true.

The interesting thing about keeping a back in good shape is that it is not just the muscles of your back that need to be strengthened. So do the muscles of your abdomen. Two large-scale studies involving some 10,000 patients with backache have confirmed this. Researchers discovered that people with recurring back pain usually have stomach muscles that are less than a third as strong as their back muscles. When abdominal muscles are weak, the body then tends to fall backward. To compensate for this one's sense of balance causes a shift in body weight, tilting the body forward and allowing the weight around the middle to hang on the muscles of the back. The result is overload, fatigue, tension, and pain—usually in that order. Then if you are overweight this only puts more strain on the inadequate muscles and makes matters worse.

When muscles either in your back or abdomen are not well toned they lack the natural resilience they are meant to have, so if you make a sudden movement or lift a heavy object, fibers of muscle can become fatigued, go into spasm, or even be ripped off the bone to which they are attached. The resulting pain is not always felt at the moment when the tear occurs. Often you can be engaged in an activity such as gardening and tear a few muscle fibers, yet not notice any pain until a day later. Ligaments and tendons can be similarly torn. All these occurrences are usually grouped under the heading "muscle strains," and almost all can be prevented by strong healthy muscles and proper movement.

HOW STRONG ARE YOUR STOMACH MUSCLES?

Most women become aware of the poor condition of neglected muscles when a strain occurs, but there are various tests you can run on specific muscles to find out how strong and resilient yours are. One in particular probably gives more indication than any other of how susceptible you are to back pain. It is used by one of Europe's top back experts, who taught it to me. And it is particularly useful for women after childbirth.

Lie flat on your back on the floor. With one hand stretched out and fingers together, press the tips of the fingers against the center line of the abdomen at the navel. Now raise your head off the floor. If the rectus abdominis muscle (the long, flat muscle on the front of the abdomen) parts, allowing your fingers to press easily into the abdominal cavity, then your abdominal wall is definitely *not* strong enough.

You can also use another test: lie flat on the floor, fingers intertwined behind your head and knees bent with your heels on the floor, as close as possible to your buttocks (you can ask someone to hold your ankles so your heels stay flat on the floor). Now try to roll yourself up to a sitting position. If, like most people, you can't, you can also be sure your stomach muscles are not strong enough to protect you from back troubles no matter how strong the rest of the muscles in your body may be.

The answer is exercise, but specific exercises—jogging and tennis, though they are great for the rest of you, won't do the trick. Swimming, however, particularly backstroke, is terrific for the prevention of back troubles because it brings into use just the muscles necessary to give good support to the spine.

LET'S GET TO WORK

If you exercise regularly, doing both an aerobic activity and also some yoga or stretching exercises, you will probably not have to worry much about your back. But in order to be sure, here are a series of movements you can do on the bathroom floor in five or ten minutes before a bath. They will strengthen and tone all the muscles of the back and abdomen, so you never need suffer the ravages of back ailments. Used regularly three or four times a week they will also help realign your posture and find your center so you will move more freely and easily and feel lighter. Finish them off with a rubdown all over, using a loofah, and then get into a lukewarm bath and relax.

Upper Back Strengthener

This exercise is great for relaxing neck and shoulder strain too. Sit in a straight-backed chair with your arms in your lap. Allow your head to drop forward gently, raise it again, let it drop backward, then raise it once more to the normal position. Then, without moving your body, turn your head as far as it will go to your right. Gently and slowly return to the center and turn it as far as possible to the left. Return to the center. Now, letting your head drop forward, roll it around slowly first to the left all the way around and back and then to the right all the way around and back, returning after each movement to the original upright position. Go through this whole series six times.

Bend-overs

Standing erect with your feet apart and legs straight, clasp your hands behind your back and bend forward as far as is comfortably possible. Then return to the starting position. Repeat five times.

Windmills

Standing erect, feet apart, legs straight and arms at your sides, tip sideways as far as you can go comfortably then return to normal, keeping the spine on the same plane (neither bending forward nor bending backward). Then go as far as you can the other way. Return to starting position. Now, with your arms outstretched at shoulder level, twist your torso around to the left keeping arms out. Go back to starting position, then twist to the right. Go through the whole series of movements six times.

Pelvic Tilt

Lie on the floor on your back with arms at your sides, completely relaxed. Tighten the muscles of the buttocks, pulling stomach muscles in hard at the same time, and flatten your back against the floor. Hold it for five seconds and then let go; relax for five seconds and repeat. Don't worry if your tummy muscles quiver—this is normal when they are weak.

Walking in Place

This exercise is especially useful for menstrual pains and stiffness. Lying flat on the floor, arms at your sides, relax completely and then tighten your muscles as in the pelvic tilt exercise and hold. Flex your toes up and elongate first one leg and then the other, alternating them by pushing one hip down and letting the other come up. (The movement itself is slight—the heel will only travel through a couple of inches—but the exercise puts the neglected muscles in the sacrum to good work.)

Head Lifts

In the same position on your back on the floor, but this time with knees bent, tighten the buttocks and pull in the stomach muscles as in the pelvic tilt, at the same time raising your head toward your knees as far as possible without straining.

Knee Touch

Lying flat on your back with arms at your sides, once again tighten the muscles of the buttocks, pulling in tummy muscles and flattening your back against the floor. Raise your head and one knee off the floor, at the same time trying to touch your knee with your forehead (or at least bring them as close as possible). Return to the starting position and do the same with the other knee.

Advanced Knee Touch

When you have mastered this, try the advanced exercise in which you lift both knees off the floor, at the same time pulling them toward your forehead with the help of your hands on your calves. Hold for a count of five, then release.

Sit-ups

Lie on the floor on your back, arms at your sides, legs straight, and feet tucked under a bed or sofa. Curl yourself gradually up to a sitting position, raising first your head, then your shoulders, then your chest off the floor and going only as far as you find comfortable. Hold for three seconds, then gradually return to the floor (the movement must be smooth with no jerks). Tummy muscles have to be strengthened progressively by making this exercise increasingly more difficult. When you can do it easily with arms at your sides, try it with your arms bent at the elbow and each elbow held with the opposite hand. Then try putting your hands on your hips. Finally, clasp them behind your head and bring your elbows as far back at each side as you can.

WATCH HOW YOU GO

Other things contribute to back troubles too—like poor nutrition, which results in stored waste in the tissues and the accumulation of fat, which puts far too much strain on heavily taxed muscles. You shouldn't sleep on a bed that is too soft either—it won't give enough support to your spine and there is always the danger of hanging on to muscle tension left over from the daytime or putting too much of an unnatural curve in your spine during sleep. But you needn't go out and buy an expensive orthopedic mattress. A simple, firm mattress on top of a board will do fine.

How you sit matters too. Most chairs are made to show off the designer's virtuosity rather than being orthopedically designed to give adequate support to the spine. Most chairs don't support the spine—the depth of the seat is too great. When you have to sit for any length of time, choose a chair that has a high back. As you get into it, lower your body gently, bending at the hips and keeping your spine straight, instead of letting your head jut out in the process as most people are inclined to do. Snuggle your back well into it and put your feet flat on the floor, letting your arms and shoulders hang easily from your erect spine. If you have to do close work like reading or sewing, bring your work up to your face instead of bending over to meet it. Also, don't assume just because you are sitting in some kind of official chair like those in airplanes and trains that it has been designed with your back in mind—airline seats are some of the worst offenders. And when you drive, make sure that your spine is well supported all the way down, even if you have to use a cushion or blanket or anything else that is handy to fill in the gap behind you. Never sit hunched over the wheel and always put your feet firmly on the floor of the car.

If you have to bend over to pick up something, bend at the knees, never from the waist, which puts far too much strain on the back muscles and not enough on the legs which are equipped to take it. Keep your back straight and bend your knees and hips, squatting to get under the package you are lifting; then, when you have it firmly in your grasp, straighten your legs and raise it up with you. When you have bags to carry, try to distribute the weight as evenly as possible between your two hands, and carry them freely so your shoulders rather than your arms take the load without tensing. Tense shoulders only lead to fatigue. When you stand at a workbench or kitchen counter, if it is low for you get down to it by bending your knees rather than your back.

Finally, when you are standing or walking, if you become tired or notice yourself curling over, remember what it feels like to be "suspended between heaven and earth," take three deep breaths, and get back the feel of being centered. You will look better, feel better, and your flagging energy will return almost as if by magic.

IF TROUBLE STRIKES

No woman should try to diagnose her own backache—leave that to a physician—but even a severe attack of back pain can usually be relieved by a combination of simple home treatments. The immediate cause is most often muscle spasm. This happens when a muscle or a group of muscles is overstrained. In fact, a spasm is a kind of safety device the body has, keeping a strained muscle contracted in order to protect it from further damage. But when muscle spasm occurs it interferes with circulation in the area, so muscle fibers are refused adequate nourishment and can't eliminate cellular waste products properly. This results in pain, which leads to more spasm, which quickly leads to more pain in a vicious circle.

To relieve an acute back problem, one has to attack both the pain and the spasm at once. An analgesic like common aspirin or a similar pain-killer prescribed by the doctor can help combat the pain, while heat or a cold compress is applied to the painful area to reduce the spasm. Then go to bed and rest, applying a hot-water bottle or heating pad to the area for periods of half an hour at a time. For some people, cold applications seem to work faster; try ice cubes in a plastic bag laid on the skin, being sure to keep the body warm so there is no danger of a chill. Massage with a muscle pain-reliever can also help—but *gentle* massage, not the kind given to football players before a game. If you can get in and out of the bath, try lying quietly in a hot bath for twenty minutes as this will also help relieve the spasm. Then, as the pain begins to disappear, start to move your arms and legs gently and to arch your back and tighten your tummy muscles. In a few hours, or the next day (as soon as the pain is better), get into the exercise program. It will put right underlying muscle weakness so you needn't suffer such a painful bout again.

ASCORBIC ACID HELPS

Vitamin C can come to the rescue of back troubles as well. Neurosurgeon James Greenwood at Baylor College of Medicine has had excellent results giving large doses of ascorbic acid—vitamin C—to patients with back pain. It is well known that besides being of great importance in the building of bones, blood vessels, and cartilage, vitamin C assists in the formation of collagen for the maintenance of strength and elasticity in the body's connective tissues, including the muscles. Greenwood gave vitamin C to 500 patients suffering from back pain, and they reported gratifying results even in cases where the pain was the result of a slipped disk. He recommends 250 milligrams a day for prevention and 1,000 to 2,000 milligrams a day if there is any discomfort or if you are going to exercise heavily.

12

Head for the Wilderness

There is something transforming about climbing a rock, particularly if
you have never climbed one before . . . or abseiling deep into a cave . . .
or shooting rapids in a canoe . . . or winding your way laboriously up a
great mountain. It is something about being in the air, about coming
close to the earth again—even more important, about the totality of the
challenges you face that makes you realize that the limits you unconsciously place on yourself have no meaning. These physical activities tell
you that you can do *anything* if you need to. The top of a mountain
with the wind blowing is one of the few places in the world where one
can discover that.

OUTWARD BOUND BEAUTY

Probably the last thing you would ever consider doing for the sake of
your health and beauty is going on an Outward Bound course. What has
Outward Bound (the province of eager children and macho men out to
prove their mettle) to do with being a woman anyway? I think just
about everything.

Living in the wilderness even for a day or two presents you with an
intense awareness of what really *is*, quite apart from the usual thoughts
and concerns around which we mold our lives. It also brings you a powerful sense of your own physical, emotional, and spiritual strengths. You
are faced with specific challenges—challenges on which your very survival can depend. Meeting them can be a source of pride, satisfaction,
and wonder. For what you are able to accomplish is invariably far
greater than what you expect. Finding this out can have a profound impact on your everyday life.

Women, I believe, often have a particularly difficult battle to fight in just being women. So many of our cultural roles demand that we adjust ourselves and our lives to the needs of others and to the demands of our society. A woman is brilliant at doing it because of her basic nature. The trouble is that in the process many women find that they themselves get lost. I have spoken to dozens of women from all age groups and social classes who have experienced this. They feel as though they have become the *roles* that they fulfill—mother, wife, lover, businesswoman or whatever—but when the roles are suspended by a holiday, an infidelity, or the nest is suddenly empty when the child goes off to college, there often seems to be nothing left except a hollowness. What, we wonder, ever happened to the *person?* Or was there ever a *person* there at all?

THE FEMALE ETHOS

To some extent the angry liberationists are right. We as women *have* been raised to believe that we are dependent, selfless, sweet and passive creatures. The cultural roles handed down to us from generation to generation demand the needs of others. By learning to conform to these feminine roles, although we may not be consciously aware of it we suppress natural qualities within us that don't fit into the notion we have of "feminine"—such things as physical strength, independence, pride, and anger. For in our culture these qualities are traditionally labeled "male," although, in truth, both male and female qualities exist in all of us and need to work together if we are to use our potential and are to express our wholeness and individuality as a human being of whatever sex.

As women we have developed the qualities allowed us to an extreme: we have enormous capacity to nurture, to be receptive, to empathize, and to be dependent. By nurturing I mean caring for the physical and emotional needs of others—supporting life. It is an enormously valuable trait, but the exaggerated degree to which we have developed it means that we remain to a large degree dependent on men to *do* and to *make*. By being receptive, I mean our ability to lean back passively and adjust ourselves to whatever comes. This is valuable, but it has to some extent deprived us of the ability to act when we want to. We should be able to choose. By empathizing, I mean the ability to identify emotionally with others and to be sensitive to what happens to them—another gift of primary importance, so long as we are able to maintain a sense of *separateness* and *self* along with it. Finally, by dependence I mean that we have learned the ability to trust and rely on somebody else. But there are two types of dependency—that which exists because one is weak and *has* to depend on another and that which is chosen out of strength, chosen because intimate relations *are* mutually dependent relationships; that's the way we want them to be.

I believe the extent to which we have developed our nurturing, receptive, empathizing, and dependent roles often stifles us. We as women tend to feel too passive, even though sometimes this is masked by the liberated assertiveness common to successful women. We have tended to consider ourselves helpless and to need and expect men to do things for us. We have been trained to hand over our power to men. In return we nurture the unspoken demand that someday we will find Prince Charming, the man who will bring us to life, shape us, and affirm our existence —our *self*. Except that, alas, somehow he never comes—or if he does come, he is never quite right, never quite everything that we feel he should be, and so once again that feeling of emptiness arrives.

A great deal of anguish in relationships, many unhappy marriages, and much disillusionment on both sides can be avoided if a woman finds ways of helping herself reclaim the human qualities traditionally considered male and integrates them together with her female capacities. For the more a woman comes to feel herself a separate and independent person capable not only of nurturing, receiving, empathizing, and being depended on, but also of *acting, doing, making, creating, directing,* and being physically strong, the greater is her capacity to share herself openly and freely with a man—or with her woman friends as well, for that matter—and the more alive, exciting, and fulfilling her relations become.

Because the "male" qualities are a part of every woman, they too have to be actualized for her person to become whole. Just as much, it is important that every man be capable of acknowledging his tender, receptive, nurturing, and caring impulses without feeling he is somehow emasculating himself. I do not know what possible tools there may be for helping to bring this about for men. I do know that heading into the wilderness, either in an organized group with a professional leader or with a friend, can be a big step toward freeing a woman's hidden potentials, which otherwise lie stifled behind her cultural roles. This is why I believe that taking up an outdoor activity such as climbing, canoeing, sailing, or cross-country skiing, in which one is committed to being in the wilderness for a day or two (or better still a week or two), is so important. And the more those hidden potentials are released, the more fun she will have and the richer and more creative her life will become.

Rock climbing, mountaineering, and caving may seem like activities that require special skills and extraordinary strength, but it is not so. Anyone who is reasonably fit can take them up. If you have no previous experience, it is usually best in the beginning to go on a course. There are many available, they are not expensive, and they have the advantage of supplying you with the equipment (from climbing boots to canoes) needed for the activities.

The Outward Bound movement started in Britain in 1940 with an aim to provide a range of outdoor activities like rock climbing, sailing and skiing and canoeing for young people. Participants were sent into the open air in situations that demanded learning physical skills and called forth the character to carry them out even in the face of danger or whatever odds the elements could throw up. Not only did they learn these new skills which helped to strengthen and develop bodies, in the process they acquired self-confidence and a sense of self-reliance which went far beyond their ability to climb a rock or jump off a cliff into a cave—a self-confidence which could be carried back to their life situations. So successful was the Outward Bound idea with young people that soon the very same principles were being applied to adults. Now there are courses for men and women of all age groups which stretch you beyond your usual limitations and give you an opportunity to have an enormous amount of fun, and get fitter in the process.

Whether or not you decide to put yourself through the paces of an organized Outward Bound course or simply to take up on your own an outdoor activity such as sailing or climbing, you'll never know how much it can do for you all over until you try it. The exercise you'll get is invaluable for toning muscles, improving skin, and bringing you a new sense of vitality whatever your age. Fresh country air and pure water can revitalize you and, equally important, can take you away from your everyday problems which, building up on top of you, cause stress and nervous tension. Instead you find yourself faced with totally different, unknown and unforeseen tasks to solve. On a course, the itinerary is usually full and you are kept on the go the whole time—mentally with discussion groups and physically with outdoor activities. On some courses, for one full day and night you have twenty-four hours of total solitude; this part of a course is called "solo." Hours to think and to contemplate, to fend for yourself, set up camp, and learn to live with silence. For some people it is frightening but for most it is a unique and valuable experience, an adventure in living both inwardly (for solitude is a rare commodity in the world in which we live) and outwardly in relation to the land around you.

There is no competition involved in outdoor pursuits, as there is in most sports. You are never given marks on how well you do, for the only thing you are working against is yourself—bettering previous attempts, becoming more skilled, gaining more confidence in your judgment and yourself. This alone is what matters, and there is virtually nothing beyond your grasp.

You can write to the Outward Bound Trust, 165 W. Putnam Ave., Greenwich, Connecticut, for information about the courses they offer.

Here are some of the different activities you might try:

SAILING

Sailing is a delight for the freedom of moving with the wind in the fresh air, but it is more often than not a lot of hard work too—both mentally and physically. Problems appear from nowhere and you have to cope—and you do. It is a demanding, rigorous sport and it gives you a great sense of achievement every time you do it. You can be any age to learn to sail, and you don't have to be fit in order to take it up. Start either by joining a club where you can get instruction or by crewing on friends' boats. If you don't know any sailors, look at the advertisements in one of the yachting magazines; there are always people looking for crew, either experienced or inexperienced, and it costs you nothing—they get help on the boat and you get experience.

It is best to begin sailing with a simple dinghy if you can, because on a small boat like that you can learn all the principles of handling sails, wind, and water. The clothes you wear depend on the season, although a nylon windbreaker is useful all year round to keep off wind and water. Wear rubber, canvas, or rope-soled shoes on board or no shoes at all. Ordinary soles damage decks. There are many courses available on the coasts or at lakes and reservoirs where you'll spend a week learning the principles of sailing. They are not expensive.

ROCK CLIMBING

Probably the most frightening thing you will ever do, and valuable just *because* of this fear, rock climbing puts much more emphasis on mental and emotional strength than on physical prowess. Because of this I think it may be the most valuable of all the outdoor sports activities for women. Most of us could make a list a mile long of things we are unable to do. Rock climbing has a remarkable way of shortening that list tremendously, simply because a woman who has scaled 100 feet of sheer rock straight up rapidly comes to know there is little she can't accomplish if she sets her mind to it. Most climbers will agree that rock climbing is far more than a mere sport. It is a perpetual challenge to climb better, faster, and with more agility than before, and soon you develop more skills than you ever thought you'd have. There is also something special about the relationship between you and the rock which is impossible to describe—you have to experience it. There is a definite sense of closeness that develops between the two of you, and when it is established you experience the most extraordinary sense of "flowing over" the rock—almost like a dance. But it is a relationship that demands *all* of your attention, for while you are on the rock face there is absolutely nothing in your mind except how you are going to move, to find your way, to keep going. This is an experience which somehow sets your spirit free.

Rock climbing seems a dangerous sport, and because of its inherent dangers safety rules and equipment are so excellent that, provided you use them, you are safer on the rock face than you would be on the highway. Yet there is something about the feeling of danger when you are climbing a rock or abseiling down from the edge of a cliff that is very valuable in terms of breaking through "female" limitations. You are safe and yet you are presented in an immediate way with the idea of death.

You do not have to be fit to begin climbing if you take it slowly, although if you climb regularly you will rapidly become fit. Sheer face climbing demands more skill and finesse than brute force. To learn, you can either join a club or go on a course where a guide teaches you. The best climbing gear is a pair of riding breeches with long socks, although a pair of straight-legged jeans or trousers will do just as well in the beginning. The equipment itself—ropes, belts, helmets, and shoes—is usually supplied by the course.

MOUNTAINEERING

Mountaineering has ceased to be a sport for the elitist few and become a popular recreation for many. Every year more people discover the freedom, pleasure, and sense of renewal that can come from walking over vast expanses of wilderness.

Mountaineering is a first-class physical activity. It develops muscles, improves the function of your heart and lungs, and makes every vital function of your body more efficient. It also makes use of your mental faculties because it demands reasoning, critical decision making, planning, and navigation.

There are many courses available for the beginner that give you information about mountaineering and teach you the skills needed. But probably the best way to learn is simply to go out with an experienced mountaineer, for you need to get out in all weathers and over different terrains. Get the feel of the hills, learn how to cope with the unexpected, and learn attitudes that can be lifesaving.

The proper clothing is essential for mountaineering because you will be exposed for a long time to weather and conditions underfoot that can injure your health and sap your morale. Boots come first. Money spent on good ones is money well spent. They should have thick commando-type soles, good ankle and instep supports, and one-piece uppers with bellows tongue. Then they will be waterproof. Good mountaineering shops stock a wide range of boots and have experienced assistants who can give good advice.

The outer shell of clothing is made up of a water- and wind-proof jacket or parka, waterproof pants and boots. This "shell" forms a barrier between the weather and the microenvironment created by your body heat and contained in woolen clothing. A pair of riding breeches with long socks is far better than long trousers, because it keeps dry and gives you greater freedom of movement. Then you will need a backpack. The size depends on the length of your walk and the season. It needs to be large enough to contain contingency supplies—an extra sweater, woolen hat and mittens, first aid kit, compass and maps, food, and anything else you may need in an emergency.

CROSS-COUNTRY SKIING

Cross-country skiing bestows exhilarating fun and physical fitness and demands speed and endurance as you set off in crisp fresh air over tracts of snow-covered country. It is becoming increasingly popular and it attracts people of all ages, from those who can barely walk to athletes who race for miles over severe mountainous terrain.

The boots you use for cross-country are light and flexible and the skis are long and narrow. The bindings permit your heels to rise up so you can push one foot easily in front of the next—quite a difference from the tight, immobile feeling of being on slalom skis. Cross-country skis are made for ease of movement. They allow you the freedom to climb gradients.

You can ski cross-country in almost any weather provided you know your route well and are dressed for it. Your clothes need to be warm and windproof and you need a pair of dark glasses to keep from being dazzled by sunlight reflected from snow.

The Fourth Dimension
Stillness

❦

Introduction

Just as stretching your body to its physical limits through exercise is a way of *widening* awareness of what is possible for you, so practicing conscious relaxation or meditation is a key to your *depths*. Like exercise, it will uncover physical and mental potential you didn't know you had. Like both exercise and optimum nutrition, it will also increase your energy enormously. And, of course, conscious relaxation is the single most effective antidote to stress.

Learning a few techniques for letting go and practicing them daily can do something else even more important: it can help you get in touch with the very center of your being, which is probably more important to the discovery of your own individual beauty than any other single thing. Here at the center is where the discovery of your *self* begins. And this discovery and the expression of this self in how you move and talk, think and feel, work and relate to others is what real beauty is all about.

Relaxation or meditation practiced daily can also unlock new ways of responding to what happens at home, at work, and in relationship to the rest of the world. It can help you discover new, more creative ways of looking at things and free you from mechanical patterns of thinking and living which—although you may be unaware of them—destroy your feeling of aliveness. Finally, it can bring you a delightful sense of serenity. These are just a few reasons why stillness plays such an important part in health and beauty and why it forms the essential Fourth Dimension of lasting health and beauty.

First, we'll take a look at how stress and relaxation relate to each other and at how to make stress work *for* rather than *against* you. We will also see how the way you breathe affects how you feel. Then we will look at how much energy you have and how changing it can bring you a sense of being centered, which makes it possible to remain calm within even when you are involved in the most demanding activity. We'll look at some of the things yoga has to offer. We'll examine why sleep is important to health and beauty and how to make sure you get enough of the right kind. And, finally, we'll look at some simple techniques for meditation or deep relaxation that should become as much a part of your routines for health and beauty as brushing your teeth every morning. When they do, then you will know for yourself the countless benefits of relaxation far better than any book could explain them.

13

Stress and Relaxation: Two Sides of a Coin

It is now common knowledge that uncontrolled stress can trigger a great many diseases and disorders—insomnia, gastric ulcers, high blood pressure, asthma, and migraine, to mention just a few. But for a long time these ailments were treated like something over which we had no control. It was assumed that one could only treat their symptoms with drugs, treat the stress that triggered them off with more drugs, and hope for the best. Now, thanks to research into altered states of consciousness and work done with biofeedback, studies have shown that every human being *can* exercise a high level of conscious control over his nervous system. They have shown that we do indeed have the ability to release excessive nervous tension provided we train ourselves to do it. They have also shown that when this excessive nervous tension is released, the physical and psychological effects of stress are significantly reduced. The key to this control is relaxation. It can eliminate digestive disorders, lower cholesterol levels in the blood, improve sleep, make reducing easier and even speed up healing in your body.

THE NOT-SO-INVOLUNTARY NERVOUS SYSTEM

Most of the automatic, or involuntary, functions of your body are governed by a part of the nervous system known as the autonomic nervous system. It looks after the changes in the rate at which your heart beats. It regulates your blood pressure by altering the size of veins and arteries. It

stimulates the flow of digestive juices and brings on muscular contractions in the digestive system to deal with the foods you take in. It makes
you sweat when you're hot and is responsible for the physical changes in
your body that come with sexual arousal. This autonomic system has two
opposing branches: the sympathetic and the parasympathetic.

The sympathetic branch is composed of a group of nerve fibers radiating from the spinal cord and is linked with the catecholamines or adrenalin class of hormones. It is concerned with energy expenditure—particularly the energy involved with stress. It spurs the heart to beat faster,
makes you breathe hard, encourages you to sweat, and raises your blood
pressure. It also inhibits the secretion of gastric juices and digestion and
sends blood to the muscles to get you ready for action.

The other branch of the autonomic nervous system—the parasympathetic—is made up mostly of nerve fibers from the vagus nerve, or
tenth cranial. Its activity is linked with the acetylcholine class of
hormones, and this system is concerned with *rest* rather than action.
In fact, the workings of the parasympathetic branch are more or less
in opposition to those of the sympathetic branch. The parasympathetic branch slows your heartbeat, reduces the flow of air to your lungs,
stimulates the digestive system, and helps relax your muscles.

GETTING THE BALANCE RIGHT

When you are in a state of stress, the sympathetic nervous system has
precedence over the parasympathetic. When you are relaxed, the parasympathetic branch is dominant. A good balance between the two is the
key to enormous energy and continuing health. Balance makes it possible
for you to go out into the world to *do*, to *make*, to *create*, to *fight*, and
to *express* yourself as well as to retire into yourself for regeneration, rest,
recuperation, enjoyment, and the space to discover new ideas and plant
the seeds of future actions. Unfortunately, few people get the balance
right.

Instead, there is the dynamic liberated woman who is ever seeking
greater challenges and heights of personal achievement and who seems to
have endless energy—until she discovers in a few years that she is suffering from high blood pressure and is told either to ease up or to go into
long-term drug therapy for hypertension. At the other extreme is the
beautifully feminine, quiet, sensitive lady who luxuriates in physical com-
forts, dreams beautiful dreams, and impresses everyone by her serenity
but who never seems to be able to put any of her ideas into effective action.

The first is a sympathetic-dominated person and the second is parasympathetic-dominated. To make the most of your potential in action in the world and still remain well enough and receptive enough to enjoy the fruits of your labors, you want to be neither. You need to be *balanced*. That's where learning the art of conscious relaxation comes in.

For, like the sympathetic and the parasympathetic branches of the autonomic nervous system which oppose each other, there is nothing vague or unclear about what constitutes a state of stress and its opposite, a state of psychophysical relaxation. These states are like two sides of the same coin. The biochemical and psychological changes that accompany each can be accurately measured in a laboratory.

For instance, under stress your body consumes more oxygen, its metabolic rate increases, your arteries contract, the concentration of lactates in your blood goes up, and your heart beats faster. During stress, cortisone levels in the body are increased. Over a long period of time this tends to block out the immune response; this is one of the main reasons why you become less resistant to disease when you are under constant stress. All these changes are reversed when you go into a state of psychophysical relaxation: cardiac rate decreases, lactate levels fall, there is a decrease in oxygen consumption, and your body returns to a regenerative state. Here are a few of the measurable differences between the two states:

IN STRESS	IN PSYCHOPHYSICAL RELAXATION
The action of the sympathetic branch of the autonomic nervous system is dominant	The action of the parasympathetic branch of the autonomic nervous system is dominant

raised	heartbeat rate	lowered
increased	blood flow to muscles	decreased
decreased	blood flow to organs	increased
increased	demand for oxygen	decreased
increased	cortisone output	decreased
increased	blood pressure	decreased
increased	muscle tension	decreased

THE RESULT	THE RESULT
Readiness for action	Proper functioning of body's organs and systems

The secret of getting the right balance between stress and relaxation, between the sympathetic and parasympathetic branches, is twofold. First, you need to take a look at the stress in your life and discover new ways of using it positively. Second, you need to learn a technique for conscious relaxation and practice it daily until it becomes second nature. Not only will this help your body stay in balance and increase your level of overall vitality, it will also give you a profound sense of control over yourself and your life that is hard to come by any other way. Let's look at stress first.

MAKE FRIENDS WITH STRESS

Long-term stress can destroy your good looks, your vitality, and eventually your health. But contrary to popular belief, that doesn't mean there is anything intrinsically dangerous in stress. On the contrary, stress is the spice of life—the challenge just waiting to be met, the excitement of something new and unknown, the wonderful, exhilarating feeling when adrenalin flows through your body and makes you feel ready for anything. It only means that if you do not know how to move from the active, stressed state of mind and body into the passive state of psychophysical relaxation at will, then you, like most people (for few have this skill naturally), are likely to find yourself stuck in the stressed state for long periods. And if it happens often enough and lasts long enough, you can become physically or mentally ill.

The Fight or Flight Mechanism

Human beings are natural seekers of challenge. In primitive times the challenge was one of survival, and this gave a certain rhythm to the working of the body. When in danger from some external cause—say, a wild animal—the body reacted instantaneously, providing the energy resources to fight or flee. The physiological changes brought about in the body by stressors are described as the "fight or flight mechanism." Adrenal secretions flash into the blood and bring strength in the form of fat and sugar energy to the brain and muscles. The pulse races, blood pressure increases, and breathing speeds up. Within seconds the body's full energy potential is realized, so one can deal effectively with the threat—either by fighting and destroying it or by running away to safety. Both actions use up all the chemical by-products of the stress reaction—the sugar, the adrenalin, and the increased muscle strength that accompanies them.

When the danger passes, the body relaxes. The production of adrenalin slows to a trickle and heartbeat and breathing decrease. The body returns to its vegetative rhythm, restoring normality to physiological processes and bringing a sense of mental and physical well-being.

We are biologically the same creatures as those who dealt with wild animals. Our bodies still react to danger in the same way, but now our sense of danger comes from different threats. They can be the pressure of deadlines for work, the fear that someone is trying to take your job from you, or worry about losing the closeness of the man you love if you do what *you* really want to do instead of what *he* wants. All these and many other things too cause a woman to move into the danger rhythm state without suffering physical or mental damage.

The trouble is that modern life, with its noise, quick pace, social pressures, environmental poisons, and our orientation to sedentary mental work, presents many of us with almost constant threat situations. This is particularly true in the business world where a woman, instead of moving rhythmically out of the danger state into the vegetative one, remains for long periods (in some cases, all her waking hours) in the danger state with all the internal physical conditions that accompany it: her blood pressure rarely goes down to normal, her pulse remains rapid, and her muscles and brain are activated by the production of adrenalin but she has no physical outlets for this increased energy. Sooner or later, unless she is moved out of the threatening situation, she, the predator who at one time preyed on the wild beast, begins to prey internally on herself.

STRESS MANAGEMENT

One of the most serious by-products of this kind of stress is the tension it produces. When you are under prolonged stress, you unconsciously tense different parts of your body. This affects not only the muscles, but also the organs themselves—gall bladder, liver, kidneys, even the area of the heart and lungs. In time this kind of tension restricts circulation to the organs and also prevents proper nutrient assimilation by the cells, encouraging their breakdown and early aging. This, and the fact that increased cortisone levels that accompany stress tend to knock out the body's immune response, is why stress is at the very least a contributory factor in many contemporary ailments including ulcers, high blood pressure, arthritis, constricted blood vessels, and heart disease. Recently it has also been linked with cancer.

Because everyone's stress level is different, and because stress taken to extreme depletes your body not only of its resistance but eventually of its life energy, stress is also a major factor in aging. In fact, one of the main theories of aging states that the body is able to withstand only so much stress and no more, and the faster this is used up, the faster it ages.

STRESS CAN BE WONDERFUL

But the idea that all stress is bad is patent nonsense. As human beings we would be little more than vegetables without some stress in our lives. Also, and most important, the more committed we are to the lives we are leading and the more right they are for us, the less likely we are to suffer the ravages of stress.

The women most susceptible to stress damage include those inclined to psychosomatic illness resulting from the constant conflict between what they are by nature and what, as a result of social and cultural pressures, they try to appear. This seems to me to be a particular problem for the twentieth-century woman. For the cultural and psychological stereo-types of femininity and womanliness can be heavy burdens to bear. They often have little to do with the true character of a particular woman— little to do with the *self*—although conditioning and the will to please have often made women accept them. But it works the other way too: many of the more dynamic, aggressive women who have striven to shed these stereotypes have their own burdens to carry in the image of the hard-driving, liberated female always eager for new challenges and al-ways moving forward. For like a piece of elastic constantly stretched, they can eventually snap or only partly return to normal. So even those who by their nature seek out challenges eventually wear out. Nobody can live under constant strain. And *any* image one is forced to uphold only strains a person unnecessarily, not to mention what it can do toward destroying one's ability to enjoy and find meaning in one's life.

MAKING STRESS WORK FOR YOU

So in personal terms, for the sake of mental and physical health and beauty it is important that every woman develop an awareness of her own personal relationship to stress and come to terms with it. This is all part of what is known as "stress management." There are many different methods of going about it. If you are familiar with them you can choose which ones work best for you and you will be able to live with your own stress, an inevitable part of every human life, and enjoy it instead of allowing it to turn to *distress* and make you miserable, ill, and old before your time.

1. Realize That You Are the One in Power

You have all the inner resources necessary to deal with any situation that may arise. But do you know it? Stressors are neutral, neither good nor bad. They simply *are*, and they call for some kind of action. Your response to them and the stress they trigger in you is entirely dependent on you. It is inside you, not the result of some outside force. And it is in your power to decide clearly whether you are going to face the challenge and see it through, so that stress becomes a stimulus to your well-being, or you are going to allow yourself to shrink from it and let it turn to distress. Marcus Aurelius put this very well when he said, "If you are distressed by anything external, the pain is not due to the thing itself but to your estimate of it." This you have the power to revoke at any time. Taking stock of your own power and realizing that you alone have the ability to control whether your stress responses will be positive or negative can lead you to look at stress in a positive way, so that instead of succumbing to misery and despair in which you experience biochemical reactions that are harmful to your body, you can, each time you face a stressor, be strengthened by it and find it an exciting challenge.

2. *Know When Enough Is Enough*

Many women who appear to deal with stress well and face stressors positively make the mistake of carrying things too far. You can enjoy the "high" of the flow of adrenalin, but you can also become addicted to it. And no one can live forever under stress. Not only will it age you and eventually make you ill, but long before then it will also distort your perceptions of your world and your sense of values so that you become mechanical in your thinking and irresponsible toward other people as well as toward the needs of your own inner being.

You have to know when to take it easy. And you have to learn how. If you happen to be a dynamic type, you also need to learn deliberately to stop yourself sometimes and temporarily give up your challenge. Everyone needs to plunge herself regularly and deeply into a state of deep psychophysical relaxation. For there, biochemical reactions are reversed, the mind in its active, outer-directed mode changes to its passive, receptive one. You are able to see things from a different perspective and you emerge from the experience not only renewed in energy and clearer in your perceptions, but also freed from the automaton-like behavior that comes with stress addiction. For everyone, stopping and letting go is difficult sometimes. For some, it is very hard indeed. For unlike those who shy away from stress for fear of its disturbing their peace of mind, some women shy away from stillness as though they fear it will make them see something in their exciting lives that needs to be changed. For you can hold on to stress as a way of hiding from yourself. But for these women, as for everyone, some form of regularly practiced deep relaxation or meditation can be the key to yet greater enjoyment, commitment, and excitement in the never-ceasing world of challenge which they love so much.

3. Get to Know the Physical Antidotes to Stress

And use them when you need to. Besides a nutritionally adequate diet that includes plenty of fiber from whole grains and raw fruits and vegetables, you can take supplements of vitamin C, the B complex, lecithin, calcium, and vitamin E. The classic anti-stress supplement formula available from health food stores is 500 milligrams of vitamin C, coupled with 100 milligrams of pantothenic acid, 20 milligrams each of B_6 and B_2 and the rest of the B-complex range in the same tablet or taken in the form of brewer's yeast. Vitamin C and pantothenic acid help protect the adrenal glands from damage. Liver is an excellent food to eat when you are under particular stress, both because of its B-complex content and because it is rich in vitamin A, another substance known to strengthen the body's resistance to illness and allergic reactions that can be induced by stress. As we said in the section on nutrition, the need for vitamin C and the B-complex range increases manyfold when you are in stressful situations of any kind, whether caused by emotional strain, excessive exertion, fatigue, internal pollution by poisons or drugs or alcohol, illness, or even falling in love. Vitamins C and E are also useful in detoxifying your body and protecting it from the potential harm of stress-generated chemicals. And it is important that you don't let yourself get overweight, which reduces your capacity for dealing with stress, that you take regular exercise, which helps burn up the by-products of stress in the body so they are rendered harmless, and that you take a holiday "away from it all" often enough.

4. Discover Your Own Guidelines

Find out how many different principles and ways of managing stress you can successfully incorporate into your life. Then do it. Stress in a relationship can be a way of improving not only the quality of the relationship but also the value that one places on it. This demands facing discontent clearly and squarely and expressing it in a way that doesn't try to make someone else responsible for it. For instance, there are two ways of complaining when your mate squeezes the toothpaste in the middle. One is, "My God, you did it again. What's wrong with you?" and the other, "You know, *I* have a problem. I am really bothered by people squeezing the toothpaste in the middle. I can't seem to get over it. I'd be grateful if you didn't do it. It would help me a lot."

Another thing it demands is looking at every relationship as it really is, rather than as you would like it to be; also it means being aware of your own needs and expressing them clearly and openly instead of being quietly resentful that they are not met automatically by others.

It will help protect you from stress if you learn to deal with one thing at a time—living in the immediate present which, after all, is the only time you can really know, rather than worrying about the future too much. The past is completely dead. Only *now* exists. Knowing this can immediately transform a lot of distress into simple, exhilarating stress.

5. Learning to Turn Off

There are scores of effective techniques for quieting the mind and re-creating the calm serenity that puts you more and more in touch with your own creative center. They include autogenic training in self-hypnosis, yoga, biofeedback, transcendental meditation (TM), zazen, creative imagery, movement, exercise and breathing techniques. Learn about them and then make them part of your life—and, most important of all, enjoy doing them. Of course, they are doing you good and you should do what does you good, but they can also be a lot of fun. And no matter who you are, they can lead you into realms of awareness you have never lived in before, literally opening up whole new worlds of possibilities in your life, your relationships, and your work.

6. Take a Look at Your Life and Throw Out the Chronic Stressors

Every stressor—every situation that triggers off the stress response in you—is like a challenge. And one way of dealing effectively with long-term stress is to take a good look at what continues to trigger the stress response in you and to ask yourself the question "Is this particular thing a challenge I really want to meet, or is it something I would be better off eliminating from my life?" The question is an important one. Many stressors provide challenges from which one can grow, but some are simply habitual, rather like the treadmill in a hamster's cage. They lead nowhere and they bring you little in terms of increasing awareness or an ability to make better use of your life and energies. If there are habitual stressors in your life, then consider eliminating them.

For instance, take a look at the work you do and ask whether it is really satisfying to you. What about the financial demands you have taken on—are they *really* necessary? If so, is there a way you haven't thought of to reduce them? If not, have the courage to drop them and accept the changes which doing so will bring about. We all have a tendency to hang on to the status quo at all costs—and usually the cost is the loss of a lot of our energy and life. Even if you learn the finest techniques for meditation and stilling the mind, if you are in a job year after year which you hate, or if you are faced with a relationship that no longer has meaning for you, they will all do little good. For while they may protect you from serious illness, you will still be banging your head against a brick wall. It is not only important to take responsibility for facing up to the demands of stress instead of trying to avoid it, it is also important to take responsibility for *removing* stress where it is no longer useful and relevant to you.

7. *Develop Your Own Personal Ways of De-stressing*

Explore them all, not only the meditative techniques—try a walk in the woods for clearing consciousness (something quite specifically ordered by Tibetan doctors for patients who suffer from worry and rapid swings of mood), sailing, running, dancing, gardening, listening to music, or a hobby.

14

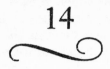

Learning to Let Go

We live in a world of constant activity. It is a world of striving and goals, of planning and remembering—a world of never-ending sensory stimulation, of exciting new ideas and discoveries. Yet amidst all this activity somewhere inside you is a center of stillness—a wordless, formless space where the seeds of creativity are sown that later become your ideas and your accomplishments. Here in the silence and the darkness you can hear your own "inner voice." You can come to know the difference between what you really want, feel, and think, and what has been programmed into you by habits, false notions, and values that are not your own. This space, a woman's center, is also a place of safety and security for her; she can move out of it as she chooses, to meet the outside world, to form friendships, to love and to learn. It is a permanent sanctuary to which she can return when she feels overburdened, tired, confused, or in need of new vitality and direction.

Locating this center within yourself, recognizing its value, and then living your life more and more from it are an essential part of staying well and being beautiful—in short, of becoming what you are. The key that opens this particular door for most people is *relaxation*.

PASSIVE AWARENESS

By relaxation, I don't mean sleeping or flopping down on a bed when you feel you can't go on, or losing yourself in a mindless state in front of the television—although sleep is certainly essential and the other two states have many things to recommend them too. I mean something more: learning to move *at will* into a temporary state of deep stillness or meditation in which your usual concerns, your habitual thoughts, and the never-ending activity of your daily life are replaced by a kind of alert, yet totally *passive*, awareness. The relaxed state permits some of the physiological changes normally experienced during sleep to take place to revitalize your body and mind simultaneously. But it is different from sleep. For while your body is deeply passive, your mind is very alert.

For some people this state occurs spontaneously, often between sleep and wakefulness. It is then that their best ideas come or that they experience a sense of harmony in themselves and in relation to the rest of the world. Scientists studying this state of psychophysical relaxation find that the brain wave patterns in it are very different from those of the normally awake state. After tens of thousands of hours of observation of the changes in brain wave patterns in subjects hooked up to EEG equipment, researchers have been able to analyze and describe a number of interesting altered states of consciousness during relaxation, each with its own brain wave patterns, objective physical manifestations, and subjective feelings. They have discovered that there is an increase in overall awareness and creativity as a person moves from one level of relaxation into the next deeper one.

This is interesting, for most people have a fear of letting go, thinking that if they give up control of things they won't be able to think clearly and independently or work well, or that someone is likely to put something over on them. In fact, just the opposite is true. When you are able to enter a state of deep relaxation at will, this *frees* you from patterns of living and thinking to which you tend to be a slave (although sometimes an unconscious one). It enables you to think more clearly and simply and to act more directly when action is called for.

RELIEF FROM STRESS

Relaxation is also the most important key to freedom from the damaging effects of long-term stress. This is something which by now has been well established scientifically. Many studies have been made of people taught a relaxation technique and then monitored as to the psychological and physiological changes that take place after fifteen or twenty minutes of practicing it. These studies show that relaxation techniques bring the parasympathetic branch of the autonomic nervous system into play, calming you, reducing oxygen consumption, lowering blood lactates (high lactate levels are associated with anxiety, arousal, and hypertension), slowing your heartbeat significantly, and changing brainwave patterns. They have also shown that repeated practice can lead to improved memory, increased perceptual ability, and a subjective feeling in participants that their work and their lives are somehow more creative than they were before.

Another interesting benefit from the daily practice of deep relaxation is a reduction of negative habit patterns such as drug taking (of both prescription and mind-altering drugs), alcohol consumption, and cigarette smoking. For instance, research in the United States involving 2,000 students between the ages of nineteen and twenty-three who had practiced a form of meditation for periods of from a few months to a couple of years showed that their dependence on alcohol, drugs, and cigarettes dropped sharply. The number of smokers was reduced by half in the first six months of doing the practice. By twenty-one months it was down to one third. And these changes were entirely spontaneous—at no time was any suggestion made that relaxation or meditation would change any of these habits.

Cardiologist Herbert Benson did the first studies into the effects of Transcendental Meditation with Keith Wallace many years ago at Harvard, then continued on his own to investigate this state of relaxation. He believes that each of us has what he calls the "relaxation response"—a natural ability to experience the relaxed state with all its benefits—and that all we need to bring it about is some kind of tool to turn it on.

The possible tools are many. They range from Transcendental Meditation, yoga, breathing exercises, zazen, silent repetition of a word, and autogenic training to long-term strenuous exercise and biofeedback—the list is almost endless. Each can be useful as a tool for silencing everyday thoughts and for temporarily shutting off habitual ways of seeing the world and doing things—for creating a pathway between your inner and outer world. All of them are different, and for you some will work better or be more enjoyable than others. That is why it is worthwhile to try a few different techniques until you discover which ones you prefer.

Practicing one or two techniques every day will make you aware of the enormous power your own mind has—power to alleviate suffering and bring a sense of well-being, power to change those things you want to change but which seemed impossible to change before, power to expand your whole awareness of your world of work, pleasure, and relationships. Meanwhile, almost automatically you will reap the well-documented physical and psychological benefits of stilling your mind. But regular practice is important.

DISCIPLINE FOR FREEDOM

We live in an age where discipline is often looked down upon as something that impedes spontaneity and freedom, something old-fashioned and stifling to life. We all tend to rebel against it. But it has been my experience, and the experience of a great many professionals working in the field of humanistic in-depth psychology, that the kind of discipline needed for daily practice of meditation or deep relaxation tends not to stifle one's ability to be involved in the spontaneous business of life but to free it. This is something you will have to find out for yourself. At first it may take a little effort to get up the fifteen minutes earlier each morning to practice a technique and to take fifteen minutes out of your busy afternoon or early evening to practice again, but you will find it is well worth it. The most common excuse is that you don't have time. The reality of the situation is that practicing twice a day for fifteen to twenty minutes will *give* you time, not take it from you, for you will find that you do everything with greater efficiency and enjoyment, that far less of your energy is wasted in fruitless activity. Every minute you spend in a deeply relaxed state will yield a fourfold return in the energy you need in your outer life.

Here are a few useful techniques to try. Some are oriented more toward the body, such as Jacobson's progressive relaxation and many of the breathing techniques in the next chapter; others, such as Benson's relaxation response or zazen, focus more on the mental processes. But it is important to remember that there is no real separation between the two; mind and body are not different entities, they are merely different ends of the same continuum. Each technique affects both. It could not be otherwise.

PROGRESSIVE RELAXATION

A technique based on the work of Edmund Jacobson, this is an excellent way to begin if you have never done any sort of relaxation or meditation technique before, because it gives most people some sense of what relaxation feels like even the first time they try it. As you repeat the technique over and over again (it is best done for fifteen minutes at least twice a day), you will find you enter a state of relaxation that is progressively deeper and deeper.

You might find it helpful to have the instructions read to you by a friend, at least until you get to know them yourself, or to make a cassette recording of them to play while you are relaxing. Remember to leave enough time after each instruction for you to carry it out. The whole practice demands about fifteen minutes with a break of from two to five minutes of stillness while you experience the relaxed state you have achieved.

The first few times you try the technique, you may find you have trouble picturing all the images as they come or preventing your mind from wandering. It doesn't matter if you don't "see" anything—some people are more visual in their imagery and others more feeling; both work superbly well—just approach the exercise from your own point of view. When you find your mind wandering (which is a common occurrence because one's concentration is not used to focusing so intensely, or because its being a new technique or a new feeling causes a little anxiety) ask yourself *why* is my mind wandering? Pursue that thought for a couple of minutes, then go back to the exercise and continue to go through it as best you can. All difficulties will iron themselves out automatically after you have practiced the technique often enough.

1. Find a quiet room, preferably one without too much light, and sit in a comfortable chair that gives support to your back. Place both feet flat on the floor and close your eyes.

2. Become aware of your breathing and just watch the air come in and go out of your body without doing anything.

3. Take a few deep breaths, and as you breathe out each time slowly repeat the word "relax" silently to yourself.

4. Focus on your face and let yourself feel any tension in your face or eyes, your jaw or tongue. Make a mental picture of tension—you could picture a clenched fist, a knotted rope, or a hard ball of steel—then mentally picture the tension going and everything becoming relaxed, like a limp rubber band.

5. Feel your face and your eyes, your jaw, and your tongue becoming relaxed, and as they relax, experience a wave of relaxation spreading through your whole body. (Each step takes about ten seconds.)

6. Tighten up all the muscles in your face and eyes, squeezing them as hard as you can. Then let go and feel the relaxation spread throughout your body again.

7. Now apply the same instruction to other parts of your body, moving slowly downward from your head to your neck, shoulders, and upper back, arms, hands, chest, mid- and lower back, your abdomen, thighs and calves, ankles, feet and toes, going through each area until every part of your body is relaxed. With each part, picture the tension in it mentally and then picture it going away; each time, tense the muscles in that area and then let them go and feel the relaxation spreading.

8. When you've relaxed every part of your body, sit quietly in this comfortable state for up to five minutes.

9. Now let your muscles in your eyelids become lighter . . . get ready to open your eyes and come back to an awareness of the room.

10. Open your eyes. Now you are ready to go about whatever you want to do.

This technique can also be done lying down if you prefer. It is particularly useful when combined with creative imagery (more about that in the next section), which is an excellent tool for rediscovering health if you are ill, also for self-discovery and for making positive changes in other areas of your life.

ZAZEN

One of the simplest ways of meditating, this technique involves nothing more than just being aware of your breathing. But don't be deceived by its simplicity. It is a potent tool for stilling the mind and regenerating the body. And concentrating your awareness on the breath is not as easy as it sounds.

1. Find yourself a quiet place where you will not be disturbed. You can sit cross-legged on the floor with a small cushion underneath you or you can sit in a chair if you prefer, but your back should be straight. (This straight-back position is a requirement for many meditation techniques since it creates a physical equilibrium which makes calm mental focus possible.) Let your hands rest quietly on your lap.

2. Close your eyes. Take several long, slow breaths, breathing from your abdomen so it swells out with each in breath and sinks in again when you breathe out.

3. Now rock your body from side to side and then around in large, gentle circles from your hips to the top of your head. Rock in increasingly smaller circles until you gradually come to rest in the center.

4. Now breathe in and out through your nose quietly without *doing* anything to your breathing (that is, don't try to breathe deeper or slower or faster; just breathe normally). With each out breath, count silently to yourself. So it goes: in breath, out breath, "one"; in breath, out breath, "two"; and so on up to ten, counting only on the out breath. When you get to ten go back and begin again at one. If you lose count halfway, it doesn't matter. Go back and start the count at one again. Counting isn't the whole point, but only a tool for focusing your mind on your breath.

If you are like most people, the first few times you do the exercise you will find you lose count often and you are often distracted by thoughts or noises. Each time some random thought distracts you, simply turn your mind gently back again to counting the breaths. Distractions don't change the effectiveness of the meditation.

5. After fifteen minutes (sneak a look at your wristwatch if you must), stop. Sit still for a moment, then open your eyes and slowly begin to go about your everyday activities again.

The exercise, like most techniques, is best done twice a day, morning and evening. A beginner will usually notice positive results by the end of a week but they become increasingly apparent the longer you go on doing it. Some Buddhist monks do this exercise for two or three years before beginning any other form of meditation.

BENSON'S RELAXATION RESPONSE TECHNIQUE

Herbert Benson, who wrote *The Relaxation Response*, discovered that the same measurable physical benefits that accrue from practicing Transcendental Meditation, which depends on the silent repetition of a mantra (a word sound), can be had by repeating *any* word over and over while the eyes are closed and the body is in a quiet state.

Meditation by concentration on a mantra or word sound has a long tradition. Some mantras are said to be sacred words that have particular sound vibrations which transmit particular powers. Each tradition has its own mantras such as *Guru Om, Om mani padme hum, La ilaha illa 'llah*, or in the Catholic religion, "Hail Mary, full of grace, the Lord is with thee." Whether their magic aspects are true or not, the technique works beautifully to replace the habitual chatter that runs through one's mind, such as worries about things past and things yet to come.

Benson suggests you find a word that is pleasing to you. It could be anything—say, "flower," "peace," or "love." He likes the word "one" as it is simple and has the connotation of unity about it. (The teacher Krishnamurti once remarked that *any* word would be better than the fruitless and often destructive thoughts that normally run through our minds; then he wryly suggested "Coca-Cola.") Here's how:

1. Find a quiet place where you won't be disturbed for fifteen to twenty minutes and a comfortable chair that supports your back.

2. Sit down and close your eyes. Give yourself a moment to settle in and you are ready to begin.

3. Simply sit there, feet on the floor and eyes closed, quietly repeating your word over and over to yourself: "one . . . one . . . one . . ."

4. Whenever your mind wanders or you are disturbed by a sound or thought, simply turn your mind gently back to repeating the word again.

5. That is all there is to it. After fifteen to twenty minutes, stop repeating the mantra and get ready to open your eyes.

6. Open your eyes, stretch, and go about your everyday activities. This is a particularly useful technique once you have practiced it a few times because you can do it in so many different places, such as in a waiting room or on a commuter train or bus. I know a lot of men and women who have made it a part of their daily trek to and from work with tremendous benefits.

TOTAL BODY RELAXATION

Like Jacobson's progressive relaxation, this technique is useful in getting rid of physical tension rapidly as well as in preparation for using creative imagery. It is also a technique that is often used in self-hypnosis. Unlike many relaxation or meditation exercises, it is done lying down. Once you get the hang of it and have done it a few dozen times, it becomes so efficient that the whole process from alert wakefulness to deep relaxation can demand no more than a couple of minutes. This is hard to believe at the beginning, but it is so. I have used it for years in bed each morning before I get up and each evening before I go to sleep, together with imagery or visualization about things I want to change in my life (see next section). I also use it in the middle of the night if ever I am awakened instead of just lying in bed fitfully trying to go back to sleep again.

If you do it during the day, it is often useful to place a small pillow under your knees while you lie back, your arms quietly at your sides or folded over your abdomen. If you like, you can put the directions on tape for use until you have mastered the technique.

1. Lie down in a quiet, preferably darkened room. Get comfortable with a pillow or two under your head and one under your knees too if you wish. Now close your eyes and take a few deep breaths, letting them out completely before you begin.

2. Think of your feet. Forget everything else and just concentrate on your feet. Now mentally tell them to let go; say to yourself silently, "My feet are relaxing and getting heavy—heavy and warm, warm and relaxed. They are sinking into the bed."

3. Now go on to your ankles. "My ankles are getting heavier and heavier, more and more relaxed—relaxed and floppy, floppy and warm and heavy. I let them go completely." Now go on to your calves and then to your thighs—"My calves are getting heavier and heavier, warm and heavy, heavy and relaxed. They are sinking into the bed—heavy and relaxed, relaxed and floppy. I let them go completely."

4. Now you give the same directions to each part of your body, moving from toes to head, one part to the next part, relaxing each part as you go—hips, back ("I let go vertebra by vertebra all the way up my spine") —then come around to the front to the abdomen. ("My tummy is warm and relaxed, all soft and floppy, sinking heavily into the bed.") Then chest, neck, shoulders, head, face, tongue, jaw, and eyes. Now do your arms, forearms, hands, and fingers until every part of your body is given the direction to let go. "My whole body is completely still . . . warm and relaxed . . . heavy . . . quiet and at peace . . . relaxed and warm. I can feel it in my mind."

Now you are ready to use whatever visualization you want, or you can let yourself sink even deeper into relaxation by counting backward from ten to one, saying with each number, "I am sinking deeper and deeper into a state of warm relaxation . . . deeper and deeper." When you reach one, stay for a few minutes in this peaceful, relaxed state, feeling the calm all through you. Then, when you are ready to finish, say to yourself, "Now I am going to open my eyes and get up feeling pleasantly fresh and well." Open your eyes and get up.

This exercise is done entirely in the mind. No physical movements are necessary as you go through the body. You are *telling* your body to let go. That is one of the reasons it is useful for making you aware of how much of an effect your mind can exert on your body. When you begin to practice, don't be discouraged if you feel you are not really very relaxed sometimes—it works even so, and the more you practice the easier it will become. After having practiced it a few times you will feel the pleasant warmth and tingling of the relaxation. Don't try to *do* anything—just let it happen.

BEYOND RELAXATION

Once you are familiar with the practice of deep relaxation or meditation and with all the benefits it can bring you, you might be interested to go on to investigate other, more complex forms of meditation. There are many, for meditation is not a word that is easy to define. It takes in such different practices. Some forms such as zazen or vispassana (sometimes called insight meditation) demand complete immobility. You sit watching the rise and fall of your abdomen as you breathe, and whenever your mind wanders you gently turn it back to this observation. This simply concentrated attention, which can be likened to the "continuum of awareness" in Gestalt theory, is capable of bringing up many repressed feelings and thoughts that have been stifling your full expression and of liberating them. The Siddha Yoga of Muktananda and the chaotic meditation of Rajneesh where the body is let go to move as it will are examples of this sort. They often involve spontaneous changes in muscle tension and relaxation and in breathing, and they demand a sense of surrender to the physical body for the release of mental, emotional, and bodily tensions. These kinds of meditation can be particularly good for someone with a tendency to be physically rigid.

Then there are the visualization meditations such as those used in Tibetan Buddhism in which you focus your mind on a particular image, fine-tuning it to the specific beneficial energies or influences this symbol carries (the creative imagery techniques in the next section are also an example of this kind of meditation). They have been used recently to cure serious illness and also in the sports world to improve athletic performance. Another form of meditation is that of "mindfulness," where you go about your daily activities simply being *aware* of each thing that you do, as in Gurdjieff's "self-remembering," shikantaza or mahamudra. These are just a few of the possibilities worth investigating if you want to go further. Each has something worthwhile to offer and the mere act of learning a new method and the set of ideas and attitudes that go with it can be an exciting experience as well as tremendously beneficial.

15

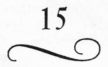

The Breath of Vitality

Even more important than the food you eat is the air you breathe and the way you breathe it. They can affect how you feel emotionally and physically, how your skin looks (for cells of the skin are dependent for their metabolic processes on a constant supply of enough oxygen), how much vitality you have, and even how clearly you can think.

Because breathing is the only one of your body's functions that can be either completely involuntary or voluntary, it can form a bridge between your conscious and unconscious functions. This makes it possible to look at your breathing to find out how you are feeling and what is happening to your body. It also means you can use breathing to change your energy level or your mood.

BREATH ENERGY

Throughout history the breath has been associated with energy, force, and power of both a physical and metaphysical kind. In the Bible, the word translated as "spirit" can also be translated as "air." It is the invisible life force, the energy the Chinese call *chi* and attempt to manipulate in acupuncture treatments. The Sufis refer to it as *baraks*. It plays an important role in their techniques of meditation. The yogis call it *prana*, and claim it is responsible for the extraordinary control they can exert over their minds and bodies. *Prana* means breath, respiration, life, vitality, wind, energy, and strength. It is also used to mean soul as distinguished from body. Yogis believe that if we are able to control our breath we can also control pain, emotions, and physical health, as well as supernatural phenomena.

The air you breathe is not a chemical compound, but a simple mixture of gases: 78 percent nitrogen, 21 percent oxygen, 95 percent inert gases, and 3 percent carbon dioxide by volume, plus a carbonic acid content that varies between .02 percent and .06 percent (when it is higher, the oxygen content is lower). In addition, it contains traces of water, a little ammonia, various mineral salts, and ozone. This curious mixture is the most necessary stuff in the world to all forms of life. You can live for several weeks without food, several days without water, but only a few minutes without air.

We tend to think that the energy we have comes from the food we eat. But as the ancient traditions teach, air, not food, is the primary fuel for driving the human engine. Without the oxygen air contains, your body would not be able to break down the nutrients you take in through your foods in order to produce energy and to nourish your cells. When air is first taken into the lungs, it fills the tiny bronchioles. Oxygen diffuses through their membranes into your bloodstream and is carried throughout your body to every cell of every organ and tissue. Your blood is capable of absorbing up to four times as much oxygen as water can, as long as there is enough iron available to produce hemoglobin which carries the oxygen through the bloodstream. One of the most important common symptoms of iron-deficiency anemia is the inability to catch your breath—you simply cannot get enough oxygen.

THE BODY'S CLEARING SYSTEM

While the act of breathing is supplying your cells with the oxygen they need, it is also removing carbon dioxide and wastes from your system. Carbon dioxide is a by-product of oxidation and energy release. If it were allowed to build up it would poison the cells and eventually kill them. So tiny blood vessels carry the waste back to the lungs, where it is eliminated when you breathe out and exchanged for new oxygen when you breathe in. At least that is how it *should* work.

In most women, however, this vital process of taking in necessary oxygen and eliminating poisonous wastes is neither as efficient nor as complete as it should be. This can be due to many things, from tissue anoxia as a result of a diet too high in fats (discussed on page 61), from insufficient iron, B_{12}, folic acid, or vitamin E resulting in anemia. But by far the most common cause is simply poor breathing. Most of us use only half our breathing potential and we expel only half the wastes, so in effect we are only getting from oxygen half the support for health and beauty that we should be getting. And because we don't exhale fully, when we take in new air the old air that is still in the lungs is sucked deeper into the sacs. This means that the oxygen level in the tiny alveoli which supply the body is far lower than it would be if the air they contained were fresh from the outside. Thus the amount of oxygen available to the blood, brain, and nerves, as well as the skin and the rest of the body, is reduced.

From the point of view of skin health and beauty alone, this can matter a lot. Seven percent of the oxygen you take in is used directly by your skin. When skin cells don't get all the oxygen they need, they are unable to carry out cell division rapidly and efficiently and the elimination of wastes is impeded, which contributes to more rapid aging of the tissues.

Less than optimum levels of oxygen in your body can also affect the functioning of brain and nerve cells. In fact, there is considerable evidence that many of the mental changes usually associated with old age, such as senility and vagueness of thought, as well as certain physical illnesses are the result of too little oxygen being available to the cells, either as a result of limited breathing or blockages in the circulatory system or both. Hyperbaric oxygen therapy, which involves giving pressurized and concentrated oxygen, has recently been used experimentally to treat a variety of ailments from osteomyelitis of the spine to brain damage.

Some researchers also believe that the air we breathe may at least be partly responsible for the subtle energy field which surrounds and pervades the bodies of humans and animals and which changes according to their state of health or disease.

On a more simple level, some physicians and therapists such as the late Captain William P. Knowles have had excellent results when treating chronic chest complaints, fatigue, depression, and nervous disorders simply by teaching patients the art of breathing fully. Making changes in the way you breathe or using specific methods of breath control can also help you do a lot of useful things such as increase your vitality, calm your emotions when they are disturbed, and clear an overtaxed mind.

THE BREATH OF EMOTION

The link between the way you breathe and your emotional state is well established. Not only do your emotions affect your breathing (Remember the last time you were frightened and you gasped for breath? How when you are excited your breathing becomes shallower and faster than usual?), but how you breathe can bring on or turn off emotional states too. Here's an experiment that shows this: Start to breathe very shallowly so only the shoulders and top of your chest show any signs of movement, and pant in and out quickly for about forty-five seconds. At the end of that time your heart will be pounding and you will have all the feelings of anxiety and fear. Or try it the other way around. The next time you are in a difficult situation and you feel you might lose control, *stop*. Take three or four long deep breaths from the abdomen and let them out slowly. Then take another look at the challenge. You'll find your mind and feelings a lot calmer.

The art of normal breathing is something I think every woman concerned with protecting her good looks and preserving her health should know. When your lung capacity is developed and used to the full, you will have more energy, suffer less from fatigue, and be able to think more clearly. It will also make your skin glow with health and your eyes shine. And it is not as difficult as you might imagine. It involves no more than learning a few new habits. Let's look at four that you can start developing right now. Then we'll go on to some specific breathing techniques for specific effects.

THE ART OF FULL BREATHING

1. When you breathe, breathe with your whole chest and abdomen too. Most of us breathe only with the top part of our body, which means we are not fully lowering the diaphragm and expanding the lungs and so are not making use of their full capacity. This kind of restricted breathing stifles emotional expression and is often linked with anxiety, depression, and worry. To check for abdominal breathing, put your hands on your tummy. Does it swell when you breathe in and sink when you breathe out? It should. Lying flat on a firm surface, practice breathing fully and gently until you get the *feel* of it.

2. Make sure that with each out breath you let out all the air you take in. By exhaling more of the carbon dioxide, you will get rid of more of the cells' waste products and you will be able to make full use of each new breath of air as it is taken down into your lungs.

3. Take up some kind of aerobic exercise—such as running, bicycling, or dancing—that demands full use of your lungs every day.

4. Use the following exercise for five minutes twice a day to increase your lung capacity, slim your middle, purify your blood, and help you learn the art of fuller breathing. You can also use it whenever you feel tense or need to clear your head:

Resting your hands on your rib cage at the sides, just above the waist, breathe out completely. Now inhale gently through the nose, letting your abdomen swell as much as it will to a slow count of five. Continue to breathe in through the nose to another count of five, this time letting your ribs expand under your hands and finally your chest too (but don't raise your shoulders in the process). Hold your breath for a count of five, now slowly let it out through your mouth as you count slowly to ten, noticing how your rib cage shrinks beneath your hands and pulling in with your abdomen until you have released all the air. Repeat four times.

Here are a few special breathing techniques for specific ends.

Sensuous Breathing

This technique, taught to me by one of Britain's top bioenergetic therapists, is a wonderful way of rediscovering the feel of your body. The therapist uses it to encourage the unblocking of any repressed emotional or physical tensions. She also claims that it increases one's ability to experience heightened sexual pleasure all over the body.

Lie on the floor on your back and relax as much as you can, letting your arms and legs flop. Close your eyes and feel your body against the floor; do you notice any tension in any part of it? Shoulders? Back? Legs? Now focus *inside* your body and ask yourself where you feel any movement in your muscles because of your breathing. Anywhere you feel tense, imagine you're breathing into that spot, imagine you can *exhale* through that part of your body and as you do, experience the breath relaxing your sore muscles as it filters through them. Then, when you are relaxed, experiment with the movements which are part of natural free breathing. They are beautiful movements.

When you breathe in, feel your pelvis tip back gently so there is a slight arch to your back while your abdomen and chest rise, ribs and back expand, and chin tilts forward just barely. Then, when you exhale, your pelvis moves down again so your spine almost touches the floor, your back contracts, and your chin and head move back again exposing the front of your neck a bit more. This natural movement is a wavelike motion that flows without hesitation from each in breath to its following out breath and so on. Practice it, exaggerating the tiny movements at first until you get the feel of it and then it will flow naturally.

The Decanter

This exercise stimulates the nervous system and at the same time stills a restless or anxious mind. I like doing it after I have been working in an immobile position for a long time—for instance, when I have been at my desk writing for several hours. I do it just before I get up to move about.

Sitting comfortably in a chair with a straight back or cross-legged on the floor, imagine that your body is like a decanter, the bottom of the decanter being your pelvis and hips and the top of it your head. Pretend that you are going to fill it with energy in the form of air. Now, breathing in slowly, imagine it filling up gradually. After you have taken in as much air as you can comfortably hold and are getting to the top, hold your breath as long as necessary to become aware of the feeling of fullness. Then exhale slowly and imagine that it is emptying as you do. Repeat this five to ten times. (If you find yourself becoming light-headed, it is nothing to worry about. This often happens if lungs are not used to being fully used. But don't ever *force* your breathing.)

Tension Taker

This exercise is useful to do whenever you find yourself under stress or feel you are getting tense.

Stand comfortably with your arms at your sides and inhale through your nose *slowly*. Hunch up your shoulders as high as you can, clench your fists and, standing on tiptoes, tense your body harder and harder, concentrating on your center—the navel area—to help you keep your balance. Hold your breath and sink back onto your feet, loosening your shoulders and letting them drop. As you unclench your fists, exhale through your nose very slowly, pushing down on your palms and on your shoulders. Do this five or six times.

Revitalizer

This exercise was taught to me by a friend who teaches yoga. It is wonderful if you are feeling drowsy from sitting too long or are very tired. It revitalizes you very quickly.

Let all the air out of your lungs—then even more—and then even more. Now take a deep breath from your abdomen so it swells as you breathe in. Exhale immediately through your nose, jerking in your abdomen quickly so it pushes all the air out forcefully. Relax your abdomen momentarily and then jerk it in again, pushing out even more air. Repeat this five times until your lungs are completely empty. Now take in a long, slow breath, retain it for a count of five, and slowly exhale it all away. Repeat the whole exercise five times.

Prana Power

This is an interesting exercise which makes use of the breath to do all sorts of surprising things such as banishing minor aches and pains caused by tension. If practiced regularly it can also help keep the skin of your face looking smooth and wrinkle-free. It is a simple yogic technique for directing prana, or breath energy, to whatever part of your body needs it.

Sitting in a relaxed position with your spine firmly supported, or lying on a firm bed, slowly breathe in deeply, imagining the life force you are taking in as you do. Hold your breath for a few seconds . . . then, as you begin to breathe out, imagine directing the energy to whatever part of your body you want to affect for the better. For instance, see the skin on your face as soft and unlined and direct the energy there, or direct it at your shoulders to make them lose tension and so forth. Repeat the process for three to five minutes at a time. If you are using it for smoothing away lines on the face, you need to do it twice a day. It is good to do just after a relaxation or meditation exercise if you can.

16

Yoga for Union

Like good breathing, yoga can also make you beautiful. And I don't mean by simply trimming a flabby thigh or flattening a neglected stomach. Of course, it will do these things too. But what I mean is more fundamental. The meaning of the word yoga is "union," or in modern terms, "integration." Practicing yoga regularly can bring a sense of calmness, poise, and detachment that eliminates the negative effects of stress and clears away tensions that stifle the full expression of your individuality—intellectually, emotionally, physically, and spiritually. It can also help bring together these four parts of a woman so she functions as a whole.

I first became aware of the potency of what is often considered a sophisticated form of physical education or rudimentary meditation—yoga—when I met a young British teacher named Geoffrey Triessman. Geoffrey, who had spent several years as a Zen monk before he began to teach yoga, made me realize that the yoga asanas, or postures, are much more than just a way of exercising the body and keeping fit. They are also a way of stilling the mind while making one aware of the particular psychic and physical energy blocks that chronically inhibit you, and then of gradually removing these blocks.

In many ways Geoffrey's approach to yoga parallels contemporary psychology. Humanistic and bioenergetic psychologists maintain that our tensions and habitual thought patterns are manifested in our bodies. For instance, chronic tension in the muscles of the lower back can often be a sign of sexual rigidity—an armoring that has grown up in the body as a result of a fear of experiencing pleasure and the full flow of orgasmic feeling.

Similarly, a fixed smile on the face can be a kind of mask which in time not only distorts someone's natural facial form and structure, but also hides her feelings and makes the face she shows the world false instead of true.

These habitual thought patterns or emotional restrictions that are locked into the body may be long-term, but they are by no means permanent. Change their physical manifestations—break down and free muscle tension, firm and tighten flaccidness through yoga practice—and you will change emotional, intellectual, and creative functions too.

THE THREE SELVES

According to yogic theory, there are three basic levels or modes of expression in human life: the subconscious or instinctive self; the intellectual or reasoning self; and the *mind* from which intuition, inspiration, and real creativity spring. In order to be healthy on all levels, these three need to be balanced. In most of us they are not; one or another or even all three are undeveloped, overactive, or uncontrolled. For instance, you've met the kind of person whose intellectual life is particularly vital and interesting, but whose emotional or instinctual life is immature. Another person has a capacity for deep feeling but is unable to find expression for it. No matter what the imbalance, it inevitably leads to feelings of frustration and dissatisfaction since part of that person's self is always lying dormant or battling against the rest of him instead of being freely expressed. Yoga works, through the body, to restore the balance, and removing energy blocks and chronic tensions is the way it goes about it.

One of the curious things about these blocks is that although we all buck against them, in a strange way we are also intent on preserving them. They seem to offer some kind of stability we can hang on to. In psychological terms they represent the bounds of our ego, which is familiar to us and, because of its familiarity, gives us a certain feeling of security. For we think we know ourselves and know what to expect. But the ego is invariably far smaller in potential than the whole person. By eliminating bodily tensions through yoga practice, one gradually enlarges the bounds of the ego so that one's awareness and experience of life—the capacity for work and play—expands enormously.

PASSIVE AWARENESS OF DISCOMFORT

In a sense this happens each time you practice yoga. You move into one of the postures slowly and calmly and you find yourself in a state of stillness. Your senses are sharpened to what is happening inside and out. It is a kind of passive concentration that is almost without thought or imagery. As you move slowly through the posture, the feeling in your stiff body becomes more intense. It can sometimes be very painful. One's natural inclination is to get away from the discomfort by coming out of the posture, but the effectiveness of yoga depends on not allowing yourself to do this. Instead of either withdrawing from the asana or struggling hard to maintain it (the ways one would usually deal with discomfort) you simply allow yourself to *go with* the pain, to be *in* it until, surprisingly, it disappears. If you can do this, if you can keep your concentration on the posture itself, accepting the discomfort, then after it is finished you will feel exceptionally clear-headed, whole, and well-balanced.

But it takes a little discipline at first. Then after you've practiced yoga for a few weeks you realize you are feeling better all the time. And the effort of getting up that fifteen minutes earlier to go through a few new postures is no longer a chore but something you look forward to. You will also find that you are thinking in new ways and that lots of the energy which was once wasted in various internal conflicts is becoming available for you to use as you wish.

It is important if you take up yoga seriously that you find yourself a good teacher, someone who has a personal understanding of the richness and potentials the practice offers. And good yoga teachers, although more prevalent than they once were, are still not always easy to come by.

Meanwhile, here is a series of simple postures which Geoffrey taught me and which anyone can do at home even without previous experience of yoga. They will give you a feel for what yoga is all about and help you decide whether it is something that will be useful to you. In the process they will also help you sleep better, deal better with stress, improve your all-over physical condition, and help any menstrual troubles you may have. They are safe for anyone who is in reasonably good condition and not suffering from a slipped disk, but if you have any doubts, consult your doctor first. If you set aside about twenty minutes a session to practice them, they will also leave you revitalized. But as with all the tools for health and beauty, the secret of success is perseverance—repeating them day after day is what brings the real rewards.

THE ASANAS

Every woman has two kinds of energy, male and female. Male energy is like the sun—invigorating, stimulating, creative, and powerful. The male postures in yoga call forth this dynamic energy and release it.

Female energy is recuperative, calming, nurturing, and gentle. The female postures are restoring to body, mind, and spirit. Yoga attempts to release male and female energies and ultimately to fuse them in union—to integrate the person.

The first four postures are male. They are done standing and they re-vitalize you. The last four are female and calming. In order to achieve the best balance and effect, it is best to do them in the order in which Geoffrey recommends them.

Do each posture slowly and deliberately, taking note of how your body feels with every movement. Never hold a position if you feel real strain, but do expect to feel some initial discomfort as your body stretches and loosens. The discomfort will pass.

Revitalizing Stretcher

Stand with your hands at your sides, palms open, feet together so you are well balanced. As you *inhale* slowly, raise your arms above your head until your palms come together. *Exhale*, keeping the arm position and rise up on your toes. Now *inhale* again; be aware of the stretch in your spine. Hold your breath for a few seconds. Now *exhale* slowly, bringing your arms down to the starting position and coming down from your toes. Repeat this three times. This exercise is particularly good to do when you get up since it stimulates the whole system and gets you ready for the day.

Shakedown

Standing with your feet a comfortable distance apart, start the exercise by shaking your hands loosely from the wrists as vigorously as you can, then work up the arms and shoulders, shaking them too until you are shaking your whole body vigorously. Then lift up one leg at a time and shake it too. The idea is to shake throughout the whole musculature of the body and get rid of all excess tension. The whole process should take about twenty seconds. This exercise is fun to do and its invigorating effect lasts a long time afterward.

Thigh Stretcher

Standing with your hands on your hips, your heels together and toes apart in a "V" shape, *inhale* slowly, at the same time rising up on your toes. *Exhale* slowly, coming all the way down to a squatting position and keeping your back straight. *Inhale* and come up very slowly, pushing down on the balls of your feet. (It helps to keep your eyes fixed on something steady to balance.) With feet flat on the floor, *exhale* again, resting in the standing position. Repeat three times. This exercise tones the thigh muscles and the ankles, as well as improving your poise and balance.

Windmill

Stand with your feet about three feet apart, arms hanging loosely at your sides. *Inhale*, raising your arms to clasp your hands above your head. *Exhale*, bringing arms down, with hands still clasped, in a circle to one side and then right down toward the floor. Go around three times in each direction, inhaling on the upward swing, exhaling as you come down. Feel the twist in your torso at the side each time you start another circle as you exercise muscles not normally used. Finish by bending forward from the waist and letting the arms and torso hang loose, imagining that all the tension in your body is draining to the floor. This exercise loosens your spine and trims your midriff.

Knee Touches

Lying on your back, *inhale*, bringing one knee up to your chest. *Exhale* and bring your forehead up to meet your knee. Return to the starting position without inhaling again until you raise the other knee to repeat the movement. Repeat the exercise until you have exercised each knee three times. This exercise is particularly good if you suffer from digestive problems.

Double Contractions

Do the preceding exercise with the same breathing pattern as before, but pulling up both knees at once and lifting your head to meet them with your forehead. Finish by rocking back and forth on your back like a rocking chair. Go through the routine six times. This loosens up the spine and the muscles deep in the back as a preparation for more advanced postures.

Tummy Twists

Lying flat on your back on the floor with your arms spread wide to each side from the shoulder, *inhale*, bringing knees up, feet flat on the floor. Keeping knees together, *exhale*, twisting to the right and lowering knees to the floor, keeping shoulders flat and head straight. Hold for ten seconds, breathing normally through the nose. Then *inhale*, bringing knees back up again slowly, and *exhale*, this time lowering them to the left. Do the exercise twice, alternating from side to side. This posture stretches and brings back blood to the intestines, improves lumbar back conditions, and promotes a strong spine, as well as tightening stomach muscles and stretching the sides of your body down to the hips.

The Corpse

Lying on your back with your arms at the sides of your body, palms facing upward, let your feet fall open and your body go completely limp. Close your eyes. Take four deep breaths through your nose, saying to yourself, "As I breathe in I take in healing energy, and as I breathe out I breathe out all the tension and all the anxiety and all the pain and negativity from my body." Now gently direct your thought to your feet and be aware of them. Tell them to relax and free them of all their tension. Move up slowly and gently, directing your ankles to relax, then your legs, your thighs, your hips. Let them sink heavily into the floor. Then concentrate on your spine, letting each vertebra go one after another, then the neck, head, face, eyes and on through the shoulders, arms, hands, across the abdomen and chest. Become aware of the feeling of complete overall relaxation and stay in this state for thirty seconds to one minute (longer if you can). This posture is an excellent way to begin and to end a session of yoga.

17

Beautiful Sleep

Sleep is a great healer. It regenerates your body, rejuvenates your skin, clears emotional conflicts, and helps you think and work at top efficiency. It is another form of relaxation essential to health and beauty. In many ways, though, sleep remains a mystery in spite of all the elaborate research that has been done into how and why we sleep and dream.

Most of the common notions about sleep are untrue. For instance, sleep is not some kind of "little death" from which you are rescued every morning. Nor do you go to bed to fall deeper and deeper into sleep until you reach bottom somewhere after midnight, after which you come closer and closer to consciousness until you finally awaken. Also, deep sleep is not any more beneficial than light sleep. And we do not necessarily need the obligatory eight hours a night to remain well and fresh-looking.

THE TWO FACES OF SLEEP

There are two kinds of sleep: orthodox sleep, which is dreamless—sometimes called "synchronized slow-wave sleep" (S) because of the brain wave patterns that accompany it—and is vital for physical restoration of the body, and paradoxical sleep, during which dreaming occurs along with rapid eye movement (REM)—sometimes called desynchronized sleep (D)—and which is essential to your mental and emotional stability. Research into sleep measured by electroencephalograms has shown that all of us spend our sleep time in and out of the two stages in a predictable rhythmic pattern. If for any reason this pattern is repeatedly disturbed, we suffer.

There are four levels or depths to orthodox sleep. When you fall asleep you move into the first level, characterized by low-amplitude fast-frequency brain wave patterns. (Sometimes sleep starts with a sudden twitching movement that is called a myoclonic jerk. This is the result of a sudden flare-up of electrical activity in the brain, as in a minor epileptic seizure.) Then, as you move to level two and even deeper into levels three and four, there is a general slowing of the frequency and an increase in the amplitude of your brain waves. All through each night you move in and out of these levels in your own characteristic pattern.

Normally one falls off to sleep and remains for a short time at level one and two and then plunges into levels three or four to stay there for seventy to one hundred minutes. At that point comes the first period of REM or paradoxical sleep when dreams begin. This dream period of REM lasts only ten to twenty minutes. It is repeated again at about ninety-minute intervals throughout the night, with orthodox, undreaming sleep in between.

During orthodox sleep your body is quiet. Heartbeat slows down, blood pressure falls slightly, and your breathing gets slower and more regular. Even your digestive system slows down. In the deeper levels of orthodox sleep, brain waves gradually become more synchronized, as if everything in your body is at peace. During these times, your body's restorative processes come into their own, rapidly repairing damaged tissues and cells, producing antibodies to fight infection, and carrying out a myriad of other duties necessary to keep you healthy. Without orthodox sleep in all its different stages, this important vegetative restoration does not take place properly and you become more prone to illness, early aging, fatigue, and muddled thinking. Orthodox sleep is the master restorer.

REM sleep, which is diametrically opposite to orthodox sleep in many ways, is just as vital. It more than earns its name "paradoxical" by being a mass of contradictions: although the body is virtually paralyzed during the REM state, the fingers and face often twitch and the genitals become erect. Breathing speeds up to the level of your normal waking state. Heartbeat rate, blood pressure, and temperature rise and adrenalin shoots through the system. Beneath the lids, eyes move rapidly from side to side as though you were looking at a film or tennis match. And this is exactly what is happening—you are viewing images that come rapidly in succession. Your brain waves in the REM state show a marked similarity to the rapid, irregular patterns of being awake.

The first REM period of dreaming usually happens after you've been asleep for ninety minutes and lasts for about ten minutes. After that they occur regularly throughout the night, culminating in the longest period (usually about half an hour) just before you wake up.

Although the exact purpose of REM sleep remains somewhat a mystery, researchers know that it is essential for maintaining one's mental and emotional equilibrium. The need for paradoxical sleep also varies from one person to another. How much you will need is related both to your personality and your general psychological state. Longer periods of REM sleep and more of them throughout the night take place in times of psychic pain, or when your defense patterns are being challenged by new demands. Women tend to have increased REM periods during the premenstruum—the three or four days before the beginning of a period. For most women this is a time of increased anxiety, irritability, mood changes, and unstable defense patterns.

But there is a lot that is still not known about the function of paradoxical sleep. Well-known French researcher Michel Jouvet, who has done extensive studies of the REM state in animals and their unborn young (in which it occurs as well), believes it is a kind of practice of the genetic code in which lower animals run through their instinctive behavior patterns. In mammals and man, he thinks, it is a time when we are probably practicing our learned behavior as each night we go through the process of integrating new information with the knowledge we already have.

When animals are deprived of REM sleep they become increasingly excitable, appetite soars, a perverted sexuality appears, and eventually they suffer a nervous breakdown. So far, studies show that too little REM makes them more and more restless and anxious. Their short-term memory starts to fail and they suffer from poor concentration and other unpleasant symptoms. Sleep researchers have discovered this by watching carefully, and each time subjects enter the paradoxical stage of sleep (indicated by rapid eye movements clearly visible beneath closed lids), they awaken them.

This aspect of REM sleep is particularly interesting, for when scientists disturbed sleepers in the orthodox state, they found that deprivation of orthodox sleep doesn't lead to any psychological disturbances. But after being deprived of REM sleep for several days, sleepers become desperate for it. Their normal sleep patterns alter so that they slip into REM immediately on falling asleep and then experience twenty to thirty periods of it each night instead of the usual three. Psychologists refer to this phenomenon as "REM rebound." It is often accompanied by fierce nightmares as psychic imagery, too long repressed, seeks strongly to reassert itself.

BEWARE OF SLEEPING PILLS

Sleeping pills repress this REM phase, and repression may result in lasting psychological damage to the pill popper. After taking sleep-inducing drugs regularly, when you come off them you may fear you are going crazy as you start to experience the REM rebound. Vivid and frightening hypnagogic images and nightmares appear as the body hungrily tries to make up for what it has been denied.

There are other reasons to steer clear of sleep-inducing drugs. Both barbiturates and nonbarbiturates prescribed for sleep are physically and psychologically addictive (barbiturates to an even greater degree than heroin). They can also be fatal, even at low dosage, when mixed with alcohol in the bloodstream. Finally—something that few people realize— they are also not very effective over the long term. Sleeping pills can be successfully used to bring on sleep only for the first week or two. After that dangerously increased doses are needed to work.

For many women who rely on sleeping pills, the power of suggestion brought about by putting one in the mouth and swallowing it is far more useful than the drug in introducing sleep. The drug itself can only do harm, in the long run. There are other, safer, and more effective ways of getting to sleep.

HOW MUCH SLEEP DO YOU NEED?

The amount of sleep you need varies tremendously from one woman to another. It also varies from one day to the next. There is no truth in the idea that you need eight hours of sleep to stay well and feel energetic. You might need ten hours, while another woman gets on very well with four and a half. One study showed that short sleepers tend to be active, outgoing people who are sociable, flexible in their personalities, and more conformist socially. Those wanting longer periods of sleep are more introverted and creative and are particularly good at sustained work. Often the more stress-filled your day, the more sleep you will need to recover from it.

As people get older they tend to sleep less. Many sixty- and seventy-year-olds get by on a mere three or four hours a day. Occasionally you meet someone who sleeps as little as half an hour to an hour each night, yet appears to be perfectly normal. The amount of sleep you need depends so much on your biological and psychological individuality that you can't make hard and fast rules about it. Many high achievers and great minds throughout history—Napoleon, Freud, and Thomas Edison, for instance—have been poor sleepers while others like Einstein could sleep the day away.

But the idea that you need a certain amount of sleep each night to stay well is a powerful one. For many people it is so embedded in their unconscious that if they only get seven hours one night instead of eight, they are convinced they will be tired the next day and soon develop all the signs of it. If you are one of these people, try reexamining your premises, and experiment—sleep less and see what happens. You may find that how you feel after a certain amount of sleep depends more on your own choice than on the time spent in bed. Try sleeping less for a few days. Many women find when they do, they actually have *more* energy.

STOP WORRYING ABOUT INSOMNIA

A lot of so-called insomnia is nothing more than the result of worrying about getting to sleep. Many people who consider themselves insomniacs are really victims of general propaganda about sleep rather than non-sleepers. And many women seek treatment because they can only sleep four or five hours a night, although that may be all they need. There is nothing more apt to cause sleeplessness than the worry that you won't be able to drop off. Sometimes, too, sleeplessness is normal. After all, we all experience a sleepless night now and then, particularly if we are over-tired, worried, or excited about some coming event.

Real, chronic insomnia is less frequent. A major research project into long-term insomnia turned up some interesting facts about sufferers. Over 85 percent of the 300 insomniacs studied had one or more major pathological personality indications, such as depression, obsessive compulsive tendencies, schizophrenic characteristics, or sociopathy. For them, their insomnia was a secondary symptom of a more basic conflict; it was a socially acceptable problem they could talk about without fear of being judged harshly. Insomnia like this is little more than a mask for whatever is really bothering the non-sleeper.

Occasionally the inability to sleep can be a manifestation of a nutritional problem—often a deficiency of zinc coupled with an excess of copper, which produces a mind that is overactive intellectually and won't wind down—or a deficiency of calcium or vitamin E, which can lead to tension and cramping in the muscles and a difficulty in letting go.

The more easygoing an attitude you take to sleep, the less likely you are to have any problem with it. If you miss an hour or two, or if you are not sleepy, simply stay up, read a book, or finish some work. Believe it or not, one of the best times for coming up with creative ideas is in the middle of a sleepless night. And chances are that you'll more than make up for it in the next couple of days—provided you don't get anxious about it.

HOW—AND HOW NOT—TO GET TO SLEEP

1. Get more exercise regularly during the day. This helps burn up stress-caused adrenalin buildup in the brain, which can result in that tense, nervous feeling where you're "up" and you can't seem to get "down." But don't take strenuous exercise before going to bed, as it can set the heart pounding and stimulate the whole body too much.

2. Don't go to bed when you are not sleepy. Instead, pursue some pleasant activity, preferably passive. Television is not the best choice, for rays emitted from the set disturb your nervous system when you least need it.

3. Don't drink coffee, alcohol, or strong stimulants at dinner. This isn't just an old wives' tale. One researcher looking into the effects of caffeine on human beings recently showed that total sleep time is decreased by two hours and the mean total of intervening wakefulness more than doubles when patients are given three milligrams of caffeine, the equivalent of a couple of cups of coffee. Alcohol may put you to sleep but it tends not to keep you there, awakening you instead in the early hours of the morning.

4. Don't let anyone smoke in your bedroom. Stuffy air can prevent you from sleeping.

5. Stop worrying about getting to sleep. Just let it happen. If it doesn't tonight, so what? It will tomorrow night. Or the next. Lack of sleep is not going to kill you, but worrying about it long enough just might.

NATURE'S SLEEP AIDS

1. Milk. It is an old-fashioned remedy, maybe, but it is scientifically sound that drinking a glass of milk before bed helps you to sleep. Milk contains tryptophan, an amino acid that is converted in the body to serotonin, a brain chemical that sets off the deeper levels of sleep. High in calcium, it is often referred to as the slumber mineral because it induces muscle relaxation.

2. An ionizer. A little contraption beside your bed that sends negative ions into the air and is a godsend to anyone who has the kind of nervous system that tends to go "up" and doesn't want to come "down." Although not cheap, it is an excellent investment for you can use it at a desk when you have a lot of work to do. Or, if you buy one of the portable varieties, you can also take it in the car on long trips to keep from

going to sleep (it magically works both ways) and on airplane trips to minimize the effects of jet lag. Negative ions also stimulate the production of serotonin in the brain.

3. Take a lukewarm bath, submerging yourself as much as possible for ten minutes. Then, wrapping a towel around you just long enough to get rid of the drips, pop into bed immediately. Lukewarm water is the most relaxing of all temperatures on the body. A hot bath before bed is a mistake. It is far too stimulating to the heart and gets your motor running.

4. Get into a rut, going to bed as far as possible at the same time every night and developing a routine or simple ritual about it. Doing the same thing every night before bed quickly accustoms the mind to accept sleep.

5. Practice a relaxation or meditation technique twice a day. A valuable tool for insomnia, it will lower elevated blood pressure and help you cope better with whatever stress you tend to carry off to bed with you.

6. Get to know the natural tranquilizers and herb teas and whenever you feel the need use them, sweetened with honey if you like, as a bedtime drink. Peppermint, camomile, skullcap, catnip, and vervain are renowned for their relaxing effects. Or you can try some passiflora (passionflower), which is probably the best-known of herbal soothers. Many health food stores carry it in tablet form.

Book Two
Maintenance

The Body

Introduction

Beauty also depends on form: the curve of your body which is nothing less than the physical expression of *you*, the flow of your movements when you walk and speak, the sheen on your skin. To an astute eye, your body can reveal almost everything about you. It can tell how you think and feel, how you eat, how you exercise (or don't!) and how much physical care you give yourself.

Every woman has her own perfect form. She has a natural shape of body and face that is unique to her. When this perfect form has not been obscured by excess weight, poor muscle condition, blemished skin, or such things as cellulite that develop when toxic wastes and fat are stored in the body, it is a true expression of you. If, however, your body has been ignored, treated carelessly, or is distorted by excess weight and general neglect, then the form that should be expressing you in all clarity serves only to obscure you.

This is the case with many women. They are carrying too much weight, or they have neglected themselves, believing wrongly that to look after their skin and nails, hands and feet, is a useless self-indulgence. This section is all about the things that can help you rediscover your own unique form if you have lost it—cellulite treatment, breast care, slimming, and massage—as well as what will help you keep it if you haven't—nail care, foot care, bathing, and aromatherapy. In short, it's all about looking after your body. And caring for your body is caring for your *self*.

18

The Psychology of Slenderizing

Lean is supposed to be beautiful. As a result, some women spend most of their adult lives trying to get thin and stay that way. For, in our society, thinness has become a symbol of loveliness, success, self-control, and social acceptability—and being overweight the twentieth-century bête noire of womanhood. You know the kind of thing: "Lose that nasty twenty-five pounds with our super new slenderizing regimen and it will transform your life into a wonderful world of bliss." Well, don't believe it.

From a health point of view, of course, there is every reason not to be overweight. Overweight women die earlier and are more subject to such illnesses as hypoglycemia, heart disease, and diabetes than their lean sisters. They also tend to have less energy. But the on-again-off-again dieting women go through to try and lose weight and keep it off is far worse than the extra few pounds.

Losing weight depends on restricting calories, but successfully restricting calories depends on your attitude, your habits, and your mental and emotional states. The psychology of weight loss can be just as important as the physical facts of it, if you are going to lose excess pounds permanently. First, it is helpful to have some understanding of why you overeat, if you do, and what things trigger it in you. Second, you can benefit from using some simple behaviorist techniques to alter your eating patterns. Finally, practicing a deep relaxation or meditation technique coupled with the use of creative imagery can make the whole process of weight loss much simpler and more fun as well as bringing you other benefits, such as an improved self-image and a greater sense of control over your life.

THE PSYCHOLOGY OF OVEREATING

There are a million reasons why people eat too much. Psychologists have at times explained chronic overeating by such phrases as "oral dependency," "incorporate cannibalism," a "compensation for loss of security" —you've probably heard them all. They sound interesting and may well be valid, too. But they usually do little to solve the problem. It is so easy to dismiss yourself as a compulsive eater, using this as an excuse for being overweight, thereby relieving yourself of the responsibility for it, and making yourself miserable in the process. But it is not very helpful.

There are some things, however, that researchers studying chronically overweight people have discovered that can be useful. For instance, Dr. Hilde Bruch at Baylor University in Texas has observed that abnormal eating patterns are usually "a failure in self-experience." She and other researchers have studied people with weight problems and found that often as children they failed to develop a strong sense of personal identity or a feeling that they have much control over their own lives. Grown-up, these people often appear to lack initiative. They also have trouble differentiating between hunger and other states of discomfort like anxiety and unhappiness. When they were young, Bruch believes, many of them were treated in such a way that they came to think their own sensations—whether they were hunger in the body or feelings of like or dislike of an experience—were unimportant. In fact, they were made to feel their perceptions were so unimportant that they gradually got out of touch with them altogether, so that now they are unable to disinguish between hunger, for instance, and anxiety, fear, or a need for comfort. Many chronically overweight people rarely experience sensations of true hunger at all. Some cannot even tell when they are hungry and when they are not. This phenomenon has been observed and confirmed by a number of studies. Researchers at Columbia University discovered that where normal-weight people tend to eat when they are hungry, the eating habits of overweight people are often controlled by the clock. They found that when they altered the hands of a clock so that overweight people thought it was mealtime, the overweight people would eat more. The appetite of the group of normal-weight people remained unaffected by the clock alteration.

Another study, by R. E. Nisbett, showed that overweight people are also more affected by the sight of food than normal-weight people. Researchers took thirty-three subjects who believed they were taking part in research into psychophysical responses, put them through a complicated but bogus series of tasks during which their responses were supposedly being carefully recorded by the tester, and then finished by offering them a plate of either one or three roast beef sandwiches and a bottle of some soft drink. The testers told participants they were sorry the experiments had made them miss lunch and that they were welcome to as much food as they wanted, since there were more sandwiches in the refrigerator. Then the subjects were left on their own. Surprisingly, the overweight people ate more sandwiches than the normal-weight control group when there were three sandwiches on the plate in front of them, but less when there was only one sandwich there. In other words, their appetite depended on what they saw. Where the normal-weight group would go to the refrigerator for more when they wanted it, the obese group simply ate what was put in front of them, whether it was a lot or a little.

Such things—the fact that overweight people tend to eat what is in front of them and not what they do not see, and the fact they tend to eat not from signals of hunger but from internal signals of anxiety and other things, or from habit, depending on the time of day and so forth—can actually be put to practical use in a weight control program. This is what the behaviorists have done.

THE BEHAVIORIST THEORY

Behavioral psychologists begin with the notion that eating behavior is learned and maintained as a result of interaction between you and your environment. And their definition of environment includes everything around you—people, events, things you see and respond to. These psychologists are not very interested in deep-seated motives for compulsive eating and they acknowledge that there is nothing you can do to change your genetic inheritance. But what you can do, they say, is to get to grips with overweight by looking at it as a voluntary disorder brought about by habit and environmental stimuli (remember how the habit of eating at certain times or the sight of food triggers hunger in overweight people). Change your environment, they say, and you will alter your habits and your eating patterns so you lose weight and keep it off.

Although the behaviorists tend to be somewhat simplistic in their approach, they emphasize quite rightly that the woman who wants to lose weight has to take responsibility for herself. It is a down-to-earth approach that offers a lot of help to dieters. It gives you things to do that help break through unconscious eating habits, and makes use of all that is known about overweight people and the triggers that spur them to eat. It also teaches you that you can have control over your own eating instead of letting it control you. And for many women who have long struggled with the battle of the bulge, finding this out also makes them aware that they have control over their own lives—a kind of magic wand that gives them entrance to all sorts of places and pleasures they never thought possible.

Behaviorists dismiss the idea that willpower is an important part of weight loss. They claim that a lasting change in your food habits is brought about not by willpower (the "should I or shouldn't I eat that delicious-looking pastry" syndrome) but by awareness of your behavior patterns and conscious decisions about how you can change them for the better. Here's how to put their techniques into practice.

Step One: Take a Look at Where You Eat

Most overweight people are stimulated to eat by external factors such as the time on the clock, the sight of food, or habits such as always having a snack when the television is on. So the first thing you need to do is limit the number of places you eat and cut out other activities such as talking on the telephone or watching television while you are eating. This eliminates much unconscious eating right away. It also forms new habits so that instead of being reminded of food every time you turn on the television or pick up the telephone, you will simply carry out these activities on their own. And it eliminates the cook's tasting of foods that can add many hidden calories each day.

So: *Decide to eat in one room only.*
       Decide to eat in one place in that room only (such as at the table).
       Decide to do nothing else while you are eating.

Step Two: Take a Look at What You Eat

Every woman has her favorite temptations. The shops are full of them, fattening goodies that manufacturers have cleverly produced and packaged to be eaten at first temptation. Convenience foods like pastries, cakes, and cookies and other snacks are a constant source of temptation for women on a weight-loss diet. Not only that, but most of them are nutritionally inadequate and only rob you of the space you need to take in more complete foods that provide you with everything you need for lasting health and beauty. So when you head for the market, make a careful list of what you will buy and then stick to it. Do not keep temptation foods in the house and you will not be faced with the problem of having to resist them. Another helpful tip is always to go shopping just after a meal. Studies of women's food buying habits show that they spend almost 20 percent less on food when they shop after a meal than when they shop on an empty stomach. When you are at home, let the sweet-toothed members of the family stick to their desserts at mealtimes while you have your own, and do not leave high-calorie garnishes such as mayonnaise or sour cream on the table at all. Finally, after meals, be sure to empty all the leftovers directly into the garbage can or compost heap so you are not tempted to pick at them.

So: *Decide to eliminate high temptation foods from your shopping, table, and cupboard.*

Step Three: Consider How Your Food Looks

It matters. Research has shown that the overweight woman is strongly affected by her visual contact with food and it is important to take care how your food is served and prepared. One researcher, Richard E. Stuart, a behaviorist psychologist and adviser to Weight Watchers International, carried out an interesting experiment with plate size. He asked one group of women to serve measured amounts of food on small plates while the other group served exactly the same amounts on ordinary dinner plates. Seventy percent of the women in the small-plate group reported a feeling of greater satisfaction than those in the large plate group, even though all the women knew how much food was there all along. Researchers have also found that more satisfaction is felt (and therefore the need to eat to excess is reduced) when food is attractively served.

So: *Decide to use small plates.*
     Decide to use measured quantities of food.
     Decide to make your food look as attractive as you can.

Step Four: Take a Look at How Fast You Eat

Overweight people tend to eat much faster than their slimmer friends. When you eat too fast you bring about two negative effects, both of which should be eliminated from any weight-loss diet. First, eating fast makes you unaware of both the taste of what you are eating and also how much of it is going down. You eat a lot simply because you have no real idea of how much you are taking in. This, and the fact that you will not be able to digest fully the starches you eat unless you chew them thoroughly, make it important that you slow down.

So: *Decide to put your fork down after each bite.*
     Decide to chew each bite twenty times.
     Decide to take no more food into your mouth until what you have in it has been swallowed.

Step Five: Investigate Ways of Keeping Up Your Spirits

Overweight women who lean on food to boost them up emotionally and physically, for example by turning to food when they are tired or a bit blue, often get into the habit of skipping meals. It is not always a good habit to get into. When you skip a meal you feel deprived. This lends itself to a familiar rationalization like, "Well, I skipped breakfast, I've been very good, so I can have just a bit more now." Don't let yourself fall prey to this. Plan a regular timetable for your meals and then stick to it. A second danger to guard against is letting yourself slip into a state of depression, for it is then that any reducing program seems meaningless and you are apt to slip back into your old careless habits of eating that got you fat and kept you that way in the first place. Feelings of deprivation also come with exhaustion. One of your prime objectives when slenderizing should be to see that you don't get overtired. Fatigue can easily and quickly lead to depression and to rationalization. Get enough sleep, regardless of what you have to forego in your social life to make this possible. Also, set aside fifteen minutes every morning and evening to practice a relaxation or meditation technique, which will not only refresh and renew you, but also will help work against any addictive patterns in your life such as smoking or overeating. This kind of practice brings with it a sense of physical and psychological well-being and an awareness of personal autonomy so that you know you can rely on yourself to do what is best for you. It will greatly enhance your self-esteem. Then you won't have to turn to food so often as a crutch.

The third danger to dieters is boredom—this is an all-too-familiar cue to head for the cupboard or refrigerator. So make plans for work and plans for your social life that keep you busy and make sure they have nothing to do with food. Change the lunch dates for a trip to a gallery, sewing, browsing through shops (not the delicatessens), theater-going, or whatever. When you plan to see friends, let them know in advance that you do not want a meal. If you are firm and serious, they will soon get the idea without being offended. The more interest and satisfaction you get from activities that are not connected with food, the more you will be able to develop the new habits that will keep you slim once the weight is lost.

So: *Decide to eat regular meals on a timetable.*

Decide to get enough sleep and regular deep relaxation.

Decide to increase your participation in activities not connected with food.

Step Six: Keep a Record for Improved Awareness

The behaviorist method of weight control demands awareness and participation from you. The more you give it the more successful it will be. Get yourself a notebook and make a chart on each right-hand page that includes such things as what you ate, when, how you felt before and after, what else you were doing at the time, and so forth. Before begin-

ning your weight loss program, just eat as you have been, eating whatever you normally eat and whenever you do it, but this time write down
the information. On the left-hand page write down anything else that
seems important, including your weight, your ambitions about being
thinner, any feelings of worry or anxiety about it all, and anything else
that seems relevant. After a week of this, you will be able to look back
and see the different things that have triggered your eating (perhaps a
telephone call that upset you, or perhaps you tend to eat mostly in the
evening when you are bored, or during the day when you become fatigued and need a break). Then you can take action to provide the things
you need, such as a rest or amusement, instead of taking out everything
on your stomach. Record as well your exercise program: when you exercise, how you find it, and how you feel about it. The more aware you
become the easier it is to use food for what it is intended, namely to
nourish your body, instead of for other reasons. After you have begun
your weight-loss regimen, continue to write in the journal—each time you
eat and also to record your feelings about weight loss, your foods, and
yourself. It will lend a great support to the whole program and be an important key to your coming to know and understand yourself better.

THE GENTLE ART OF MIND-BENDING

Where behaviorist techniques can help change the outer things that
affect your appetite and eating patterns, creative imagery can help your
inner attitudes. And attitudes are important. For how you see yourself,
how you think of yourself, and how you think of food, day after day,
has a great deal to say about what you become—fat or thin, in control or
out of control, truly responsible for yourself or at the mercy of others
and circumstances.

In recent years, many useful techniques of meditation, often coupled
with guided fantasy or creative imagery, have been developed. They can
be helpful to the dieter in three ways. First, all of them demand the use
of some form of deep relaxation practiced twice a day. This, even on its
own, eliminates much of the tension-provoked eating that leads to weight
gain and gives you another (less fattening) way of coping with stress
and anxiety than turning to food for comfort. Second, many of these
mind trips give you access to information from your subconscious and to
insight, which make the process of slimming easier. Finally, directing
your imagination toward leanness and toward the elimination of whatever blocks have been in the way of it helps to bring about the change in
size you are seeking and to maintain it afterward.

There are two different approaches to mind-bending for weight loss—

meditation and creative imagery. You can use either or both. But before you do, read about how creative imagery can work for you in Chapter 2 and learn a basic technique for relaxation and meditation from Chapter 14. It is their repeated use that makes them powerful.

THE SLENDERIZING MEDITATION

Using the relaxation response technique, substitute the word "slim" "lean," "trim," or "health" (whichever sounds best to you) for your ordinary mantra. Put yourself into a state of deep conscious relaxation for fifteen minutes, twice a day, preferably right before a meal. The best time is usually when you get up in the morning (even if you have to get up fifteen minutes earlier to make it possible). Then again just before lunch or dinner. If you can't manage it then, take time out in the middle of the day, or do it in the evening after dinner.

This has the effect of stilling your mind and instilling the idea of slimness so that eventually it becomes second nature.

The body image of most overweight women is quite distorted. They think of themselves as overweight and picture their physical form as very large and bulky and without grace. This unconscious picture only further contributes to the condition of being fat. Used regularly, meditation technique slowly and steadily helps to alter this image for the better. Gradually you begin to see yourself as thin rather than fat. You begin to behave as thin people do in their eating habits and in how you dress and you find it easier to *be* thin than fat. This is something that you have to experience to appreciate but it is extraordinarily worthwhile and an essential part of any well-designed program for weight control.

BODY IMAGERY

Your unconscious mind is tremendously powerful. It is a source of energy and creativity which—provided you can get in touch with it and turn it toward your desired ends—will work wonders for you. The use of creative imagery specifically geared to slimming can help you harness your own power. Following the principles of creative imagery (outlined in Chapter 2), here are a few imaginary trips you can take to help you slim. Some will bring insight and increased self-awareness, others will help you get accustomed to yourself as a healthy, lean woman, still others can help you shed old, no longer useful thought patterns that have been hampering you.

It is useful to read each exercise through three or four times before you begin your relaxation, to get familiar with it. These are only examples. Once you get used to using the technique, you can make up your own mind trips. You can practice creative imagery any time but it is often easiest to do when you have just awakened in the morning and are still lying in bed, just before you go to sleep at night, or if you lie down for fifteen minutes during the day. It can be done sitting or lying (whichever you prefer). Begin each exercise either by doing fifteen minutes of meditation or by taking yourself quickly through the progressive relaxation techniques until you have worked through all the different areas of your body. Then go on to the guided fantasy.

The Dungeon

Aim: to make you aware of things that will help you lose weight.

Eyes closed, imagine yourself locked in the dungeon of a castle, deep in the earth with hard stone walls and only one tiny window high in the wall for light. This is a dungeon you have made for yourself by eating too much, too fast, the wrong things, and too often. It stands for all the many times you have failed in the past and all the unpleasant feelings, like frustration and despair, you get when you think about being overweight. Stay in the stone room for a while and look at the walls around you. They are hard and imprisoning but they are entirely your creation. You have made them yourself and you can choose to leave them. As you look around the room notice that there is a large old trunk in one corner. See it. Feel yourself going over to touch it. What is the texture like? Hard? Smooth or rough? Is it bound in metal? Now reach down and open it.

It opens slowly to reveal a bunch of large, old keys. Attached to each key is a tag on which is written something. The keys will open the great door to the dungeon that you have made and set you free. Pick one, read what is written on the tag attached to it. It will tell you something you can do to help solve your weight problem. Now take the key to the door and unlock it. Feel yourself doing this as the metal key turns in the lock and presses against your hand. Watch yourself go out of the door and climb the winding stone steps to the courtyard and the open air. Now open your eyes.

There are many keys because there are many different things that together will help you overcome your weight problem and set you free from imprisonment. Each time you do the exercise you will probably find a different one. This technique can also help when you feel stuck with a problem of any kind. If you let yourself visualize a key attached to a tag on which the answer is written, you can often find the way out.

The New Body

Aim: to accustom you to what it will feel like and be like to be leaner, healthier, stronger, and to encourage a transition from your old body to your new one.

Imagine yourself in a large store with beautiful high ceilings and carpeted floors. It is Sunday and the store is closed so you are alone and free to wander about looking at things and testing things as you choose. What does the room you are in look like? Are there pleasant smells in the air of perfume or cosmetics? Feel the soft pile of the elegant carpet beneath your feet. Now wander about the store until you come to the clothes department. Here there are mannequins wearing all different styles of clothes, some for evening, others for sports, other daytime dresses, suits, slacks, sweaters, and shirts. All of them are lean as you will be. Look at all the clothes. Go along the rails and touch different garments, smell and feel them so they really come alive for you.

The garments in this store are not ordinary garments, they are magic. They have the ability to change the shape of the woman who wears them. The moment you pick out a suit or dress, a swimsuit or a pair of slacks and start to put it on, your body changes shape to suit the garment, and all the garments are in small sizes. Your waist becomes thinner, legs leaner, arms slimmer so that when you look at yourself in one of the many different mirrors around the walls, you see yourself immediately slim and beautifully dressed in whatever you have chosen to wear. Try a swimsuit or a pair of shorts and see how good you look, then think of all the fun you will have in them. Now put on something else, whatever you would like to own, and see how different you feel in it. Now leave the store wearing the new garment. It is yours for the taking. Walk down the street. Notice how the people react to you. Is it different? What do they say? What do they do? Now return to the big store, go back to the place where you found the garment and take it off, placing it on the rail. Dress yourself in your own clothing and leave the store knowing that you can return at any time to try on other garments and the new body that goes with them—the body that you, yourself, will have before long.

This exercise helps you get the feel of getting thinner. When you repeat it again and again it helps you also to begin to think of yourself as lean rather than overweight and to make the important mental and physical transition from one to the other. Finally, it helps eliminate that feeling of being trapped in the same shape and size forever.

Have a Chat with Food

Aim: this is a Gestalt technique designed to increase your awareness of how you feel about food and why the desire to eat has always seemed so compelling.

Picture a food which you think has a particular hold over you and which has contributed to your being overweight. See it in front of you and be aware of how it smells and feels and tastes. Now imagine that it can talk to you. Ask it questions like, "What are you doing?" and "What do you want from me?" Listen to its reply. You may have to speak to it several times. Then let it speak and pay attention to what it says. Do you agree or disagree? Carry on a dialogue with it and listen to all it has to say about itself and you. Continue with the conversation until you have said all that needs to be said and heard all it wishes to say to you.

This exercise can reveal a lot about one's compulsive eating and what it is all about for the particular person involved. It is worth repeating several times because important information that is helpful to weight loss tends to emerge bit by bit.

Positive Reinforcement

Aim: to reinforce positively the idea of getting slim and staying slim and to break down negative thought patterns that lead to wrong eating and overweight.

After practicing meditation for fifteen minutes or putting yourself into a state of deep relaxation, choose a phrase that appeals to you and each day repeat it over and over several times in a row. You need to do this regularly for results. Here are some simple phrases, or you can make up one of your own. But it must be positive in form. It is no good using something like "I won't eat too much any more"—only a positive phrase will give the strength and reinforcement needed to break down the mental resisters and bring success.

Try one of these:

1. I love eating and I eat to live. But I do not live to eat.

2. Every day I am getting slimmer and slimmer.

3. I have a new, controlled relationship with food, so I am every day coming closer to my perfect weight.

4. I patiently and happily accept my new approach to food and to my life.

When you are using creative imagery or positive reinforcement you need never be concerned if you seem to get stuck somewhere. If, for instance, one of the keys you pull out of the box doesn't have a tag on it or the food you speak to doesn't answer you sensibly at first, it will be different the next time. In fact, it is different every time and any kind of block only means that your unconscious isn't quite ready yet to deal with that particular challenge or problem. Just be aware of it and continue with the exercise. When your subconscious is ready it will give you the information. At the end of every exercise, open your eyes, take three deep breaths and let your air out completely each time, and sit up. A combination of meditation and creative imagery with growing self-awareness and a few behaviorist techniques makes a complete package deal to lend psychological support to a weight-loss regimen. It is every bit as important as the diet itself and the regular physical exercise that should go along with it.

WHAT IF YOU'RE TOO THIN?

Are you really? In an overweight society someone who is lean can feel like a freak when there is nothing wrong with her. And there can be real advantages to being thin. For instance, you are likely to live longer, be healthier, and excel in sports that demand skill. You also probably look great in your clothes.

If you are genuinely underweight, gaining weight is not just a matter of eating more jelly doughnuts. Many factors figure in why someone is excessively thin and all of them must be taken into account if you are going to do something about it.

Many thin women do not realize how little they actually eat. They assume that because they sit down at the table three times a day like everyone else, they should look nicely rounded too. But they are often more interested in conversation than in the food and, without realizing it, eat very little. Thin women also tend to skip meals.

Before you do anything to change your eating habits you need to be sure of just what they are and how much in a week you actually do eat. Carry a notebook around with you and record in it each snack or meal, what and how much you ate, how you felt and what you thought before and afterward, what things distracted you, and so forth. This will make you aware of what needs to be changed. It will also give you a clue as to what things may be worrying you. For worries, anxiety, and other stress-related thoughts and feelings play a large part in chronic underweight.

When a woman's body is in a state of stress as she sits down to a table two things happen: first, her mind is taken away from the task at hand, namely eating, to conjecture about the past or future, and she loses interest in eating at all. Second, blood is drawn away from her internal organs that concern themselves with digestion—the liver, stomach, and intestines —and channeled into the muscles. In order to digest and assimilate food properly the blood supply has to be directed away from the muscles and into the digestive system, so that it will secrete the enzymes and digestive juices essential for normal processing. This will only happen if the stressed state is replaced by a state of relaxation—only then will you get the full nutritional benefit of the food you eat. For although many underweight women actually eat plenty, much of what they eat passes right through them instead of being assimilated.

Physiologically, the two most common reasons for excessive thinness are an overactive thyroid, coupled with weak, underactive adrenals, and an inability to digest and absorb food properly because of long-term stress, which inhibits the digestive and assimilation processes. In the first case, excessive eating of high calorie foods like sugar and concentrated starches only tends to stimulate the thyroid and make matters worse. Overindulgence in fatty foods is little better. It results in indigestion, which prevents you from eating a normal amount of any sort of food afterward. Eating excess protein from foods or liquid or powdered supplements may help temporarily to fill you out. This is why they give it to athletes who want to build their muscles. But when you tail off from the protein gorging, the new flesh is likely to disappear.

What does help is well-planned, regular meals, eaten slowly, quietly, and chewed thoroughly to aid the digestion of starches. Supplementary digestive enzymes with bile, hydrochloric acid, and lecithin taken temporarily can also be useful for underweight people whose digestion and assimilation is not functioning well.

And a relaxation or meditation technique practiced twice daily, preferably before meals, will do wonders to improve both appetite and assimilation.

Exercise helps too. Most underweight people get nowhere near enough because they fear it will make the problem worse. But half an hour's walking morning and evening in the open air or running a mile or two a day not only improves the general physical condition but also releases tension and adrenalin buildup in the brain and heart, which can bring a hearty appetite.

Finally, take heart. Many lean, racehorse type women lose their excessive thinness in middle age as the activity of the thyroid subsides naturally. Then they begin to put on weight, sometimes far too easily.

19

The Physiology of Slenderizing

Going on and off fad diets is an ineffective way to lose weight. It can also be dangerous, for you risk creating subclinical vitamin and mineral deficiencies that will not only affect your physical well-being and your emotional stability, but in the long run can also make your weight problem even worse. Fad diets upset your health in another way as well—because of the inevitable weight gain that follows each. When your weight seesaws up and down your skin ages more rapidly and serum cholesterol builds up in the cardiovascular system, making you more susceptible to heart disease.

According to statistics, the average fad diet lasts from one to three months and the woman following it is off the diet for about half the time. She goes on one and a quarter of these diets a year, usually seasonally. Sales of diet products climb in January and February when the post Christmas guilt arrives and again in May and June when thoughts of bikinis begin to raise their ugly heads. Then sales sag in October each year, reaching their nadir over the Christmas period. It is all part of the elaborate and amazing game of so-called weight control, in which the poor overweight woman more often than not is the pawn.

Believing that the loss of that ten to twenty-five pounds with which she has been struggling will transform her life, she goes on one diet after another, suffering guilt, loathing, and nutritional deficiencies when she fails and experiencing a kind of hollow victory if the weight does come off, because it usually brings with it a sense of disappointment, fatigue, and more nutritional deficiencies. For a while she may find that getting thinner makes her look better in a pair of slacks, but it will do nothing to change her attitude toward herself or to make her, fundamentally, any happier.

If you are someone who has long struggled with excess weight and is still struggling, stop for a moment and do something: take a look at yourself and decide if you truly want to lose weight or not. Many women find that, although they may not even know it consciously, they really don't want to be thinner and the so-called struggle has been nothing more than a way of defeating themselves. Extra pounds may offer them a feeling of security and protection, which they fear slimming down might take away. For other women, this battle with the scales represents a way of rebelling against a set of conventional values about sexiness. It is a way of saying, "I will be accepted for myself, fat as I am, or not at all." Examine your feelings about thinness and ask yourself what reasons you might have for being fat.

You may be surprised to find there can be advantages to it. For instance, some women feel they could not cope with the sexual advances that their thinner body might engender. Still others simply feel better when they are slightly overweight. The fatty tissues act as a buffer and their own biochemical makeup provides them with energy stimulants that help them lead extraordinarily productive lives. All of these things are important to consider. Being aware of your feelings about them and facing any that may apply to you is far more important than starting another crash diet to lose fifteen pounds, only to mess it all up again by going on an eating binge. Not everybody should be thin.

Lean may be beautiful. But lean is not enough. For real beauty your muscles need to be elastic, your skin smooth, your circulation good so every cell of your body gets all the nutrients it needs to function well, and your gait must be free and graceful. While some of these things may be helped by losing excess pounds, none of them is dependent on your looking like a bean pole, no matter how much advertisers in glossy magazines would have us believe otherwise. Beware of that universal dictum that you have to be thin to be beautiful. You do? Who says so?

If, after taking everything into account, you decide you do want to lose weight, take heart. It is not as difficult as everyone believes. Lasting weight loss depends on two things: first, the true wish to be thinner. And second, a genuinely adequate low calorie diet that provides you with all the essential minerals, vitamins, and trace elements as well as enough protein, unrefined carboyhdrates, and the essential fatty acids that you need to ensure you have no hidden nutritional hungers.

FIRST LET'S EXPLODE SOME MYTHS

A lot of nonsense is talked about weight control. Many false statements are made that do little more than worry would-be dieters and lend support to a multimillion-dollar industry in diet foods, books, devices, and drugs—the existence of which is entirely dependent on failure. If they all worked, then overweight women would use them, get thin, and never need them again. But no. Slimming is made to seem a great struggle in which every woman needs a lot of paraphernalia for support. Here are a few commonly accepted false notions about slenderizing: "Diet pills make you lose weight." "Specially designed diet foods and breads provide all the nutrients you need to keep you healthy and make you lose weight fast." "You should not get too much exercise if you are trying to lose weight or it will increase your appetite." Not one of them is true.

Diet pills do not make you lose weight. For a time amphetamines may decrease your appetite but this effect is lessened with each passing day you take them. There is also considerable risk of becoming psychologically and physically dependent on appetite suppressants. As far back as thirty years ago, amphetamines and placebos were tested on two different groups of children and the placebo groups showed the greater weight loss of the two. But old myths die hard. So do amphetamines, even though addiction to them can lead to psychosis-like states. The cellulose tablets designed to create bulk in the stomach and therefore to make you want to eat less are not dangerous, but they are not very useful either. The best way to find out for yourself is to try them and see.

Most specially made diet foods fit into the category of overprocessed, overrefined foodstuffs that are best avoided. For, in spite of their being enriched with some of the vitamins and minerals that were removed in their manufacture, valuable nutrients have been destroyed in their making. A dieter needs all the benefit of truly wholesome foods, not twentieth-century "plastic" copies. Artificial sweeteners such as saccharin, the cyclamates, and others are safe if you use them in small quantities, say to sweeten a couple of cups of tea a day. But if you take them in larger doses in the form of diet foods, dietetic sweets and cookies, and no-calorie colas while on a nutrient restricted diet, the long-term effect on your health is not predictable. They are artificial chemicals and are best used only sparingly, if at all.

WHY ARE YOU OVERWEIGHT?

About 5 percent of overweight is considered to be the result of a metabolic disturbance. But most often the cortical or hypothalmic dysfunctions on which overweight is blamed are the *results* of overweight rather than the cause. Sometimes a tendency to be fat originates in infancy. Bottle feeding and the early introduction of solid foods often result in overfeeding, which probably sets up eating patterns that are carried over into childhood and adult life. Some authorities believe too that when a baby is fed too much, it develops an excessive number of fat cells and from then on will always have a tendency to be fat.

Epidemiological studies of primitive peoples in underdeveloped countries point to our consumption of refined carbohydrates such as white flour and sugar and convenience foods, which tend to be high in hidden fats and sugar, as an important cause of obesity. It is interesting to note that in societies where the people eat a simple diet of unrefined grains, legumes, and fresh vegetables—such as the Lifestyle Diet—with or without meat and fish, obesity is rare. But when Western food technology comes into their countries they rapidly develop weight problems along with many of the illnesses that have come to be known as the diseases of Western civilization, such as diabetes, heart disease, peptic ulcers, arthritis, and cancer.

LET'S LOOK AT THE "BIG DIETS"

You probably know them all—the cider-vinegar, kelp, and B_6 regimen, the Stillman Quick Weight Loss Diet, Dr. Atkins' Diet Revolution, the macrobiotic diet, the Drinking Man's Diet, the protein sparing fast, and the Mayo Diet (which incidentally has nothing to do with the famous Mayo Clinic). There is a new one almost every year.

The Cider-vinegar, Kelp, and B_6 Diet

The cider-vinegar, kelp, and B_6 diet, popularized by Mary Ann Crenshaw, who claimed to have lost twelve pounds in two weeks on it, is unlikely to do you any harm providing, as Miss Crenshaw suggests, you ensure that along with the B_6 supplements you take supplements of all the rest of the B complex too, and provided the 1,000 calories you are eating come from a wise choice of foods including whole-grain breads and cereals, raw fresh vegetables and fruits, and some of the special "Super Foods." Vitamin B_6 is known to help eliminate water retention so to this extent it can be helpful. It also plays a part in fat metabolism, as do many of the B group of vitamins. It is doubtful whether the cider-vinegar or kelp will do much, although kelp is a good source of important minerals for the health of hair and nails as well as overall fitness—provided, of course, you take enough of it. This usually means a small handful of dried tablets per day rather than three or four.

Mayo Diet

Grapefruit, which is one of the so-called keys to successful dieting in the Mayo Diet because of its supposed fat-dissolving abilities, will do nothing more than provide some good vitamin C with bioflavonoids (provided you eat some of the white pulp of the skin at the same time). It has no fat-burning abilities regardless of how many women believe otherwise.

Precocious Protein Diets

The high-protein, low-carbohydrate regimens such as the Atkins and Stillman diets work on the principle of inducing ketosis—the presence of excessive quantities of acetone or ketone bodies in the urine, which indicates that stored fats are being burned off as fuel. On the Stillman regimen you eat only lean meat, fish, poultry, and low-fat cheese and you take a vitamin supplement, plus eight glasses of water a day. You will get rapid initial loss of weight but in a test where one set of dieters was put on this regimen and the control group on a balanced low-calorie regimen, that was the only benefit, besides a decrease in appetite as a result of increased ketone bodies.

But the ketosis on which the diet depends induces a metabolic state which can result in permanent cell damage. Some carbohydrates are necessary in order for the body to regulate its protein and fat metabolism and to support the health of nerve cells and brain tissue. The diet can also be extremely hazardous to anyone with a hidden kidney or liver ailment. And research shows a 33 percent average rise in serum cholesterol levels in people kept on the Stillman diet for between three and seventeen days.

Less drastic, but formulated along the same lines, the Atkins diet puts you on a no-carbohydrate regimen at first to stimulate the use of stored fat as energy and allows you to eat all the fat and protein you want. The diet is very high in saturated fats and tends, when the body weight stabilizes, to increase B-lipoprotein and serum cholesterol levels, which may contribute to atherosclerosis and heart disease. Both regimens can lead to serious nutritional deficiencies unless the proper vitamin and mineral supplements are taken. It is true that both the Stillman and Atkins diets will help you lose weight, but at a cost in terms of long-term health and beauty. And because they are so eccentric, many dieters stay on them for only a short period of time before they are forced to revert to their usual habits of eating too much of the wrong kinds of foods.

Other Fad Diets

Other more esoteric regimens, such as the rice diet or macrobiotic diet and the protein-sparing fast, can be extremely dangerous leading to serious nutritional deficiencies, hypoproteinemia, hypocalcemia, and kidney and liver troubles. Long-term fasting (from two weeks to several months) can be an excellent way of reducing weight if you have a lot of weight to lose and if it is done wisely under the supervision of a doctor who knows about fasting. A doctor can advise you as to which nutritional supplements you need to take and also keep track of important physiological changes that indicate that your fast should be broken. On your own, you should *never* fast for more than a couple of days although, once your weight has been reduced to normal, a day's fast every week can be an excellent tool in ensuring that it stays there. The other ways of weight reduction, such as bypass surgery, wiring the jaws together, and staying on foolishly long unbalanced diets, are best left alone.

GETTING IT RIGHT

The only way to lose weight is to change your eating habits permanently so you follow a life regimen of eating moderate quantities of good, wholesome food, which provides a full complement of nutrition for lasting health and beauty. This means reeducating both your palate (to expect different tasting, lighter foods) and your appetite so that you lose weight gradually. This way you also do not have any of the diet shock that leads to going off a regimen and defeats its purpose. Two pounds a week weight loss should be your goal, not more. Then you can keep it off.

The diet you choose should be one that fits in reasonably with your daily relationship to food. For instance, it is worthwhile, if you have to cook for a family, to incorporate your own needs for raw vegetables, low calorie cheeses, low-fat yogurt, lean fish, and liver into the menus for the rest of the family, so you are not cooking two separate meals every time you go into the kitchen. It is not necessary to follow stringently a specific regimen where you eat exactly what is written for the meal and day. What is necessary is that you restrict yourself to a level of calories that will make it possible for you to continue with your daily activities without fatigue and that you make every calorie count in terms of nutrition. For many women, simply changing to the Lifestyle Diet brings about a steady, slow, consistent loss of weight without any restrictions even if they have been unable to lose weight before.

The idea that you can eat a candy bar or anything else you like a day and still lose weight, provided you don't eat more than your calorie allowance, is foolish. Certainly it is possible for you to lose weight, but you will lose it at a cost. The candy bar will rob your system of precious vitamin B necessary for the health of the nervous system and to resist stress. It will supply you with empty calories instead of contributing to your daily intake of important minerals and trace elements. It will also go none of the way toward enlightening your palate so you develop a taste for fine fresh foods that will help keep you slim forever.

Every food you eat needs to count. Following the guidelines in the nutrition section, put together a balanced diet for yourself that adjusts itself to your lifestyle and your needs but stays within your calorie allowance.

Buy a little calorie counter and read it. Get to know the number of calories in the foods you eat. Also buy a notebook small enough to slip into your pocket or handbag and carry it with you. In the beginning, after each meal that you eat, record the number of calories you have consumed. Set yourself a limit. If you are not particularly active, 1,000 calories a day should be plenty provided they are well spent for nutritional efficiency. If you are more active, or if you have a lot of weight to lose, you are probably better off on a 1,500 calorie regimen.

Think of it as so much money in the bank. If you have 1,200 calories to spend in a day, you can spend them as you please, saving them for use at an evening meal, or spending them in the morning or at lunchtime, if you feel more energetic during the day that way. You can even work it out on a weekly basis to take in special occasions. For instance, if you know you will be out to a meal on Saturday night, you might eat only 700 calories on Thursday and Friday and only 400 during Saturday morning, in order to create a credit of 600 calories to spend in addition to your other 600 for Saturday, thus making it possible to eat a 1,200 calorie meal on Saturday night without interfering with your weight loss. But try to see that whatever you do eat at the dinner party is within the bounds of the Lifestyle principles; low in fat, no refined carbohydrates or sugars, and at least 50 percent of it taken raw.

EATING PATTERNS

Everyone has their own. There is no sense in forcing down a breakfast if you never feel well in the morning when you eat. On the other hand, you may be in a state like this from overeating regularly at night so your body is not ready for food when you awaken. Most authorities on weight loss advise that you eat three regular meals a day. This helps women who are unconscious pickers at food to break the habit. It also gives the digestive enzymes a rest, for if the enzymes are in constant demand as a result of continuous nibbling on high fat or sugary foods, this can lead to enzymic insufficiencies or depletions that may result in food allergies, hypoglycemia, or other mental and physical problems. There are many healthy and lean men and women who remain so by eating one nutritionally sound meal a day. Others do better on several small meals. You have to discover what works best for you. But don't assume you know. Experiment within your calorie limit and find out. If you suffer from low blood sugar, try taking six small meals a day instead of two or three main ones. Carry around snacks with you—raw vegetables, whole-grain crackers, a hard-boiled egg, cottage cheese, sunflower seeds (all of which have been accounted for in your calorie allowance for the day) so you can munch whenever you feel the need. This will eliminate much of the impulse to overeat if you find yourself facing a restaurant meal or tempting high-calorie low-nutrient snacks. For most women a breakfast with some protein food in it, a salad for lunch, and a low-calorie dinner with another salad is ideal.

HOW TO MAKE IT IN A RESTAURANT

It is easy. First of all, just because you order something doesn't mean you have to eat *all* of it. Also, there are lots of low-calorie and high-nutrition foods on menus provided you know what they are and provided you ask for them. If you know the calorie values of food from your calorie chart (which you will learn very quickly if you are keeping that record properly) and you occasionally order something that is high in calories, eat only part of it, then compensate by making whatever else you order low in calories. Also get away from the idea that you have to eat a three-course meal every time you sit down at a restaurant table.

Here are some of the good bargains for dieters in restaurants: oysters, crab with a twist of lemon, shrimps, tomato and fresh basil salad, grilled liver, poached fish with lemon, poulet au pot, clear soup such as turtle, chicken, or beef consommé, jellied bouillon, an artichoke with French mustard and lemon juice instead of oil and vinegar, a little caviar on celery sticks, melon, and crudités.

My favorite is a salad made from everything raw in an Italian restaurant. Italians understand fresh vegetables better even than the Chinese. They have a real feel for selecting them for their freshness and fineness and are usually most conscientious in preparing a salad for you that isn't on the menu but which in flavor and looks far surpasses most of what is. For dressing, try some lemon juice and fresh herbs (particularly basil) or mild French mustard mixed with lemon juice. A drop or two of Tabasco juice can add zest to a lovely fresh salad.

USEFUL TOOLS FOR WEIGHT LOSS

Instant broth cubes are superb for quelling an appetite and they cost you only about twelve calories a cup. You can also carry them to work with you or, if you don't have boiling water available, make them up in a thermos to take along. They are also nutritious whereas coffee and tea will do nothing for you in terms of building health and beauty. Herb teas (no calories) are also excellent although they don't give you the same full feeling that broth does. They can be sweetened with a teaspoon of honey, which is an excellent source of essential trace elements such as zinc, copper, iron, manganese, and chromium—often in scarce supply in ordinary slenderizing regimens. My favorite drink is Perrier water, chilled if you wish, but it doesn't taste the same. Perrier or soda are also nice mixed with fresh fruit juice (half and half). Water can help you not to be hungry too, for it flushes out the acid from your stomach and helps wash out excess salt from your system, which can contribute to water retention.

Creating some new eating habits will help your weight loss too. Chew all your foods very slowly. The slower you go the better will be your digestion and the fuller you will feel from everything you eat. Don't drink alcohol. Don't put any extra salt on your foods at the table. Five minutes before sitting down to a meal, try drinking an eight-ounce glass of ice water. It will help eliminate the feelings of hunger so you will want less when you actually begin to eat.

DO YOU NEED TO TAKE SUPPLEMENTS?

Probably. Unless you are in the country and practically live on fresh vegetables from an organically grown garden and untreated meats and poultry from the local farms. A multipurpose vitamin tablet is useful. It can be bought from your local health food store. It should not have minerals in it, however, for multimineral tablets contain copper, which is not usually needed in supplemental doses and can cause harm in excess. And do look carefully at the vitamin section to see what your personal supplementary requirements might be.

A group of supplements for "rebuilding" such as the one on page 126 is useful on a weight-loss regimen. In particular, zinc and B_6 are important.

Brewer's yeast and yogurt are musts for dieters because lots of B-complex vitamins help to maintain your mental equilibrium and keep your energy level high. Eating yogurt—provided too you get plenty of roughage in your diet from raw fruits and vegetables or bran—promotes the health of intestinal flora, which produce the important B groups of vitamins in the body. Liver is another useful food for dieters. It is high in vitamin A, the B group, and many minerals. Eat it often in small quantities. Finally, sprouted seeds and grains eaten raw are the supreme diet food of all time. They are totally alive, full of vitamins and minerals in a concentration you won't find in any other food, and a wonderful source of the eight essential amino acids in a high-quality form. One of my favorite meals is a bowl of low-fat cottage cheese on which is sprinkled a mixture of sprouts; mung beans, lentils, alfalfa, wheat, or whatever I have, topped by a shake of garlic powder or a couple of drops of Tabasco or fresh herbs. It is completely satisfying and such a concentrated source of nourishment that it is hard to believe it is so low in calories.

GET INTO AN EXERCISE PROGRAM

Not all slenderizing is a question of eating less. Exercise plays an important role too. Regularly indulged in, what exercise does do is decrease the appetite. Britain's most well-known researcher in obesity, Dr. Gaston Pawan, has also found that, "with regular exercise not only does energy expenditure increase and all-over bodily functioning improve, but the metabolic substrata shifts so that you are able to mobilise fat quicker." Exercise also helps reduce anxiety and improves your mental state and helps you stop thinking about food all the time. Numerous experiments with overweight people have shown that a reducing diet plus a program of regular exercise make a far more effective weight control program than diet alone. Spend half an hour a day on your own exercise program —running or bicycling, swimming or dancing, or even simply stretching exercises done on the floor of your bedroom.

FOOD ALLERGIES CAN BLOCK WEIGHT LOSS

They do exist, particularly among women who have been on the weight seesaw for many years through crash dieting. Sensitivities to specific foods such as milk and milk products or grains (the two most common culprits) can make reducing almost an impossibility, for in the allergy-prone woman, the foods to which she is sensitive are invariably those that she craves and also those that, when she eats them, increase her appetite and lure her into giving up her weight loss program. For instance, I knew one woman who was allergic to wheat (although she wasn't aware of it at the time). She would go on a reducing diet and stick to it conscientiously until the third day, when the diet called for a piece of toast. She would eat her piece of toast and then find she could not stop there. One piece of toast would turn into two or three and four and by now she would feel so depressed and angry with herself that she would give up her diet again in despair. Once she discovered she was sensitive to wheat (a discovery she made by going on the *Rohsäfte-Kur* for three days and then eating a piece of bread, to which she reacted by feeling depressed and increasingly ravenous), she designed a diet for herself that was altogether free of wheat and other grains but which included yogurt and the stress supplements of B vitamins plus zinc (all of which are particularly useful in the case of food allergies as well), which she found easy to follow. The excess weight came off steadily bit by bit.

If you are overweight, have cravings for particular foods, or find it difficult to control your appetite, it may not all be your fault. You could be suffering from a food sensitivity, be allergic to a particular protein, or have a body that seems unable to deal effectively with certain metabolic wastes that themselves set off allergic-type reactions. The overweight overeater who chides herself and feels ashamed of her lack of willpower may well be doing herself an injustice. Overweight is not simply a lack of willpower, as some women's magazines and advertisements would have us believe. Neither is compulsive eating necessarily entirely psychological in origin. Clinical ecologists (who look at how factors in the environment can trigger off symptoms by inducing sensitive or allergic reactions that involve the central nervous system), allergists, and psychiatrists, examining the physical causes behind much illness, have recently found that many psychological moods, and even appetite itself, can be sparked off by chemical states in the body. Alter these chemical states through vitamins, minerals, diet, or by removing an offending substance from the environment and you alter the response of a person, eliminating his symptoms. In recent years such thinking has been successfully applied to the treatment of serious mental illness such as schizophrenia and physical ailments such as migraine, high blood pressure, and intermittent abdominal pain. For many who have unsuccessfully fought the reducing battle, it can also be applied to overweight. You may be able to get rid of an insatiable appetite and shed resistant excess pounds by changing what you eat and drink or altering the combination in which you take your foods.

To understand how, let's take a look at what is known about food allergies. The question of how and why certain foods set off sensitivity reactions in some people as yet remains a mystery. Very little is known for sure except that a food allergy is much less likely to occur when foods eaten are completely digested. Fatty acids, simple sugars, amino acids, and glycerin, the products of normal digestion, won't usually cause any problems. But for complete digestion to take place, a large number of specific chemical products and enzymes need to be present in the body in sufficient quantity. When, for any number of reasons, the supply of these is deficient, digestion of foods remains incomplete. This is often the case with proteins. Proteins incompletely broken down instead of becoming simple amino acids—their proper end products—are split into intermediate or large molecules that leak through the lining of the intestines and enter directly into the bloodstream. These incompletely digested particles are toxic to the cells. For instance, the amino acid histidine can be changed into a toxic substance called histamine, which is responsible for allergies such as hay fever.

Other incompletely broken down food products can also irritate cells. Such leakage occurs in most people to one degree or another but in some it is very prevalent. It causes no problems if one's body is easily able to eliminate these toxic products. But when, for any number of reasons, they are too prevalent or can't be eliminated quickly, a person is likely to show signs of food sensitivity. This kind of sensitivity is curious in that a certain food can not only cause specific reactions such as headache, depression, and increased appetite; when eaten it can also spark off a craving for more of the same food. But if you continue to eat the offending food your symptoms get better rather than worse, for the sensitivity is masked behind the craving. Later, if for any reason you stop eating the food, within a few hours to three or four days you can experience temporary but unpleasant withdrawal symptoms. These can be headache, emotional upset, increased appetite, or any number of other things.

To locate possible food allergies, clinical ecologists usually fast a woman for five days (to take her through the withdrawal stage) and then test specific foods one by one for reactions by placing a couple of drops of the food in aqueous solution (dissolved in plain water) under the tongue. If there is a sensitivity the woman will, within a couple of minutes, show an emotional or physical reaction to it. Then by eliminating the offending food or foods from her diet, she is able to remain free of whatever symptoms made the doctor suspect a food allergy in the first place.

Such an approach has proved successful in the treatment of any number of illnesses from migraine to gastric ulcers, high blood pressure, depression, and severe anxiety neurosis. These same principles can also be applied to overweight and to a tendency to compulsive eating.

Have you ever gotten up from a meal only to find instead of feeling satisfied you wanted to eat more? Or had a craving for a certain food and when you started to eat it found great difficulty in not stuffing yourself? Or found after eating something you feel high, tired, depressed, worried, or very hungry indeed? Or have you been unable to follow a reducing diet for more than a few days without suddenly going on a binge and stuffing yourself, then felt guilty and ashamed because you apparently had no willpower? If any two of these things are true of you, you might be one of the many who is prone to food sensitivities. Then, either by changing the foods you eat together at each meal (food combining) or by testing for and then eliminating a few foods that are troubling you from your daily fare, you may find that it will make all the difference in helping you get slim and stay that way.

LET'S LOOK AT FOOD COMBINING

First developed by Dr. William Howard Hay, the theory behind careful food combining is simple: don't mix protein or acid fruits with carbohydrates at the same meal. If your enzyme system is not as good as it should be, eating concentrated proteins and starches at the same meal can play havoc with digestion, increasing the number of incompletely broken down food particles that find their way into the bloodstream to cause trouble. Concentrated proteins such as cheese, eggs, fish, and meat need an acid medium for digestion. If there are any concentrated starch or sugar foods in the stomach at the same time this can interfere with or even neutralize the acid medium so that the proteins are incompletely digested.

Carbohydrates are different. They need an alkaline medium for digestion. Normally, the acidity of the stomach isn't high enough to interfere with this process. Just how much acid is released into the stomach depends on the amount of protein present in the digestive tract. In the presence of acid fruits, meat, or other protein foods, the breakdown of starches can be greatly interfered with in someone whose digestive enzymes are already inadequate. This can result in quantities of incompletely digested food particles that pass directly into the bloodstream and can cause sensitivity reactions. Some of the most common reactions in overweight people are feelings of increased hunger, fatigue, or anxiety, or food cravings, all of which lead you to eat more and gain weight instead of losing it. If you have difficulty with compulsive eating or trouble losing weight, it is a good idea to apply the food combining principles to whatever slenderizing regimen you choose to follow.

Eat one protein meal, one starch meal, and an alkaline-forming meal a day. For instance, take meat, fish, or poultry together with a tossed salad or root vegetable and fresh fruit at one meal. Then your whole-grain cereal, whole-wheat or rye toast, plus natural sugars such as figs or raisins or dates at a second meal. Finally, have an alkaline-forming meal of, say, fruits and milk or yogurt at the third meal.

DO-IT-YOURSELF ALLERGY TESTING

The second approach depends on testing yourself to see if you have any particular foods that may be producing sensitivity reactions that can result in tiredness, increased appetite, or depression, which spark you to eat more than you should. This means sitting down and making a list of the foods you eat every day, those that you crave, and those that, after you eat them, make you feel more hungry, tired, nervous, or depressed, and those that you use to improve your mood. (Chocolate can cheer up lots of people, or bread, cookies, and cheese.) Once you've made your list (and it may mean keeping a record for several days of what you eat, what time, how you feel afterward, and so on), you can see clearly the foods most likely to be troublesome to you. They are almost always those you crave the most, eat most often, or use to boost your morale when it needs it. Some of the most common offenders are grains such as cereals or breads, milk and milk products such as cream, yogurt, and cheese, and packaged, processed foods that contain monosodium glutamate or chemical colorings, flavorings, and preservatives. Put yourself on a diet *free* of all these things for a week by sticking to fresh meat, fish, and poultry with fresh fruits, salads, and fresh vegetables. Or, better still, go on the *Rohsäfte-Kur* for five days. Then see how you feel.

Have you lost some of your insatiable hunger? Have you also lost weight? Now, one by one, reintroduce these foods—slowly and carefully, only one at a time. Eat cheese, for instance, a moderate amount at a meal, and then don't eat it again for four days. Then test another food in the following four days. Did you experience any kind of withdrawal symptoms such as headache or increased hunger during these days? Did you get a lift from eating the food or any immediate reaction to the food? If not, then you are pretty safe with it and can introduce it back into your diet. If you did, it is likely to be a trouble-causer for you and is best completely eliminated. Food allergies and how they can affect us can be enormously complex, but these two methods are very simple things to try if you suspect a food allergy could be behind your problem in losing weight. For anyone who has repeatedly suffered with overweight, they are certainly worth experimenting with. Whichever method you choose, drink a lot (eight to ten glasses a day) of pure water (not coffee or tea) to help eliminate toxic wastes before they can cause trouble, stop using extra salt on your foods, and eliminate white flour and sugar from your diet.

DESIGN YOUR OWN REGIMEN

It is important that every woman develop her own slenderizing regimen to suit her needs and her tastes within the bounds of good nutrition, but there is one particular regimen that I find extremely useful, and which I offer as a possibility, called the Breakthrough Diet. It was worked out with the help of Dr. Dagmar Leichti, director of the Bircher-Benner Clinic in Zurich. It is designed to get you into a slenderizing program with a bang and into a new way of eating and also to help you reeducate your appetite quickly and remove all the by-products of stimulants such as coffee, alcohol, and pollutants from your system. But it demands you spend the first day of the regimen in bed if possible, or at the very least, resting quietly. Sunday is a good day to start. Many women who have tried it find it is just the impetus they need to get them going.

ONE-WEEK BREAKTHROUGH DIET

Night Before

A cup of blood-cleansing herb tea from a health food store to clear out the digestive system

Day 1: Bed/juice day—400 calories

BREAKFAST

7 ounces fruit juice, made fresh if possible (orange, apple, grape, etc.)

LUNCH

7 ounces vegetable juice

DINNER

Same as breakfast
Throughout the day you may have solidago (goldenrod) herb tea (available only from herbalists), which acts as a natural diuretic and helps you get rid of excess fluids from waterlogged tissues.

TREATMENT

Relaxation exercises and breathing exercises morning and evening. This is an important start to your diet. Bed/juice days are the cornerstone of healthy weight control, to be used once a week after first week. This day should be spent quietly in bed, resting, reading, listening to music, at home. Bed early, no distractions, a day of contemplation.

Day 2: Juice or fruit fast—550 calories

BREAKFAST

7 ounces fruit juice or 9 ounces any fresh fruit

LUNCH

7 ounces vegetable juice or 9 ounces any fresh fruit

DINNER

Same as lunch
Throughout the day you may have solidago tea and bottled water if thirsty.

TREATMENT

Relaxation and breathing exercises morning and evening. Warm bath. Early to bed. Should you experience insomnia, see under general directions below.

Day 3: Jucies and supplements—800–1,000 calories

BREAKFAST

5 to 7 ounces fruit juice and 5 ounces natural yogurt

LUNCH

5 ounces fruit juice and 5 ounces mixed vegetable juice and 5 ounces almond tonic

DINNER

Same as breakfast

TREATMENT

Begin your exercise program, five to ten minutes, but do it slowly and gently. Use a loofah to rub your body for three minutes morning and evening. Take an hour or two to rest in the middle of the day. Go to bed early. First thing in the morning walk for fifteen to twenty minutes in the open air.

Day 4: Raw food—1,300–1,400 calories

BREAKFAST

5 ounces diet muesli; 3 to 7 teaspoons minced nuts; herb tea (choose from rose-hip, linden blossom, and peppermint) with a little fresh milk, if desired

LUNCH

A piece of fresh fruit or 5 to 7 ounces raw vegetable salad (one root, one leaf, one bulb or "fruit") with low-fat dressing, seasoned with fresh or dried herbs, garnished with three teaspoons of minced nuts

DINNER

Same as breakfast, or yogurt and fruit instead of muesli

TREATMENT

First thing in the morning walk for thirty minutes to one hour in fresh air. Rub skin twice a day. Take a pine oil bath and soak for twenty-five minutes. Exercise for fifteen minutes. Go to bed early.

Day 5: Raw food with supplements—1,750 calories

BREAKFAST

5 ounces muesli, 1 piece of whole-wheat bread or pumpernickel or crispbread spread with 4 ounces of cottage cheese, one cup of herb tea with a little milk, if desired.

LUNCH

A piece of fresh fruit, a salad of root, bulb or "fruit," and leaf vegetables garnished with herbs, garlic, and a non-oil dressing or lemon juice.

DINNER

Same as breakfast or salad as at lunch, or fruit and flatbread with 2 ounces cottage cheese

TREATMENT

Same as for Day 4.

Days 6 and 7: Full diet, but low in salt and fat—2,000 calories

BREAKFAST

Same as fourth day but also add 5 ounces of low-fat yogurt and 1 teaspoon of wheat germ

LUNCH

Same as fourth day, but add 2 ounces of cottage cheese and 1 medium potato baked in its skin (eat skin too), or 2 steamed vegetables garnished with herbs

DINNER

Same as fourth day, but add 1 slice whole-grain bread or crispbread, spread with 2 ounces low-fat cottage cheese

TREATMENT

Walk two hours. Brush skin morning and evening. If possible follow with alternate warm and cold shower. Exercise for twenty minutes. Go to bed early.

General Directions

Check your weight daily. Eating snacks between meals is forbidden as are sugar, alcohol, ordinary tea, and coffee. Drink only herb teas and spring water. Always sip your juices from a teaspoon. End your meals before you feel completely full. Take no medications during the diet, including appetite depressants. The first week is the most difficult. After a few days a natural feeling of well-being and vitality becomes such a source of satisfaction, along with your knowledge that you have become master of your eating habits, that you are on your way to fulfilling your beauty potential.

Should you experience any adverse reactions, remember that they are a result of your body throwing off toxins at an enormous rate and will quickly pass. Headaches and nausea, for example, usually come on the first day, if at all. Retreat to a dark room. Don't eat until your discomfort has passed. Take camomile tea, fennel tea, or lemon juice in water. For insomnia take lemon peel tea and honey. Eat a dozen raisins in the evening before you go to bed. Take a long lukewarm bath in the evening.

TWO-WEEK FOLLOW-UP DIET

DAY 1   Bed/juice day
DAYS 2, 3   Raw food
DAYS 4, 5   Full diet
DAY 6   Fruit fast
DAY 7   Full diet

RECIPES

BIRCHER-BENNER DIET MUESLI

1 tablespoon rolled oats
7 ounces grated apple
1 tablespoon honey
1 teaspoon lemon juice
3 tablespoons natural yogurt
1 tablespoon minced hazelnuts and almonds

Soak the oats overnight in 3 tablespoons water. Just before serving, add apple, honey, lemon, and yogurt. Top with grated nuts. (For variety, use berries, oranges, or raisins with or instead of apple.)

ALMOND TONIC

6 fresh almonds
1 tablespoon honey

Blanch almonds by pouring boiling water over them and letting them stand for 3 minutes. Remove skin. Liquidize with honey and 7 ounces water (preferably spring or bottled water).

LEMON PEEL AND HONEY TEA

1 lemon
1 tablespoon honey

Thoroughly scrub lemon. Slice peel finely with potato peeler. Simmer in a pint of water for 5 minutes. Add honey. Let it stand for 10 minutes. Strain.

MIXED SALAD

To make a healthy salad you need fresh vegetables—ideally sun-ripened, organically grown ones. They should be prepared just before serving so that no loss of juice occurs and they don't wilt.

The vegetables should be carefully mixed so that every raw dish combines a root vegetable, a bulb or "fruit" vegetable, and a leafy vegetable. Ideally for digestion, not more than three different vegetables should be served at once.

Leafy vegetables include cabbage, lettuce, endive, Romaine lettuce, red cabbage, spinach, lamb's lettuce, dandelion greens, watercress, sprouted seeds and grains, and corn salad.

Root vegetables include carrots, beets, turnips, radishes, kohlrabi, celeriac, and salsify.

Bulb or "fruit" vegetables include tomatoes, cucumbers, zucchini, green and red peppers.

Wash vegetables. Slice or grate them fine (always use a stainless steel grater so the vitamins are not destroyed). Toss in dressing, if required.

Dressing
1 tablespoon oil (e.g., sunflower)
1 tablespoon lemon juice
Pinch fresh or dried herbs
1 teaspoon onion or garlic (optional)

MIXED NUTS

Handful each of almonds, hazelnuts, and brazil nuts
1 tablespoon sunflower seeds

Mince in blender or coffee grinder for 30 seconds. Quantities for a few days can be made in advance and stored in a sealed jar in the refrigerator.

VEGETABLE JUICE

2 large carrots
2 large tomatoes
Juice of any other vegetables to make up 1 pint
1 teaspoon lemon juice
Pinch fresh or dried herbs

Prepare vegetables in juice extractor. Add lemon juice and herbs for flavor. If you can't make your own, vegetable juices made from organically grown vegetables are available from health food stores.

20

Tissue Sludge and Cellulite

The enormous fuss that is made about cellulite always surprises me. "Does it or doesn't it exist?" "What are its causes?" "What, if anything, can be done about it?" Such is the way women tend to treat cellulite, as if it were some kind of externally imposed curse to which they fall innocent victim.

Cellulite is the manifestation of the wrong kind of lifestyle for health and beauty: eating wrongly (or too much), living under prolonged stress, being exposed to too many pollutants, and all the other things that we tend to think we can get away with, but never really do. And no number of expensive or painful treatments is going to help the problem for long unless you change the things that brought it on in the first place.

Cellulite exists, whether or not one wishes to call it cellulite or something else and whether or not a few adamant medical voices loudly deny its existence. It is real enough for the woman who, in spite of being slim and well, reaches down and pinches her thigh only to find it puckers, ripples, and looks like the skin of an orange. Cellulite differs from normal fat in three ways:

1. It doesn't disappear when you slim down and exercise regularly as ordinary fat does.

2. Cellulite areas contain more water than ordinary fat tissue.

3. Radioisotopic examinations have shown that, while the components of ordinary fatty tissue change every eight days, gel-like cellulite remains almost stagnant.

Quite simply, cellulite is a pollution problem. It is the result of a build-up of wastes in specific areas of the body. When you examine a layer of cellulite under a microscope you find that the fat imbued with water and wastes is held there by a fine network of hard fibrous adhesions. These adhesions, a kind of sclerosis of the connective tissues, get worse with the passage of time.

There are two situations that attract cellulite. First, it occurs in parts of the body where the circulation is poor through inactivity and the muscles are flaccid, for instance, in the hips and upper thighs of women who spend each day sitting at a desk in front of a typewriter and get no exercise. Second, it appears in areas where tension has led to chronic spasm of the muscles. This not only interferes with proper circulation of blood and lymph to the cells, so that they are never properly nourished and wastes from them are not properly eliminated, it also irritates adjacent nerves and soft tissue structures, which in turn results in yet more spasm. Slowly, a congested area forms, since cell nutrients and wastes are only sluggishly exchanged and vascular dilation and constriction in the area is erratic. Gradually, wastes accumulate and a kind of tissue sludge is formed. There it tends to remain, for each condition in the area tends only to reinforce every other one in a vicious circle.

DEADENED AREAS OF THE BODY

Areas of cellulite—which occur most commonly on the hips, thighs, upper arms, shoulders, and back—are deadened areas. They have long been the concern of bioenergetic psychotherapists and Rolfers, who know that they need to be broken down and dispersed in order for the person to feel fully alive and to function really well mentally and physically. Although these professionals are in no way concerned with the beauty problems of cellulite, they know a lot about how it feels and behaves. For instance, they will tell you that often it begins as soft cellulite where the tissue is exceptionally tender to the touch and then slowly turns into the hardened variety where there is little or no feeling if you pinch it, knead it, or press it. They will also tell you that by working on it with the right kind of massage and breaking down the hardened and distorted tissue, they can break up the stasis and restore normal circulation. Then the hardness, the puckers, the orange peel quality, and the distorted sensitivity to touch disappears. And interestingly enough, where in its formation cellulite often goes from the flabby stage to the hard gristly one, in its treatment the process is often reversed, with the soft, flabby look returning again before normality is finally restored to the area.

WHAT CAUSES CELLULITE IN THE FIRST PLACE?

The wrong kind of lifestyle, of course. But what specific things in it? Three things. First, anything that puts into your system more pollutants from the air, food, and water than it can efficiently deal with and eliminate quickly. Second, poor elimination, as a result of constipation (often unrecognized constipation, for many women who have a bowel movement every day assume that they aren't constipated but they still may be only partially removing the wastes from their intestines), or poor liver, kidney, or lung function. This leads to wastes and the by-products of normal metabolism building up in the system with no possibility of efficient release. And third, the excessive production of wastes in the body that come from shallow breathing, wrong eating, too much of the wrong kind of exercise, prolonged stress, and faulty digestion or assimilation of foods, much of which shows itself as food allergies.

There are other factors that often contribute to cellulite: hormones, the long-term use of diuretics, and vertebral lesions in the pelvis or chronic constipation, both of which tend to restrict the flow of blood to the lower limbs and impede proper lymphatic drainage to the legs.

A predisposition to cellulite occurs in women with hormonal imbalances—those that produce large quantities of estrogen or whose level of estrogen is not properly kept under control by the liver or by the amount of its antagonist hormone progesterone. It is interesting, and not very well known, that 75 percent of cases of cellulite in women have started during a period of drastic hormonal change in their lives. Dr. Pierre Dukan, author of *La Cellulite en Question*, La Table Ronde edition, has compiled statistics of cellulite sufferers. He has found that:

12 percent of cellulite begins at puberty
19 percent when a woman first takes the Pill
17 percent during pregnancy
27 percent at the first indications of menopause

Women on the Pill, those who suffer from irregular periods, and those who suffer any severe or long-term stress are perfect targets for tissue sludge. The pituitary, often called the master gland, is affected both by shock and stress. Because it is largely responsible for triggering the secretion of female hormones, when its function is disturbed or upset, hormonal secretions are modified and often increased and cellulite develops.

If, after following the whole body treatment for cellulite for a month, you feel no signs of real progress, it is a good idea to have your sacrum looked at by a responsible chiropractor or osteopath. For if there is any long-term displacement in the vertebrae present, so that muscles in the lower back are in a chronic state of spasm, this will have to be corrected by manipulation and massage before you can expect lasting results from an anticellulite regimen.

HOW TO KEEP CELLULITE AWAY

The first and most important rule is don't take into your body too much of the wrong kinds of foods in the first place. This includes all forms of refined carbohydrates, all overprocessed, precooked, or pickled foods, and prepared meats. Alcohol and coffee are major pollutants. If you are really serious about remaining cellulite-free, then avoid them altogether and drink spring water or fresh, unsweetened fruit or vegetable juices, or herb teas sweetened with a teaspoon of honey.

Smoking is also taboo when it comes to the prevention of cellulite, for two reasons. It robs the system of vitamin C, which is essential for the health of collagen, the connective fibers that support muscles and skin and the circulatory system. When the collagen fibers start to go it is very hard indeed to get rid of cellulite. Also, nicotine in the system interferes with the circulation so that cellular exchange, vital to keeping the body free of tissue sludge, is drastically slowed down. This creates ideal conditions for cellulite to form.

Although proper nutrition is the single most important thing in protecting yourself from cellulite (and, incidentally, in removing it when it has formed) it is by no means everything. Getting enough regular exercise is also essential. So is learning to breathe properly, which only takes about ten minutes a day to practice and is one of the most helpful ways of clearing your system of substances that can cause internal pollution problems. And, finally, so is some form of deep relaxation or meditation practiced daily to calm your tensions and put your body and mind into the passive vegetative state in which the body can regularly restore itself from the ravages of stress. Read the sections on dealing with stress, relaxation, breathing, and exercise. But don't just take them in for interest's sake, put each of them into practice. The knowledge will be worth nothing unless you *use* it. For cellulite is not some mysterious aberration that suddenly appears. It is a *whole body problem*. And as such it requires whole body methods of prevention and cure.

WHAT TO DO WHEN YOU'VE ALREADY GOT IT

Apart from getting onto the regimens outlined above and staying on them, you should use special methods of detoxifying your system and giving the wastes stored in the tissues a chance to be removed from the body. The problem has to be attacked simultaneously from within and without. From within, put yourself on a spring cleaning regimen of raw foods to encourage waste elimination and improve the rate of cellular exchange.

Two other useful dietary tools are the water fast and the *Rohsäfte-Kur* which, in my experience, is better than anything else in helping to eliminate tissue sludge quickly. You should not stay on it for more than two or three days unless you are under medical supervision, but this is all that is necessary to get the ball rolling. Then you can go onto the Spring-cleaning Diet, or better still, alternate the two—five or six days a week on raw foods interspersed with one or two days on the *Rohsäfte-Kur* juice fast.

There is no reason why you cannot stay on a raw food regimen for quite a while, even several weeks if necessary, until most of the cellulite problem is cleared up. If you choose to do it a slower way, after a few days on the Spring-cleaning Diet, eat normally, simply avoiding the bad foods and making sure (and *this is important*) that at least half of all your foods are eaten raw. Besides providing you with the optimum concentration of vital nutrients, this helps protect you from hidden constipation, one of the main culprits behind both cellulite and varicose veins. If you happen to be on a reducing diet where the amounts of food you are eating are greatly restricted, then you should take some bran—two or three teaspoons is usually enough sprinkled on plain yogurt, on salads, or stirred into a glass of fresh vegetable or fruit juice. But you must drink lots of water with it. For bran only does its job effectively when there is plenty of water in the system to develop its bulk.

Here are some vegetable and fruit juice combinations that are particularly good for clearing tissue sludge from the system:

FORMULA 1

Carrot—4 ounces
Celery—2 ounces

FORMULA 2

Carrot—3 ounces
Beet—2 ounces
Cucumber—2 ounces

FORMULA 3

Carrot—4 ounces
Celery—2 ounces
Apple—2 ounces

FORMULA 4

Carrot—4 ounces
Watercress—½ ounce
Cabbage—1½ ounces

FORMULA 5

Orange—4 ounces

Try to drink at least two glasses a day. Also make sure you get plenty of water in order not to put too much strain on the kidneys, which will be dealing with some pretty concentrated wastes as your system begins to clear. If you are on an all raw food diet, with vegetable or fruit juices two or three times a day, you won't have to worry about taking any extra water. Raw fruits and vegetables are mostly water. If you are only eating half of your foods raw, then in addition to the two or three glasses of juice a day you should drink another pint of pure water. A

French mineral water, Contrexéville, is particularly good for cellulite-prone women because of its high mineral content and its tendency to release stored water from the tissues.

There are also some herb teas that are particularly good for cellulite sufferers either because of their blood purifying capabilities or because they are natural diuretics and encourage the elimination of excess water from the tissues.

Maté tea is a tonic for the kidneys, a tension soother, and is so satisfying to drink that you feel less inclined to eat. It is nice taken plain or with a squeeze of lemon in it.

Solidago tea (wild goldenrod) is an excellent natural diuretic and a mild stimulant. It is a favorite for spring-cleaning the system at the Bircher-Benner Clinic in Zurich.

Nettle tea is another diuretic and tonic, excellent for the lymphatic system. It doesn't taste as nice as solidago, so needs to be sweetened with a little honey.

Many experts in orthomolecular medicine and megavitamin therapy believe that food supplements can help protect against internal pollution and in elimination. Vitamin C is the detoxicant par excellence provided you take enough of it—that is, measure the doses in grams and not milligrams. Vitamin E, because of its stimulating effect on the circulatory system and because it has been shown to offer protection against pollution and some forms of irradiation, is also useful. And recent research shows that one of the finest protectors of all is dietary fiber from whole grains, bran, and raw fruits and vegetables.

GETTING TO GRIPS WITH LUMPS AND BUMPS

External treatment is almost as important as internal treatment—breaking down the pockets of cellulite physically so that stored wastes in them are released and can be eliminated from the body. There are several ways of doing it. Which you choose depends on your patience, your preference, and the state of your pocketbook. If the cellulite is hard and long-standing, if there is a lot of it—you will probably need professional help, either a beauty therapist who knows what she is doing (many unfortunately don't) or a physiotherapist trained in corrective tissue massage or Rolfing.

Properly applied, aromatherapy—the use of essential oils of plants on the skin—can be helpful too, because certain specially selected oils are useful in stimulating lymphatic drainage, while others will draw forth wastes from the skin itself. Most professional treatments for cellulite combine a number of remedies because there is no single substance that gives consistent positive results. One of the most popular is a mixture of thyroxine, an enzyme to dissolve the gel in the pockets of tissue sludge, and a mild diuretic to draw out water from the tissues. It is either briskly applied by hand to skin that has been prewarmed by infrared lamps or massaged to increase its permeability, or it is introduced into the skin with a current passing between two plates put on the body—a process known as iontophoresis.

A more drastic form of treatment is given by injection through extraordinarily long hypodermic needles inserted into and then along just under the surface of the skin, which deposit their contents as they move. This form of treatment usually demands the use of a local anesthetic as it can be very painful. Alternatively, the French have designed a special device in which eighteen tiny needles used uniformly all along the area introduce the substance and then disperse it evenly into the tissue. These treatments can be useful for some women; for others, they just don't seem to work. But they are expensive, painful, and you must never kid yourself that they are a cure for cellulite. They may help disperse it, but unless you do something to get rid of the underlying causes by changing the way you live, the unsightly puckers and bumps will return to haunt you without fail.

THE MEDIUM IS MASSAGE

Massage is important. It helps stimulate local circulation, loosen the waste products from their hold, and get rid of the pitted, orange-peel look. But it has to be done properly. A physiotherapist experienced in connective tissue massage or a Rolfer is capable of attacking an area of cellulite with what appears to be untold viciousness yet doing nothing but good. But then he or she knows what to do and has spent years using the techniques. Any woman who sets to on her own body, brutally pummeling her legs or hips in the name of self-massage, is in danger of doing much destruction to the fragile distended connective fibers and the soggy mass of tissue sludge, so that she can end up with a permanently disfigured thigh, marbled with bruises and covered with broken veins. Don't.

There is a right way to go about it. First, always use an oil or talcum powder to help your hands slide. Begin with effleurage—meaning a light stroking of the skin in the area to be treated, hand over hand, always beginning *above* the area affected (to improve the flow of blood to the area), stroking toward the heart. The only time you should work in a direction away from the heart is when you are in a very tense state, when it will help calm and relax you.

Begin with light strokes and then gradually let them grow firmer as you go until you are finally working quite vigorously on the area. This part of the massage should take about three to four minutes per area.

By now the circulation is improved and you can begin to knead the area without fear of causing damage. Work hand over hand, taking hold of your flesh with the whole palm of your hand and fingers (not *just* the fingers) and pulling it away from the bone, squeezing it rhythmically at the same time. (This is exactly like the movement you use when kneading bread.) Continue this for a minute or two and then, using the base of your thumb and the knuckles of your hands, push them gently but firmly into the troubled areas, twisting them in a circular motion at the same time. This movement helps break up the pockets of tissue sludge and release their contents into the circulatory systems, from which they can be eliminated from the body. Use this motion for no more than three or four minutes in each area or you risk irritating the tissue and undoing all the good you have done. Finally, finish off with the same sort of effleurage with which you began in order to help carry wastes away.

Massage is best done when your skin is warm and preferably slightly damp (as after a bath) if you want to get the best benefits from the oil you are using. Although there are some experts in massage who say it doesn't matter, I think a vegetable oil, such as almond, coconut, safflower, olive, or sunflower is preferable to mineral oil like baby oil. It seems to have a natural affinity to the skin and also serves as an excellent carrier for any essential oils of plants which you may wish to add for their therapeutic effects. When mixing oils, make them in quantities that you are likely to use up in a couple of weeks so there is no risk of them going rancid, particularly if you live in a hot climate. Or you can store them in a refrigerator. Here are some good mixtures for cellulite massage oil that you can mix yourself.

NASTY BUT NICE

To 4 ounces of safflower or sunflower oil (or make it 2 ounces wheat-germ oil, 2 ounces safflower or sunflower oil), add the contents squeezed from eight 100-iu capsules vitamin E that have been pierced with a pin (this will provide 200 iu of the vitamin per ounce). Then add the contents of two 25,000-iu vitamin A capsules. Shake well. Vitamin A makes the lot smell more like a medicinal than a cosmetic product, but the effect on aging or blemished skin is well worth the esthetic loss.

L'ORIGANS

To 4 ounces of safflower, sunflower, hazelnut, or apricot oil add 10 drops of oil of lavender, 5 drops of oil of juniper, and 20 drops of oil of rosemary. Shake well. Lavender is mildly antiseptic and softens the skin while rosemary has natural diuretic and stimulant properties.

IVY DOES IT

Remove the stems and crush to a pulp the leaves of half a pound of fresh ivy with a mortar and pestle. Add 6 ounces of safflower, sunflower, hazelnut, or apricot oil little by little, continuing to crush thoroughly. Put the lot into a covered glass jar and allow to stand in a cool place for two days. Strain and refrigerate.

There are also massage gloves on the market to be used with creams, gels, and soaps, most of which contain ivy, horse-chestnut, or seaweed extracts, all of which are useful in the treatment of cellulite. But the lotions and potions are not going to do you any good unless you religiously massage them in every day. This steady perseverance in the treatment of cellulite areas from the outside is the only thing that really gets results.

You may notice after massaging yourself for a week or two that the condition seems to get worse: your thighs are flabbier and your bottom more puckered than ever. Don't despair. This is a good sign. It means the treatment is working. Tissue sludge almost always goes through this stage before it is finally reabsorbed into the system and eliminated from the body.

TAKE TO THE WATERS

Another useful external treatment for cellulite is hydrotherapy. It is part of *la cure* in many of the best European spas. It works on the same principle that massage does, by improving circulation and gently but insistently breaking down the pockets of tissue sludge. There are two types. The first uses powerful jets of water directed onto the surface of the skin. The second involves the alternative plunging of the body into hot and cold water.

If you have a hose that can be attached to the bath tap or a flexible shower head with a fairly good water force you can benefit from self-treatments while you are showering or bathing every day, particularly if cellulite is on your hips, buttocks, and thighs. Direct a jet of warm water against the problem areas from a distance of four to six inches (depending on the strength of the jet), moving it systematically backward and forward across the hips and buttocks and up and down the legs in a snakelike fashion. Then do the inside of your thighs and calves and the bottom of each foot. Finish off by passing the jet, held a bit further from the skin, across the shoulders, chest, abdomen, and down the back.

SWEATING IT OFF

Another effective external method for clearing out debris from the body is a sauna. Ideally it should be able to eliminate about 30 percent of the metabolic wastes and pollutants the body accumulates through stress, diet, and unclean air. European physicians who specialize in various heat treatments claim that controlled overheating of the body also increases the rate of the metabolic processes as a whole and stimulates the functioning of the endocrine system. Artificially induced heat is one of the finest means of deep cleansing the skin as well and can even inhibit the growth of viruses and bacteria in the body.

The Finns, who are world experts on the sauna (there is one sauna for every seven people in Finland) increase the beneficial effect of the heat on the skin during the sauna by switching their backs and their limbs with birch leaves to further stimulate circulation. They claim also that the sauna makes joints and limbs more supple for graceful movements while it soothes the muscles and refreshes the mind—even increasing one's capacity for work and enjoyment. A sauna taken weekly will greatly speed any anticellulite program of massage, diet, and the rest. However, if you suffer from a serious respiratory ailment or heart disease you should use a sauna only on doctor's orders.

Rules for the Sauna

1. Give yourself plenty of time. It will benefit you most if you take it leisurely so you have time for several sessions in the heat, with short rests in between and a rest of at least thirty minutes, preferably an hour, after you are through.

2. Never take a sauna until at least two hours after a meal and never take a sauna during a juice fast. (It is excellent to use the sauna the day before you begin your fast.)

3. Never take a sauna if you have symptoms of any illness.

4. Wear little or nothing in the sauna—a towel wrapped around you is more than enough. The more you wear, the less effective will the heat treatment be.

5. Take off all your jewelery and your watch. They will become very hot.

6. Stay in the sauna room for only five minutes at a stretch. Then plunge into cold water or take a cold shower and rest before going back in.

7. Don't water the stones during your first session and be sparing with the moisture you put on afterward.

8. Lie down in the sauna room if you can, or sit quietly. Once you are used to the heat you will be able to move to a higher bench.

9. Be sure to get half an hour's rest at the end to let your body readjust to the normal temperature of the room (this is as important as the sauna itself in ensuring you get all the benefits from the treatment). Never drink alcohol just before or after the sauna.

10. Don't towel yourself dry afterward. Instead, let the air dry your skin naturally. Then you can have a shower.

PROFESSIONAL RECONSTRUCTION WORK

When there is a serious misalignment in the body, such as a chronic stoop that begins to distort the soft S-shape curve of the spine, heavy, shapeless piano legs, or twists, curves, and bulges in parts of the body, that stays there even after the loss of excess weight, cellulite treatment, and exercise, then you need professional help. There are a number of different disciplines that can be useful. Osteopathy or chiropractic, through manipulation and specific exercises, can realign spines as well as eliminate pressures on nerves or blood vessels in the spinal area. Left unattended, these pressures may result in serious back pain, varicose veins, poor lymphatic drainage to the legs, and bad cellulite. The Alexander technique can help straighten a spine bent by years of discouragement and rehabilitate the personality that carries it in the process. Tai chi and yoga work slowly and gradually, but are capable of restoring most bodies to perfect alignment and balance as well. But I've found two other techniques—Rolfing and connective tissue massage—to be especially helpful in treating body problems that, by interfering with perfect form, mar beauty.

ROLFING

Rolfing is a form of deep compression massage known as structural integration. Ida Rolf, who developed the technique which is now used widely in Europe and America, believed that the body is a mass organized in space and therefore subject to gravitational forces. It is also, she said, a physical expression of the experience and personality of the person. According to Rolf's theory, the "normal body is one in which the ear, the center of the shoulder, the hip, the knees and the ankle are all in alignment so that the body is most effectively orientated to the forces of gravity." From this balanced position you can move freely and without restriction. You can also avoid the excess stress and tensions in the muscles and tissues that occur when for any reason this natural alignment is disturbed.

By stretching and making elastic the distorted connective tissue in the muscles and skin and by repositioning ligaments and tendons which have become tightened or bunched in compensation for these distortions, Rolfing causes the joints to move more freely and the muscles and fascia themselves to take on a different quality, look, and feel. In effect, grace and economy are restored to the body as well as its own perfect form as it becomes centered along its natural alignment. This naturally helps to eliminate cellulite—it restructures the whole body.

Before and after photographs have been taken of patients that demonstrate that their natural posture has been greatly altered by Rolfing. It not only affects one's looks but also makes one feel quite different—more spontaneous, open, and responsive to the environment and more in control of one's own life.

CONNECTIVE TISSUE MASSAGE

The other treatment that can be particularly useful in treating a body that has seriously lost its form is connective tissue massage (CTM). Gentler than Rolfing and, like Rolfing, not truly a treatment at all, it can work wonders to change a woman's body distorted by misshapen legs and midriff. It can also soften and sometimes even eliminate stretch marks and it can lift a sagging chin.

First developed in Austria, CTM is a specific form of massage performed primarily with the fingers and thumbs and designed to affect total body shape by altering the structure and organization of connective tissue. Unlike Rolfing, CTM is usually not painful. It is said to restore elasticity and improve the functioning of the body's connective tissues, thereby increasing blood and nutrient supply to the cells in specific areas. This is how it is able to restore form.

Connective tissue gives structure to your body and acts as bindings and support for organs and muscles. It is usually highly vascular with a great capacity to hold water. It is made up of elastic fibers, fat cells, blood cells, collagenous fibers, and plasma. Together these components form the internal environment of the body, transporting all substances to the cells, bringing products of metabolism from blood, lymph, and tissue fluid, and acting as storage space for water, salt, and glucose.

But connective tissues can become distorted by poor alignment, injury, age, or other factors (poor nutrition among them) so that the circulation of lymph and fluids to and from the cells becomes sluggish. Then you get areas of stasis, such as cellulite, sagging muscles, and poor elimination of waste, which can lead to rapidly aging skin and bulges and bumps where they shouldn't be. CTM breaks down these sluggish areas, bringing improved blood flow and altering the physical look of skin and flesh. I have seen it reshape muscles and tendons and relieve restricted functions of joints as well as changing the contours of a face, redistributing fat deposits such as pouches under the eyes and chin, and even eliminating mild stretch marks. Physiotherapists using it claim that all these benefits are due to the simple improvement in the flow of blood and lymph to the areas and the more efficient exchange of intracellular and extracellular fluids that result from the treatment.

If you have a serious distortion of form in your body, it is important that you seek professional treatment for it. See what one of these many techniques can do for you.

21

Aromatherapy

Aromatherapy is the art of using essences of plants to treat the skin, the emotions, and the body as a whole. It is one of the most interesting areas of beauty care. For each plant essence has its own unique qualities, yet like a piece of music or a painting will evoke slightly different responses from different people depending on their personalities, needs, and tastes. Learning about aromatherapy, the essences themselves, and some of the things you can do with them is sheer delight. It is also a wonderful way of looking after your skin, calming your nerves when you are over-wrought, and creating interesting atmospheres in your living and working environment. If I were allowed only one luxury I could easily dispense with makeup and trips to the hairdresser, but I would never want to be without the beauty of aromatherapy. Let's start at the beginning.

The origins of aromatherapy, like the plant essences it uses, are still shrouded in mystery. The ancient Egyptians used these essences for their beauty treatments and to embalm their dead. Alchemists from China and Tibet used them for altering states of consciousness and the ancient Greeks and Romans turned to them for their medicinal and aphrodisiac qualities. Traditional Indian medicine, called Ayurveda, has formulas using these special volatile substances for healing and rejuvenation that go back at least three thousand years to when the "rishi" yogis, who lived in the Himalayas, wrote the Vedas: in these books you will find long and complicated formulas for treating almost every imaginable illness. In many of these mixtures plant essences play an important part.

Fascinated by what I'd heard about the powerful effects plant essences properly used could have on the mind and body, I went to India to take a look at some of the Ayurvedic hospitals that use them. I spoke to patients who had made remarkable recoveries from chronic conditions like rheumatoid arthritis, polio, paralysis, and mental illness, thanks to treatment from these plant-based formulas given merely by applying them to the *outside* of the body. In India I also met scores of women with exquisite skin for whom the use of plant essences formed the basis of skin and body care, as it had for their mothers' mothers and grandmothers before them.

ETHERIC OILS

Plant essences are the fine, light, almost etheric essential oils taken from plants in their prime of life. Although they are technically known as essential oils, they have little in common with the fatty oils we know, like olive oil or lanolin. For they are complex hydrocarbons that look more like water than oil. For centuries they have been used for blending perfumes and making incense for religious rites. They are found in tiny droplets in specific parts of different plants in a concentration of between 0.01 and 10 percent; in roots and barks (calamus and cinnamon, for instance), flowers (jasmine and rose), leaves (rosemary and basil), and the rinds of fruit (lemon and orange). Highly volatile, these substances are what give a plant its distinctive smell. They seem to contain the vital essence of the plant that is probably responsible for their beneficial effects.

These effects are so varied and so profound that it is hard to list them all. Many essences stimulate the generation of new cells. (Lavender and orange blossom are particularly good for this.) Some, like fennel, contain plant hormones similar in their chemical structure to estrogen. Mixed with a good carrier oil they make an excellent antiwrinkle treatment. Others have different phytohormones that can be of equal benefit to both dry and oily skin. Many essences profoundly affect the psyche as well, both when they are rubbed on the body and when they are simply inhaled. All essential oils are powerful and, therefore, used only in minute quantities diluted in other oils. Most are easily absorbed into the skin, probably through the hair follicles, which contain sebum, an oily liquid with which they appear to have a natural affinity. From there they can be carried either by the bloodstream or via the lymph and interstitial fluid (the liquid that surrounds all the body's cells) to other parts of the body. Experiments with animals, for instance, have shown that when an essence is applied to the skin it can reach an internal organ in half an hour.

The synthetic versions of the plant essences, although they include the main components reproduced chemically, do not have the same beneficial effect on people. Some scientists believe that this is because the components of these natural substances have a synergitic quality—they work together to produce an effect greater than the sum of each working part.

Ayurvedic doctors who use essential oils in treatments in India believe that their power depends largely on the vitamins and enzymes they contain, although they freely admit there are probably a myriad of other substances in plants as yet undiscovered that may be responsible for their potency and healing abilities too.

HOW THEIR QUALITIES WERE DISCOVERED IN EUROPE

Many years ago a distinguished French chemist named Gatfossé severely burned his hand while working in his laboratory. In a spontaneous reaction to the agony, he immersed the seared flesh in a container of pure lavender oil. He was astonished to find in a few hours that the hand had virtually healed. This led him to investigate and experiment with (and categorize) the healing and cosmetic properties of a number of essential oils. Then an Austrian biochemist, the late Marguerite Maury, who was twice awarded the Prix Internationale d'Esthétique et Cosmétologie for her work, developed a range of aromatherapy beauty treatments that consisted of applying specially selected essential oils to the skin, particularly along the nerve centers near the spine and on the face.

Maury believed that since each oil has its own special qualities and since each woman is completely individual, the mixture of oils that would treat a particular problem in one woman would not necessarily eliminate the same problem in another. So she mixed her oils on personal prescription, using a pendulum and radiesthesia to select which essences to use. Her main interest was rejuvenation. She strongly believed that aging could be retarded and the degenerative processes, which take place too rapidly in the skin because of neglect, could be reversed with the use of essential oils. She developed a remarkable reputation for her work, curing case after case of intractable acne and restoring the bloom of youth to wealthy middle-aged women in France and England. It soon became obvious that her beauty treatments were far more than skip deep. Clients left her salon feeling renewed and revitalized, a sensation that often lasted weeks or months after the treatments had finished. They slept better, their migraines and arthritic ailments disappeared or greatly diminished, and most remarkable of all, their mental state often improved dramatically, so that they felt happier, more enthusiastic, and more energetic. Madame Maury became fascinated by these psychological effects. She wrote, "Of great interest is the effect of the fragrance on the psyche and mental state, of the individual powers of perception becoming clearer and more acute, and there is a feeling of having to a certain extent outstripped events. They are seen more objectively and, therefore, in a truer perspective. It might even be said that the emotional trouble which in general obscures our perception is practically suppressed." It is the ability to affect the mental and emotional states of people, common to most plant essences whatever their other properties, that more then any other fascinates me.

MIND-BENDING ESSENCES?

Our sense of smell is still something of a mystery to science in spite of all that is understood about the olfactory organ itself. Current theories postulate that smells enter the nose in the form of tiny droplets of odorous substances that are soluble in both oil and water. Then, either by a chemical reaction on the olfactory area or through some kind of vibratory effect as yet undiscovered, the messages coming from the substance are transferred to the brain. Some scientists even believe that smells, rather like light rays, enter the senses through waves sent out from the odorous substances. And it is also not clearly understood why we have such immediate mental and emotional responses to smells, although there is no doubt that we do. Everyone has at one time or another smelled an odor that instantly brought back a feeling, emotion, or memory from long ago.

Professor Paolo Rovesti, Director of the Istituto Derivati Vegetali in Milan, has shown that smelling the oils of certain plants is useful in the treatment of anxiety states and depression and that the effect of these highly volatile substances when sprayed in the air is both immediate and long-lasting. French psychotherapist André Virel uses plant essences on small bits of cotton passed under the noses of his patients to bring up repressed memories or feelings and even to stimulate abreactions in which a whole series of events from a patient's past are relived, releasing him, claims Virel, from the stifling emotional effect they have had on him.

Researchers into the psychic properties of essential oils have also discovered that some odors, such as peppermint, rose, and carnation, have the power to improve concentration and eliminate feelings of lethargy.

Scientists using plant essences such as Rovesti in Italy and Dr. Jean Valnet in France (who prescribes them both internally in minute doses and externally mixed with other oils and waxes) have now carefully categorized the characteristics of many specific plant oils and their effects on mind and body. For instance, Rovesti turns to ylang-ylang, citrus oils, jasmine, basil, patchouli, and peppermint for treating depressive states. For anxiety or fear he recommends geranium, lavender, and bergamot.

One of the curious things about plant essences is that although a specific essence, say camphor or neroli, is known to be a good antidote to shock, or another, say peppermint or cinnamon, a good stimulant, unlike drugs, some also appear to have more than one action on the nervous system. So someone suffering from fatigue as a result of nervous tension can, by smelling peppermint, be at one and the same time both calmed and stimulated. Due to this unusual quality (which you can't believe until you have experienced it for yourself) some essences such as oil of garlic are even used to treat two different conditions. Researchers in Eastern Europe have found that garlic has an ability to lower blood pressure that is too high as well as raise blood pressure that is too low. But just how and why remains yet another mystery of plant essences.

DO-IT-YOURSELF AROMATHERAPY

There are a number of ways of using plant essences for beauty. You can dilute them in oil and apply them to the face and body for skin treatments. You can use them in the same mixture on the face, at the back of the neck, and on the base of the spine for their effect on the psyche and nervous system. You can inhale them directly from the bottle or breathe them in the form of steam from a humidifier or pot of very hot water to which a few drops of essence have been added. They can also be used in your bath but always in the minutest quantities—ten to fifteen drops. Some essences will be absorbed into the skin more rapidly than others, depending on their volatility and the carrier oil in which you have put them.

Essential oils should never be applied directly on the skin. In fact, many of them are so powerful in their action that to do so would be to cause a burn. Also, their potency is such that they actually work better in minute quantities, highly diluted. Don't think that because you add more essence you will get better results. You will only be wasting your money and you will probably get slower results—essential oils have their own gentle way of acting. They can't be *forced*.

Oils for the Skin

When making an oil to apply to the skin, you need two things—the essences which you wish to use (one or more of them mixed togther) and a carrier oil in which to put them. The carrier oil depends on your taste and pocketbook. Sweet almond oil and apricot oil are excellent. So is hazelnut oil, which gives a high degree of penetration on the skin. Less expensive, but perfectly adequate, are sunflower oil, safflower oil, olive oil, and peanut or ground-nut oil. Whatever oil you choose, it should be cold-pressed to preserve the quality of essential fatty acids it contains and it should be fresh. Once mixed, an oil should be tightly capped and kept under refrigeration. A couple of capsules of vitamin E squeezed into the oil when you mix it will keep it from going rancid quickly because of the vitamin's antioxidant properties. The proportion of essence to carrier oil should be one to fifty by weight.

Pomades

You can also make a pomade or a cream from the essences. You will need beeswax, your carrier oil, and your essences. Take half an ounce of beeswax to two ounces of carrier or to twenty drops of essence. Heat the beeswax and oil in a double boiler and remove from the heat when the wax has melted. Whisk briskly to blend the two thoroughly. When the mixture begins to solidify as it cools, add your essence (not before or too much of it will evaporate), and the contents of a vitamin E capsule. Use the same ratio of essence to carrier here (one to fifty) but include the weight of the beeswax in your calculations of the carrier.

Fragrant Waters

Finally, you can make fragrant waters by using four or five drops of essence shaken well into a pint of distilled water. Put this into one of those little spray bottles used for misting plants and you can have a room freshener or scenter far better than anything you can buy. Or splash it on after a bath.

Another way to scent a room is to add a few drops to a humidifier or to a pan of boiling water just taken off the heat.

MAKE YOUR OWN COLLECTION

It is a good idea to start with three or four essences and then experiment, each time adding more oils to your collection as you get to know them. Some of the best to start with are jasmine, sandalwood, geranium, neroli, lavender, and cinnamon.

Always keep your essences in a cool place (the refrigerator is ideal) in dark glass bottles. Essential oils are highly volatile and easily destroyed by heat and sunlight. They have to be treated like something very precious.

Here are some of the common uses of essential oils:

Skin

To improve circulation	Juniper, camphor
For broken veins	Cypress, neroli
For oily skin	Lavender, lemon, geranium, sandalwood, bergamot, cypress, juniper
For dry skin	Geranium, rose, sandalwood
For dehydrated skin	Clary sage, geranium, sandalwood
For fine, sensitive skin	Neroli, rose, lavender

Body Massage Oils

Soothers when you are tense	Lavender, geranium, camomile
Pepper-uppers when you are down	Cinnamon, bergamot, patchouli, jasmine
For mild aches and muscle pains	Lavender, rosemary

For Bathing

Add a few drops to the bath when it is being run: camomile, neroli, jasmine, lavender, patchouli, ylang-ylang, rose, sandalwood, rosemary, frankincense, cardamom, or melissa.

Psychic Essences

Dilute in the carrier and rub them on the face, back of the neck, and the base of the spine. Or put a few drops in a humidifier or pan of steaming water and let it waft into the room. Or add a few drops to water and spray like an air freshener.

To calm you when angry	Ylang-ylang
To brighten you when depressed or grieving	Lavender, geranium, sandalwood
To clear your head for mental work	Carnation
Aphrodisiacs	Jasmine, ylang-ylang, sandalwood, rose

HOW AND WHERE TO BUY YOUR ESSENCES

Herb stores sometimes sell them, as well as the carrier oils and beeswax. Some health food stores sell beeswax and most have the carrier oils. Beware of so-called essential oils that are synthetic. They are not good for aromatherapy and won't work. Neither will essences that have already been diluted in oils and which are sold in little bottles for perfumes. Read labels carefully and ask questions. Be particularly cautious when buying the following—they very often are *not* real but synthetic: jasmine, lily of the valley, lilac, frangipani, cucumber, clove, carnation, musk, orange blossom (neroli), rose, ylang-ylang, and violet.

For the addresses of suppliers in your area, look in the yellow pages of the telephone directory under these listings:

> Botanicals
> Chemists, homeopathic
> Herbs
> Oils, essential
> Perfumes, raw materials

22

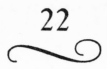

Hands and Nails

Your hands probably reveal more about you than any other part of your body. They can tell your doctor about your physical condition—whether or not you have a vitamin or mineral deficiency or an endocrine disturbance. To a psychologist, the way you move your hands betrays much of your character through body language. Your hands also communicate your immediate intentions. According to the ancient art of chiromancy, hand shape and palm lines can even reveal your innermost nature. Yet hands are often the most neglected part of a woman's body. As a result they age rapidly. And they are hard to rejuvenate once you have let them go.

Hands love moderate temperatures, hand creams, and massage. They hate water, detergents, household chemicals, harsh weather, and unprotected, prolonged exposure to the sun, which encourages the development of liver spots—high concentrations of melanin in clusters as a result of the skin's reaction to the ultraviolet rays.

Nails are made up mostly of keratin, a tough protein. But they also contain many other constituents such as sulfur. Their health depends on two things: adequate diet and protection from environmental damage.

TAKE A LOOK AT WHAT YOU EAT

A healthy nail should be strong but flexible, smooth and rich pink in color. If yours are not, the first thing to do is to revise your eating habits. Nails, like hair, need protein, B-complex vitamins, minerals, trace elements (particularly zinc, calcium, iodine, sulfur, and iron), and vitamin A to grow healthy and strong. So indicative of the body's condition as a whole are your nails that physicians in underdeveloped countries examine nails as a way of diagnosing an inadequate diet in the natives. Many physical conditions affect the look of the nails, including psoriasis, rheumatism, eczema, and heart troubles. They lead to ridges, pits, and furrows. A glandular deficiency such as hypothyroidism also shows up in the nails.

Splitting, breaking nails indicate a lack of vitamin A and protein. But don't reach for the gelatin, it will do nothing to improve them. What should help is cod liver oil or liver, or daily carrot juice. From egg yolks, cabbage, muscle meats, and onions you will also get the sulfur amino acids. Many drugs cut down on the growth of nails because of their toxic effect on the body. Growth can also be held back by stresses such as inadequate reducing diets, illness, or extreme cold. If you suffer from many hangnails, it may mean you have too little folic acid in your diet or insufficient vitamin C. If you develop a fungus condition on your hands, then you should increase your B-complex intake by taking brewer's yeast, yogurt, or acidophilus culture. Too few B-complex vitamins in the diet also causes nails to become fragile with horizontal and vertical ridges. Too little iron makes them appear pale in color instead of rich pink and can turn them dry, flat, thin, and eventually moon-shaped.

But the far most common nail problem—the white banding and white spots on weak nails—is a sign of a zinc and vitamin B_6 deficiency. This is common in women who are on the Pill. It also tends to appear the week before menstruation when copper levels in the body are high and zinc low. It is common in places where glaciers have depleted the soil of zinc, selenium, iodine, and sulfur, and white spotting and banding often occurs during days of fasting in people who are marginally zinc deficient already, as going without food only makes the condition more acute. So widespread is a zinc deficiency that although the minimum daily requirement of the nutrient is set at a mere fifteen milligrams, the average diet only gets eleven. I've seen zinc supplements (along with vitamin B_6, without which it cannot be used properly, and brewer's yeast) clear up nail problems.

A good overall nutritional program to keep nails healthy includes lots of raw vegetables and lean protein, brewer's yeast (one teaspoon three times a day stirred into half a glass of juice—tomato mixes best) plus one teaspoon of blackstrap molasses a day. It is good added to yogurt, cereal, or even herb tea. And, finally, six to eight kelp tablets taken with each meal.

ENVIRONMENTAL DANGERS

Breaking nails and unsightly hands can be caused by outside influences too—soaking your hands in detergents, bath salts, disinfectants, chlorine in swimming pools, strong lotions and soaps, cutting or filing your nails too far in at the sides, and damage done to the embryo nail (the matrix) by digging into the cuticles during a manicure. The answer to external threats is preventative care, which takes three forms: gloves (of all kinds, worn as often as possible), proper treatment, and creams.

Some hand creams are designed, like night creams, for moisturizing and treatment. Basically nourishing creams, they are usually greasy and need to be deeply massaged into the skin after hands are washed. They will work best when lathered into your hands just before bed and then covered with a pair of cotton gloves for the night. (You can also use a leftover jar of face cream for this.) Other hand creams are barrier creams, which means they are ideal protectors for daytime use. They usually contain silicone (one of the most important ingredients for protecting the skin from environmental pollution). They are water-resistant and also good for guarding the hands against chapping in cold weather. They don't need gloves to do their work, but these creams should be renewed each time you put your hands through any kind of vigorous treatment. Finally, there are the sunscreens, which, though not specifically designed for hands, are important to use whenever your hands are exposed to ultraviolet light in quantity. Many women end up with unsightly spots on their hands simply because they neglect this when they are out in the sun.

THE DO-IT-YOURSELF MANICURE

1. Take off all the old polish using an oil-based remover by soaking a large piece of cotton in the remover, placing it on the nail for twenty seconds to dissolve the polish, and then sweeping it away from the base to the tip (never the other way, as this pushes varnish and remover under the cuticle where it can do damage). If you are just touching up one nail and don't want to spoil the varnish on the other nails, put some cotton high up between your first two fingers while you remove the polish.

2. Filing is one of the most important parts of a manicure. Bad filing can cause nails to split, and good filing can actually help to stop splitting. The right way is to use the smooth side of an emery board and file from side to center, keeping the board at an angle of 45 degrees to the nail. Never saw backward and forward, as this creates heat, dries what little moisture there is in the nail layers, and can cause peeling. It is important to finish the nail well afterward. You do this by beveling it or stroking the nail lightly up and down with the emery board to coax the nail layers together. Remember that when nails are cut straight at the top with rounded or squared corners, they are less likely to split.

3. Massage a generous amount of cuticle cream or oil into the cuticle and nail area with round movements of your thumb, and then soak your fingertips in a bowl of warm water, to which you can add a little ordinary vegetable or bath oil.

4. Gently ease back your cuticles with your fingertips. Dip an orange stick wrapped with cotton into cuticle cream or remover and work away any dead skin and clean under the nail—but *gently*, never poke into the area where the nail comes away from the finger.

5. Don't trim your cuticles if you can help it. This can infect the nail unless done with thoroughly sterilized equipment and it also encourages the regrowth of thick cuticles.

6. Dry your hands and massage cream or oil well into the skin; wheat-germ oil, nut oil, and avocado oil are all particularly beneficial to hands. Start at the end of the fingers, one at a time, massaging toward the wrist. Knead the palm with the fingers of your other hand.

7. "Squeak" your nails. This means putting a little nail polish remover on cotton and running it over your nails to remove all the grease.

8. Stroke on a nail strengthener if you need one (if your nails are brittle, you don't) and leave it to dry. Then put on a layer of acetone-free base coat. This will help protect and strengthen nails from colored varnish if you want to add it later. Without it the acetone in colored varnish strips the nails of their precious oils, steals their shine, and in time can actually dye the nail plate an ugly yellow.

9. Color can change the shape of your nails dramatically. A sleek strip of dark color down the center of the nail will lengthen it. Fill the whole nail with color if it is perfectly shaped. If you have very heavy or wide nails, start at the center of the moon and brush outward and inward to the tip to give the impression of longer, almond-shaped nails. Whatever you do, start with a line of color going down the center and then one on either side. Never put too much varnish on the brush or it will take ages to dry and form ridges of color. Apply at least two coats. Once they are dry, apply a top coat of clear varnish to protect from chipping and to give a high gloss. You can also spray or stroke on some quick-drying solution to reduce waiting time. Finally, don't move! Wait until every nail is dry and while you are waiting, flex and relax your hands.

10. It is good for nails to be left without polish whenever possible. Some of the new abrasives are useful in buffing and polishing the surface so nails look polished but stay naked. But use them sparingly, for each time you use them you take off a layer of nail and weaken it.

PROBLEMS AND SOLUTIONS

1. *When nails don't grow fast enough* Exercise your hands and fingertips. Drum them on the table as if you are playing the piano. This helps improve circulation to the fingertips and carries nourishment to the nail matrix via tiny blood vessels. Open and close your stretched hands quickly. You can do this at any time of the day. To loosen your fingers, place the fingers of your outstretched hand flat against the palm of your other hand and push gently several times. Do the same with the other hand. To exercise each finger, close one hand around the other and push gently to either side. Relax your hand and take each finger at a time with the index and middle finger of your other hand. Pull gently as you slide the finger between the two other fingers. Look at your diet to see it is adequate, particularly in vitamin A, protein, and the sulfur amino acids.

2. *Nails break easily when they are brittle* Stay away from nail hardeners with formaldehyde—it will only make brittle nails more brittle. What will help is one of the protein conditioners. Leave nails free of polish and apply one of these or simply white iodine daily. See that you get adequate zinc and B-complex vitamins, particularly B_6.

3. *Nails that peel and split and don't seem to grow* Look at your diet as described above. Try a formaldehyde-based hardener, applying it carefully so you don't get any on the skin. Be sure to bevel the ends of the nails when you file them. Steer clear of water except very briefly to wash your hands—it will soften the nails too much. Wear gloves when gardening, washing, working, and out in the weather.

4. *Broken nails* There are many excellent nail-mending kits that either cover the break with fine paper and then varnish or which offer a glue that is strong enough to hold a broken tip when it is replaced.

5. *Red hands* Exercise your fingers as much as possible. Cover your hands with a rich oil or cream and alternately dip them in hot and cold water twice a day. Apply a green-tinted moisturizer over your hand cream to hide the redness.

6. *Clammy hands* Take exercises. Make dips in cold water. Use a silicone-based hand cream. Spray an antiperspirant on palms afterward.

7. *Rough hands, stained hands, and calluses* Hard lumps of skin will smooth away with a pumice stone rubbed with soap. Wash dirty areas with a brush, then rub the pulpy part of half a lemon on the skin and add loads of hand cream (the nourishing variety) before they dry completely. Repeat in a few hours and continue until they are smooth again.

23

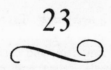

Feet and Legs

Feet are more important to beauty than most women ever realize. When they ache, not only are your posture and movements affected, so is your complexion and your energy level. Nothing brings a haggard, older look to an unlined face like sore feet. Also, one of the most common complaints with which doctors are faced is *fatigue*. And behind this fatigue lies an unnoticed foot problem.

Little wonder, when you consider that city dwellers walk an average of ten miles a day. All your weight is borne by twenty-six little bones, some of which are the most delicate in the body.

In fact, feet have a higher anatomical concentration of bones than any other part of you. They are supported by tremendously powerful ligaments and muscles (there are four muscle layers in the soles of the feet alone). Your feet are enormously complex, balanced mechanisms. If something goes wrong to upset this balance, for instance a poorly fitting shoe that puts continuous pressure on one part of your foot, you get trouble. And trouble when it arrives can be in any number of different forms: backache, pain, leg problems, irritability, fatigue, to mention only a few. Your free, graceful stride quickly becomes a restricted aging hobble. Learn to look after your feet well and you'll reap immeasurable benefits in looks, health, and high spirits. Foot care is also the first step toward having beautiful legs.

TAKE A LOOK AT THE SHOES YOU WEAR

Like fingerprints, every foot is unique. But not every shoe. In recent years, because of mass marketing and increased costs of manufacturing shoes, sizing has become more restricted than ever. Once you could easily buy a 6-D. Now even many of the best and most expensive shoes only come as wide as a B fitting. And since you can't change the size of your foot to suit the whims of manufacturers or their financial decisions, you have to find a manufacturer whose product works for you. It is not sensible to try and put a 5-C foot into a 5½-B shoe and think you are getting away with it, for width and length are not the only considerations when buying a shoe. The depth of your foot, your height, weight, and the way you spend your days, as well as the last of the shoe, also matter. The distance between the heel and the front of the arch and the length of the toes vary greatly from woman to woman. It usually takes a lot of trial and error to find a last that suits your feet. And it won't necessarily be from the most expensive shoemaker, either. Some of the manufacturers of medium-priced shoes make excellent lasts, particularly for the wider foot. Once you find a last that suits you, stick to it. You are better off passing up some new style that doesn't fit properly than suffering the long-term consequences of foot agony.

The shoes you choose affect far more than the look of your feet. Poorly fitting shoes, shoes with too rigid a sole or too high a heel, play an important part in the formation of cellulite on the thighs and in the development of varicose veins. If your shoes fit and heel height is right for you, then you stand a good chance of avoiding them. It is also a good idea to vary the height of your heel throughout the day by carrying an extra pair of shoes with you to work or shopping.

When you wear a heel that is too high you throw your posture off balance. This makes you tire more easily and tilts your pelvis in such a way that sacral muscles are forced to remain in a state of continual spasm. As a result, you can end up with a hollow in your back and agonizing backache, particularly around the time of your periods. If your heel is too low for your foot, it is not so serious, but this can result in overdeveloped calves or muscle-ache in the back of the legs.

Finding the ideal heel height for you is simple. All you need is a ruler, a flat edge (perhaps from a thin book or another ruler), and a chair. Sit in the chair and cross your legs so one foot hangs free above the ground. Reach down and put the flat edge flat against your toes and the ball of your foot, extending it horizontally beyond the arch and heel of your foot. Now measure the vertical distance between the bottom of your heel and your flat edge with the ruler and you have your ideal heel height. For most women it is somewhere between one and a half and two and a half inches.

When shoes fit well and they are the proper heel height for your foot, wearing them exercises the foot and leg muscles each time you step. This maintains healthy circulation. If you want to wear a really high or stiletto heel, or clogs, do it only occasionally. The rigid soles of clogs act as splints, immobilizing the feet so they and the legs don't get a proper workout when you walk. They are also responsible for a lot of twisted ankles and the development of deformities.

Stilettos can contribute to the enlargement of varicose veins and cause swollen ankles because the base is too small to serve as a rudder, and in order to steady the foot too much pressure must be put on the ankle. Finally, too loose a shoe of any kind rubs against the heels and toes and is responsible for a lot of corns and calluses.

LEG BEAUTY FROM THE INSIDE

Varicose veins are the most serious enemies of leg beauty. But they are not the accident of nature that many women believe. The problem is virtually unknown amongst native populations living on a diet of natural unrefined foods. But studies show that as soon as our highly refined Western diet of convenience foods arrives in a country, varicose veins start to appear. The hidden constipation that results from living on the average Western diet lacking in natural fiber from whole grains and raw vegetables is one of the prime causes of varicose veins, for uneliminated wastes in the intestines put constant pressure on the blood vessels supplying blood to and from the legs. Long-term overweight is another factor in the development of varicose veins.

So is inactivity. The small valves in the legs that open and close alternately to keep the blood flowing in the right direction between pulse beats depends on firm and well-toned muscles for support. If the tissues become weakened through lack of exercise, neglect, or poor nutrition, then a valve may not close completely so you get a back flow of blood onto the main valve below. This adds weight to the lower valve at the same time as it increases the volume and pressure within the vein. Gradually, the wall stretches and you develop a varicose vein.

To avoid the problem, follow a good diet of natural unrefined foods, don't let yourself become overweight, and get plenty of exercise—swimming is the best of all because it develops the long muscles in the legs giving them firmness without a bunched, overdeveloped, athletic look. Running, walking, dancing, and yoga are also good. They will strengthen muscles, improve circulation to the lower limbs, and also keep the blood from settling there. Exercise for legs is particularly important during pregnancy because, like constipation, the weight of the baby puts pressure on blood vessels supplying the legs. Many women first develop visible veins on their legs while they are pregnant. But with proper diet and care they can always be avoided. Everyone should avoid standing for long periods, and propping yourself up with your legs against a wall, whenever you can, will help to relieve pressure.

Nutritionally, supplementary vitamins C and E can prove useful, not only in their prevention of varicose veins but also in their treatment—C because of its anti-inflammatory quality and ability to keep collagen healthy and E because of its ability to dissolve blood clots and improve circulation. If your legs ache you can wear support stockings. But don't wear them all the time for they can only relieve symptoms—they do nothing to strengthen muscles that need strengthening and so won't rid you of the cause.

When legs ache, there are also two water treatments that can be useful for aching legs and poor circulation.

Water Treading

Run six inches of cold water in the bath. Walk back and forth in it for forty-five seconds to five minutes, as long as you are comfortable. (You can get the same effect walking on dewy grass in the morning or in a lake or stream.) Then get out and dry your legs well and put on warm woolen socks. If you can, lie down on a slant board or a bed with your feet propped up with a pillow so they are above your head for five minutes. As you get used to the treatment you can increase the amount of cold water in the bath so it covers your calves. Make sure that during the treatment the bathroom is warm and keep the top half of you dressed while you are doing it.

Cold Sitz Bath

Use this a couple of times a week. Run a bath with cold water—just enough to come up to your waist. Making sure the bathroom is well heated, and wearing something on the top half of you to keep you warm, sit down in the water for thirty seconds. Have a large towel ready. Get out but don't dry yourself. Instead, wrap the towel around you and immediately get into bed. Cover yourself warmly and rest for half an hour or simply go to sleep for the night.

ATTACKING JODHPUR THIGHS

Thick ankles and overdeveloped thighs are often brought on by an impairment in circulation in the lower half of the body. This can be the result of chronic muscle tension in the pelvis or of an injury that occurs in childhood or puberty—sometimes something as slight as slipping on a stair or tumbling from a swing, but enough to cause autonomic ganglia and nerve root disturbances from the spinal level and reduce blood flow

from the lower spine to the legs. Gradually, fluid and oil globules collect
in these areas along with uneliminated cellular waste products. Fibrous
parts of the connective tissue harden and thicken, all the while accepting
more fluid and oil globules in the pockets that have formed, until you
end up with tough, pitted areas of bulges that are far worse than the
more common cellulite (see Chapter 20).

This kind of problem needs professional help through connective tissue massage or soft tissue mobilization or Rolfing, which begins with an
examination of the whole body, its shape, characteristic folds in the skin,
posture, mobility, and color. All of these indicate to the physiotherapist
any prime areas of blockage that have to be corrected to eliminate the
condition. Most beauty therapists don't understand the importance of
finding the *primary* causes of the condition, so the massage they give either by hand or with electrical equipment can only temporarily change
the shape of the thigh. In serious cases like this, treatment by highly specialized forms of massage has to begin centrally at the diaphragm or at
the base of the spine.

Then the physiotherapist works outward toward the affected area,
sometimes using very light, feathery strokes, sometimes using immensely
powerful movements that penetrate the tissues at deep levels, depending
on the patient and on the condition of the flesh itself. The treatment is
directed toward reestablishing circulation in base drainage areas first,
then toward breaking down the fibrous structures and reestablishing circulation there. In the hands of a competent practitioner, I have seen this
kind of treatment reshape a pair of "piano" legs into their own natural
form. It is a slow process and it can sometimes be painful but it is the
only thing that really works.

There is a leg operation called a lateral thigh lipectomy, designed to
remove jodhpur thigh bulges. An incision is made beneath the buttocks
and through the outside of the thighs, excess fat is taken out, the skin is
lifted, and the incision is repaired. There is a permanent scar, but with
luck it can be hidden beneath the bikini line. The operation lasts two
hours and demands several weeks for full recovery. It is painful and unfortunately the results are not necessarily permanent, for the same
pockets can reappear in time unless the underlying blockage somewhere
in the spine or pelvis is corrected and the woman's way of life is changed
to keep her body free of pollutants. A similar operation exists for the inside of the thighs.

SMOOTHING THE SKIN

Exfoliation, the removal of dead cells from the surface of the legs and
feet, is important if you want the kind of legs and feet that can go

stockingless and still look great. Do it twice a week. You can buy a skin sloughing product with tiny grains of silicon in it to remove the rough layers (get the cheapest you can find, for they are all the same in principle) or you can use simple coarse sea salt. Rub it briskly into your legs and feet when they are damp just before you get into the bath or shower and then rinse. Afterward, apply a rich silicone-based body lotion or cream.

If you have the kind of dry and flaky alligator skin that never seems to get better, you can use this messy but effective treatment for it. In a warm bathroom, with a book to read and half an hour to spare, wet your legs with warm water, then sit on the side of the bath and rub a handful of honey or blackstrap molasses onto your legs, covering them everywhere. Stay there, all covered, for twenty minutes, then rinse the stuff off. In cases of severe dryness, you might have to repeat this three or four times—every couple of days or so—to get rid of it.

GETTING RID OF HAIR

Think hard before you decide to rid your legs of all their hair. Is it necessary? Why should women be completely free of body hair? Some, I believe quite rightly, would rebel at the whole idea. If hair is very dark, it can always be bleached by mixing half a cup of twenty volume peroxide to a paste with ordinary fuller's earth or soap flakes, then adding a couple of teaspoons of ammonia. Mix well and spread on hair and leave the paste on for ten to fifteen minutes. Then wash it off. Repeat the treatment every two days until hairs are colorless. Then do it again each month.

If you insist on being hairless, there are several ways. Shaving is the worst. It leaves an awful stubble and has to be done a couple of times a week to keep regrowth at bay. Depilatories work better, although the chemical in them can be very hard on sensitive skin. Waxing is the best method for nonpermanent hair removal. It can be done in a salon or you can buy various kinds of wax strips to put on yourself. It removes the hair more thoroughly than shaving without danger of chemical irritation, and regrowth is usually slower. But it can be quite a painful experience. There is also a Swiss method available that combines waxing with chemical treatment and is usually successful in removing leg hair permanently when given several times over a few months. The hair is waxed normally, then immediately afterward a chemical solution is patted into the skin that is designed to penetrate to the roots and deaden the follicles. After treatment, you are given a cream to massage into the legs every day until there is a sign of regrowth, at which time you go back for another session. Usually between five and twelve sessions are necessary to get rid of hair completely.

Permanent hair removal has to be done by electrolysis. It is tedious and can be painful. There are two forms: galvanism and diathermy. Galvanism, the older of the two, is very slow and laborious but has a 100 percent success rate. You are given a metal rod to hold or a metal band is put around your wrist and connected by wire to the galvanic apparatus. Then a needle, also connected to the equipment, is inserted into the hair follicle, thereby creating an electrical current. The operator turns on the current and, as a result of the chemical changes it causes at the base of the follicle, the root dies and the hair comes away from the follicle. But you can only have a few hairs per minute removed this way.

Diathermy is more efficient and faster but you get a 20 percent regrowth—all hairs are not completely destroyed the first time. A thin needle is inserted into the hair follicle to the root and then a current is passed through it so that the heat from it cauterizes the root. In a few seconds the root is coagulated and the dead loose hair is discarded with tweezers. You usually have to have electrolysis by diathermy done three times at two month intervals to get rid of all the hair. And it has to be expertly done or it can cause scarring that may never heal. Finally, there is a new method of hair removal using electronic tweezers that grasp the hair and then pass a current through the tweezers to the root. But because hair is not a particularly good conductor (you have to rely on the moisture in the hair to conduct the current and destroy the root) it is not as successful as electrolysis in permanent hair removal. It is completely painless, however, so it is particularly good for removing facial hair.

HOW TO HAVE BEAUTIFUL FEET

Wash them every day, making a rich lather and massaging it over the soles of the feet. With a loofah, gently rub the tops and soles of the feet, not forgetting the heels, to loosen the dead skin cells, and with a soft nail brush, gently brush the tips of the nails from side to side. Rinse them well in warm water and if there is any hard skin to remove, rub a pumice stone over it. Finally, rinse again in warm water and then splash with cold. Dry your feet thoroughly by wrapping them in a towel and gently rubbing and patting them, then rub dry carefully between and behind the toes until absolutely all the moisture is gone. This is important in order to protect them from infection. If your feet tend to sweat, give them a light rubdown with alcohol. If they ache, massage some cider vinegar into the soles to cool and refresh them, or make a hot and cold foot bath—three minutes of hot followed by thirty seconds of cold—and end with a good friction rub with a soft towel. Finally, dust each foot with dusting powder.

THE PEDICURE

1. Take off every speck of nail polish and soak your feet in warm water for about five to ten minutes. (Epsom salts added to the water are very soothing for tired feet; camphor is good if your feet sweat.) When the soaking time is up, dip feet into cold water for about thirty seconds. This not only relieves aches, it is also excellent for chilblain-prone feet, for it stimulates circulation. Then dry feet thoroughly and separate the toes with little balls of cotton.

2. Using either a nail clipper for toes or a pair of scissors, trim each nail straight across and no shorter than the end of the toe in order to protect your toes from ingrown toenails. Smooth the edges with an emery board without shaping the nails. Apply a cuticle cream around the nails and massage it into the skin at the sides of the nail as well as into the cuticle, then, using an orange stick, ease back the cuticles. Next, gently clean the nails using an orange stick with a tiny piece of cotton wrapped around the end and remove the cotton from between the toes.

3. Now get down to the hard skin. There shouldn't be much of it if you have used a pumice stone every day. But if it has accumulated, try a liquid hard skin remover (there are several on the market), rubbing it on and in until the rough spots disappear. If your calluses are really thick you will need to do this several times before you see any real improvement. (Or go and see a chiropodist, who will remove them with a scalpel.)

4. To give yourself a foot mask, mix rolled oats together with the juice of a lemon to a thick and sticky consistency and smooth on your feet thickly, including the soles—right up to the ankles. Rub the lemon halves against the heels to lighten and tone the skin. Leave on your foot mask for five or ten minutes, then rinse off with first warm and then cool water. Now smooth on a rich hand cream or moisturizer concentrating on the places where hard skin tends to accumulate and massaging it upward from the toes to the knees.

Rub your nails lightly with polish remover to get rid of any grease and replace the cotton between the toes. Apply a base coat to protect the nail and as a primer for the color, if you are going to use any. Let it dry completely. If you want color, choose a scintillating bold red or a soft sandy pink that tones well with your skin (orange and purple-pinks never do much for most feet) and apply two coats of it to each nail, sweeping the color from the center of the cuticle outward and inward to the center of the nail trim on each side, with a straight stroke up the center. This will give the impression of a lovely oval-shaped nail. Finish it off with a clear protective top coat to prevent the varnish from chipping and to give a strong shine. When all is dry, a splash of cologne or foot spray will add a beautifully cool finishing touch.

FEET NEED EXERCISE TOO

One of the best things you can do for your feet is to walk barefoot. Wearing exercise sandals is the next best thing. When your feet are free of shoes and hose they relax and stretch; exercise sandals are designed to let the feet do this. They follow the natural contour of the foot, imitating and slightly exaggerating the effect of walking barefoot. This is great for toes as they grip and then relax from the gripper bar with every step. But exercise sandals are just that—meant for exercise, not all-day wearing. You can tire yourself and develop bulky muscles in the calves if you wear them too much.

There are several exercises you can do for your feet that will refresh the rest of you too. They help keep feet and legs in top condition by increasing circulation, strengthening muscles, and giving joints a good workout. They are also excellent fatigue-fighters. Do them for ten minutes at the end of each day or just before a bath.

1. *Climbing the walls* Lie on the floor with legs and feet propped up against a wall. Using the toes to pull each foot up, "walk" up the wall, one foot after the other. When you get as far as you can, come down again and start over. Repeat three or four times. The last time, as you go higher, support your hips with your hands and stay there for two or three minutes with legs and feet raised high above the head.

2. *Tip-toers* Sitting in a straight chair with good posture, place feet flat on floor about six inches apart. First raise one foot from the heel and then the other, pointing toes, so only the toes remain on the floor, and then lower. Repeat ten times.

3. *Perfect pigeons* For two minutes daily walk barefoot with toes pointing inward. Try to pick up a marble with the toes and walk on the outside of the feet for another minute. (This is particularly good for slimming ankles.)

4. *Ankle twists*   Sitting cross-legged, rotate the ankles ten times one way and then the other. Change legs and repeat. (Good both for slimming ankles and strengthening them for skiing and hiking.)

5. *Cantilevers*   Stand on one foot on a telephone book or stair so that the entire weight is supported by the front of the foot, with arch and heel suspended in the air. Slowly raise the heel as high as possible (hold on to someting so you don't fall), and then down as far as you can so heel is below ball of the foot. Repeat ten times with each foot. (Another good ankle strengthener.)

6. *The shakes*   Sitting on a chair, take hold of one ankle, shake it hard for thirty seconds, keeping the foot loose, then change and shake the other one. Repeat twice. A tingling feeling of relaxation and well-being spreads all the way up the legs.

JAPANESE SHIATSU TREATMENT FOR TIRED FEET

1. Press each toe hard three times with your thumb, working down from tips of toes to foot itself.

2. Now press between the tendons on the top of the foot, grasping the foot in your hand and working up between each tendon toward the ankle.

3. Move to the plantar arch (the sole of the foot), pressing hard with your thumb and on the bottom of the foot, moving up to center.

4. Finally, apply pressure hard around sides of the ankles and on the Achilles tendon.

5. Repeat with the other foot, then put feet up on a cushion so that your legs and feet are above the level of your head and body, and relax with your eyes closed for five minutes.

PROBLEMS AND SOLUTIONS

When problems arise, deal with them immediately. A corn or a callus is a simple thing to treat if you act right away. If you wait it can turn into a serious problem in time.

1. *Calluses* Areas where the skin is hard, calluses are really a form of protection devised by the foot that is sufferering from pressure or friction. They can be removed by soaking your feet and then rubbing with a pumice stone or special foot scraper. You can also spread petroleum jelly over the callus and then wear a cotton sock over it to bed. When you get up in the morning, it will be easier to remove. Thick calloused areas will need several treatments.

2. *Bunions* A hard swelling at the base of the big toe is known as a bunion. It comes from poorly fitting shoes that push the big toe inward and sideways so that it forms a bony outgrowth at the side. A pocket of fluid called a bursa may also develop between the bone and the skin.

If you seek professional help at the first signs of a bunion it can probably be treated simply, and then corrected with exercises, but if you wait until it is fully developed, surgery may be the only answer.

3. *Corns* They are the result of ill-fitting shoes. They are another way the foot protects itself from possible damage from constant irritating friction. A callus with a cone-shaped core develops, the eye of the cone being at the deepest level of the callus. If it presses against a nerve, you get severe pain. Small corns can be rubbed away by soaking your feet in hot and salty water for fifteen minutes and then taking a pumice to them. Larger corns have to be removed by a professional with a scalpel. If you try to do it yourself, you risk causing infection. A specially designed padded ring worn over the corn in the meantime can relieve the pressure against the nerve.

4. *Athlete's foot* It is a fungus infection that usually appears first just behind and between the toes. Try not to get it in the first place, by keeping your feet clean and dry. You often pick it up at public swimming pools, gyms, and other places where you are exposed to people who have it. First there is only flaking and scaliness, then if it develops, you get cracks that can be extremely painful. Get rid of it by removing the dead skin with a pumice and then applying a fungicidal cream or powder (better both) and keeping it on the feet, which should be covered with cotton socks for the night. Expose the feet as much as you can to dry air. Always change socks, stockings, and tights daily.

5. *Verrucas* The result of a virus infection that can be picked up much as athlete's foot is, verrucas or plantar warts sometimes appear in groups on the undersurface of the foot. Occasionally, you only get one at a time. They grow downward into the foot and any pressure on them is extremely painful. Often they clear up by themselves. If not, they need medical treatment and can be removed either with Formalin, burning, or surgery.

6. *Chilblains* The painful tingling and itching and inflammation of the feet is connected with poor circulation. It can be helped by nutritional therapy—giving nicotinic acid (one form of niacin) regularly along with the rest of the B group of vitamins, particularly B₆ and pantothenic acid. Vitamin E may also be helpful. Preventive treatment is a must. This means plenty of exercise to improve circulation all over, warm socks and clothing, and no restrictions around the legs, like tight boots or garters. Soaking the feet regularly in hot water for three minutes and then plunging them into ice-cold water for thirty seconds and putting on wool socks afterward can be helpful. Arctic explorers treated them with a mixture of whisky and soap.

MAKING FOOT REFLEXOLOGY WORK FOR YOU

Feet not only affect the condition of the rest of your body, they also reflect it. A good reflexologist or zone therapist will be able to tell you just by taking your feet in his hands and pushing them what is the state of your liver, the muscles of your back, or your pituitary gland. Originally an ancient Chinese form of therapy, foot reflexology has recently become a popular form of alternative medicine. It was first developed and charted in the beginning of the century by an eminent American doctor named Fitzgerald, who described the ten specific zones of the body that are regulated by different nerve complexes. Through these zones, which go from the top of the head to the tips of the fingers and toes, so the theory goes, runs a network of nerves connecting the important muscles, glands, and organs to specific tiny points on the feet. According to the theory, when the circulation in the feet slows down because of any of many different reasons, such as badly fitting shoes, illness, a poor diet, or not enough exercise, congestion occurs and eventually crystalline deposits form around some of these nerve endings on the feet. But by deep compression massage in specific areas, zone therapists claim to be able to break up the congestion and disperse the crystalline deposits (most of which are made up of unwanted wastes locked into the tissue) and eliminate them from the body via the bloodstream. Doing this not only revives circulation and aids the feet, it also—through remote nerve connections—tones up muscles and improves blood supply to the organs and glands, relieving tension all over. This is how foot reflexology can be used to effect changes in other areas of the body within the same nerve zone.

It can also be a useful diagnostic tool, for areas on the feet that are particularly tender or hardened can be an indication of trouble else-where. Finally, reflexology is a useful preventative tool for helping to keep the body in peak condition physically. Reflexologists recommend that you massage your feet daily after washing them and pay particular attention to any tender areas on the soles or sides or the back of the heels. If you find any, give them deep friction with the tips of your fingers or thumbs until the tenderness goes away. Reflexologists also claim we would be much healthier if we went barefoot more because the natural massage our feet get when bare helps tone up the whole body.

REFLEXOLOGY TREATMENT FOR PERFECT SLEEP

1. Grasp one foot with the opposite hand, thumb underneath. Press firmly on the back of the big toe, holding for half a second, release, and repeat for three minutes.

2. Grasping the foot in the same way, press firmly against the bottom of the foot, just below the ball of the foot in the center. Hold for half a second. Release and move your thumb up the medial line of the foot toward the toes, pressing and releasing alternately for two minutes.

3. Massage the ball of the foot area and the area of the big toe firmly for a couple of minutes with an oil or cream.

24

Hydrotherapy and Bathing

Water is the finest solvent in the world. It dissolves dirt on the outside of the skin and carries nutrients to and wastes away from the cells inside. Many a fine-skinned grandmother claims her exquisite complexion is the result of washing with pure water and soap. And health spas have long relied on the magic of water—hot and cold—mixed with mud, herbs, the essential oils of plants, or carefully selected mineral salts to smooth skin, relax tense muscles, refine pores, and revitalize bodies. But there is a real art to hydrotherapy. To make the most of bathing for health and beauty, you need to know the many ingredients that go into it and why each matters.

Temperature, for instance. Most women take baths that are far too hot. Frequent hot baths (95–100° F.) have a loosening effect on muscles and skin, and cause skin to age rapidly. For a relaxing bath, the temperature should be warm (85–95° F.). For a stimulating one, make it cooler (65–75° F.). A tepid bath (75–85° F.) just before bed will help you to sleep. And cold water (55–65° F.) is an excellent tonic for skin. It has long been used by European hydrotherapists as well as Himalayan mountain people to treat respiratory ailments from minor colds to pneumonia.

In France, when a woman has difficulty losing weight (particularly when she has been on crash diets so long that her metabolism seems to have grown accustomed to them), hydrotherapists use a cold water spray up and down the fronts and backs of her legs and hips four times each morning, after which they wrap her tightly up and put her into a warm bed for an hour. Devotees swear by this treatment for stubborn cases of obesity, claiming it stimulates the metabolism and encourages the body to burn up excess fat.

There are a couple of hydrotherapy treatments that I find particularly useful.

To Get Rid of Tension and a Headache

Half fill a bath with cold water. Then, making sure you are well covered so your body doesn't get cold, walk about in it with bare feet for three minutes. Immediately afterward, put on warm socks and lie down for ten minutes.

To Quickly Recharge Yourself After a Hard Day

Fill a bath with hot water (110° F.) and soak for a couple of minutes, preferably with a towel under your head so you can lean back and close your eyes. When you have relaxed, let half the water out, turn on the cold tap, and lie back again, this time circulating the fresh water with your hands. By the time the bath is full again you will feel revitalized. And you won't be cold either. Just tingling and glowing. Now wrap yourself in a bath towel and lie down for five minutes.

Cold showers can do a lot to revive you too. First shower in hot water for three to five minutes until you are warm and relaxed. Then switch to cold and stand under the nozzle—moving about so the cold water reaches all around you—for thirty seconds to one minute, not longer. Now stop. Get out of the shower and dry yourself briskly, then dress warmly. This will protect you from a chill. The pre-shower with hot water prepared your skin for the invigorating effect of the cold. Make sure that your bathroom is well heated and that you wrap up thoroughly after any cold plunge to give your system a chance to readjust to normal temperature. This is one of the first rules of hydrotherapy.

THE BEAUTY OF BATHING

Bathing should be a pleasant ritual that should treat your mind as well as your body. There are a number of useful prebath techniques and tools. They are important because they can prepare your skin and body for taking the plunge and ensure you get more benefit from bathing.

A Loofah

A dry, rough-textured sea gourd that you soften by wetting it, the loofah is rubbed against the skin to slough off dead cells and to increase circulation. You can buy loofahs in their natural state (about fifteen inches long) or sewn into gloves and bands of terry cloth to be used as scrubbers.

A Hemp Glove

Sometimes called a *gant de massage*, a hemp glove is one of the best investments you can make for health and beauty. Not just because it will take off dead cells and leave your skin smooth and blooming, but also because a brisk rub with one improves circulation and draws out wastes that lie in the tissues near the surface of your skin—waste products that can age your body and cause cellulite and lackluster skin.

Try this test yourself. Every morning before your bath or shower, rub yourself briskly with your *gant de massage* and then take a warm, slightly damp flannel and wipe it once over the surface of your body before you get into the bath. After a couple of days you will be amazed at the unpleasant smell that emanates from the flannel. The poisons under the skin that even soap and water can't budge will have deposited themselves on the cloth.

When using a hemp glove, rub it briskly *up* from the feet to the abdomen; from the hands to the shoulders and across the back and torso. Should you get broken veins under the skin from the treatment, stop it and increase your intake of vitamin C and the bioflavonoids as well as zinc and the B complex for a few weeks to overcome the capillary weakness. Then begin again, *gently*.

Sea Salt Rub

Sea salt is a wonderful exfoliater for removing dead cells, softening skin, and removing rough, dry patches on elbows and heels. It also contains a variety of minerals that may be absorbed to stimulate skin cell metabolism. Keep a bowl of coarse sea salt by the bath. Wet your body, then rub the salt briskly all over into the skin. Now step into a bath and soak in it for ten to fifteen minutes.

Oil Massage

An oil massage just before you get into the bath works wonders on very dry skin. Rub half a cup of vegetable oil (safflower, sunflower, or corn) well into the skin of the face and body and massage it in for a couple of minutes before taking the plunge. In the warm bath, use only a mild soap to wash with or none at all. Then when you step out, briskly rub yourself dry to distribute the remainder of the oil. Indian women, whose skin is particularly lovely and young-looking despite their country's harsh sunlight, use this treatment by mixing sandalwood oil (a few drops) with the vegetable oil, which in India is usually coconut.

Relaxing Baths (85–95° F.)

Vinegar soother: Add 1 cup of cider vinegar to the bath.

Essential calmer: Add 3 drops of essential oil of basil, 3 of rosemary, and 3 of mint to the water while it is running.

Quiet calmer: Make a little muslin bag 6 inches square and fill it with a mixture of comfrey leaf, sage, thyme, lavender, and marjoram. Then sew it up. Take it into the bath with you and use it to wash yourself all over. Then let it soak under the water so the herbs infuse the bath. This bag can be used again and again before its therapeutic properties become exhausted.

Herbal calmer: Infuse a handful of camomile flowers and a handful of comfrey leaves in a pot of water just off the boil for half an hour. Strain and pour the tea into the bath and then soak.

Invigorating Baths (65–75° F.)

Pine extract: Make a pine extract by simmering pine cones and needles in a large covered pan (one part needles and cones to four parts water) for half an hour. Then strain and continue to boil the liquid until it starts to get thicker. Add 4 ounces of it to a bath and store the rest in the refrigerator for another time.

Nettle stimulator: Make a thick pot of nettle tea to which you have also added a handful of rosemary, lemon balm, and lavender. Steep for fifteen minutes, strain, and add to the bath. (You can also add a few drops of essential oil of rose, sandalwood, or geranium for a beautiful smell.)

Aphrodisia: Add two drops each of oil of basil, cardamom, jasmine, patchouli, and myrrh to the bath water when it is running. This is a particularly beautiful-smelling mixture that is supposed to have aphrodisiac properties thanks to the cardamom and jasmine.

After-sports Baths

(Start with water at 100° F. and decrease temperature to about 55° F.)

Mineral bath: Add one pound of Epsom salts to the bath. Stay in for twenty minutes.

Vinegar bath: Add one cup of cider vinegar to bath to relieve aching muscles. It can help to rub the vinegar right on the muscles themselves and then to step into the water.

Horse rub bath: Add three tablespoons of horse liniment (yes, *horse* liniment, used on horses with sprained muscles) to the bath, step in, soak.

Skin-softening Baths (85–95° F.)

Milk bath: Add two cups of instant dried nonfat milk to the water to smooth and soften skin at a fraction of the cost of buying an expensive milk bath. A few drops of oil of geranium added to the water will make it smell lovely too.

Herb softener: Make a muslin bag and fill it with camomile flowers, elder flowers, comfrey, and linden blossoms. Sew it up and use it to wash your skin in the bath and let it soak in the water.

Heat-rash bath: Infuse a handful of comfrey leaves in water just off the boil and let it stand until cool. Drain the leaves and then add three-quarters of a cup of cornstarch to the liquid. Add to the bath and soak for at least twenty minutes.

Bran wash: Bran is an excellent skin softener. Stuff a muslin bag with it, sew up, let soak in warm water, and then use the bag to wash all over with. It will last through several washes.

Oatmeal soother: Stuff a bag with rolled oats mixed with elder flower blossoms (if you have them) and use it to scrub the skin. It helps exfoliate and is an excellent soap substitute.

GO EASY ON SOAPS AND BATH FOAMS

These are not very good for your skin. Soaps are made of fatty acids taken from animals and treated with caustic soda. Many of them are also full of antiseptics that can cause irritations to the skin and be very drying. If you bathe every day, you don't need soap to get clean. If you do use it, choose a neutral soap (one that is not alkaline) or one of the pH balanced detergent bars that are mild on the skin and don't remove the natural acid mantle from it. Even then you probably only need it under the arms, around the genitals, and on the feet unless you have been out in the mud and genuinely need to wash away grime. Bath foams and other detergent-based products can contribute to vaginal infections such as trichomoniasis and candidiasis. The fungi, yeasts, and bacteria that cause them grow better in an alkaline medium, which you are sitting in when you use such products every day. Disinfectants in bath water or from vaginal deodorants and soaps can also cause irritation and soreness. If you

want sweet smells in the bath, stick to a few drops of essential oil put
into it or mix your own bath oil by combining one cup of safflower oil
or sunflower oil in a blender with three tablespoons of an acid balanced
shampoo. A good soap substitute can be made by mixing half a cup of
powdered orris root with half a cup of cornstarch and sewing it into a
bag. It can be used several times.

UNDERWATER EXERCISES

The bath is an excellent place for doing some isometrics to keep specific
areas of your body in shape. All the following exercises are done *lying* in
the tub.

Tummy Flattener

Push out your abdomen as far as it will go and hold it for six seconds.
Then let go and rest for six seconds. Now pull it in as hard as possible
again. Let go and rest six seconds and repeat. Go through the whole
series four times.

Arm Firmers

First, with your hands against the sides of the body, press as hard as you
can in toward the center. Hold for six seconds and then release. Repeat
three times. Second, with arms and hands against the side of the bath,
press out as hard as you can and hold for six seconds. Release. Repeat
three times.

Back Strengthener

With your toes against the end of the bath, press hard, curving your
neck and bringing your chin down to your chest. Hold for three seconds. Now let your back sag in the bath, let your head fall back, and
press against the end of the bath with your heels. Hold for three seconds.
Repeat the two movements in succession three times.

Leg Shapers

Press legs against the side of the bath and hold there for six seconds, then
release. Repeat three times. Press legs hard inward together and hold for
six seconds, then release. Repeat three times.

Leg Looseners

Taking one leg at a time, lift it high, bending the knee toward your face and pointing your toe. Then straighten your leg and curve your toes back toward you. Now, leg still straight, point toe again hard. Finally, return the leg to the bath and do the same thing with the other leg. The whole exercise is done to a slow count of four. Repeat six times with each leg.

Ankle Twisters

Twirl your ankles around first one way and then the other, ten times each.

Neck Looseners

Gently rock from side to side as far as you can comfortably go, ten times.

THE WONDER OF MASSAGE

What you put on your skin when you emerge from the bath is likely to do it more good then than at any other time. Your skin is warm and damp and ready to take to creams and oils. Use them lavishly, from the simplest vegetable oil such as safflower or sunflower oil to almond and apricot or hazelnut oil, or aromatherapy oils that you can mix yourself.

Massage can help eliminate tension in the muscles, make you aware of your body, and soften your skin. What it can't do is melt away excess pounds or get rid of wrinkles. But it is a wonderful tranquilizer that acts on the central nervous system, the autonomic nervous system, and the nerve endings throughout the body. You can do it easily yourself when you get out of the bath, but it is even nicer to have it done for you. And there is no great mystery to it either. Once you get the feel of stroking the skin you really can't go wrong. Practice is all you need. Although some forms of massage such as connective tissue massage, Rolfing, and neuromuscular massage are extremely specialized and have to be done by an expert, ordinary massage following the basic movements outlined by Pehr Henrik Ling, the gymnast who popularized standard Swedish massage, is simple to do.

Begin with an effleurage or stroking movement that goes from the end of the limbs up backward toward the center of the body and from the bottom of your back upward toward the shoulders. Massage the abdomen in a circle, one hand over the other, going clockwise. Then go on to friction—a harder rubbing going out in the same direction. Now you are ready for petrissage, which is kneading movement where you lift the flesh all over the body gently away from the bones and work it exactly as you would knead bread dough. This gets the circulation going and breaks up stasis in the tissues. Finally, you finish off with more effleurage, or if you want a stimulating massage as is given to athletes before they go out onto the fields, give some tapotement (tapping) against the skin with the cupped palm of your hand.

PERSPIRATION AND ODOR

There is a common misconception that body odor comes from perspiration. It doesn't. Perspiration or sweat consists of nothing more than almost odorless water plus a few mineral salts that are responsible for that slightly salty smell many find has an almost aphrodisiac appeal to it. The unpleasant smell often thought to be the result of perspiration or sweat is in fact caused by waste products from the bacteria on the skin. The smell only occurs when more water is given off from perspiration than can be easily evaporated into the air and/or when clothing—particularly clothing made from synthetic materials, which hinder evaporation—interferes with this drying out process.

The body's perspiration comes from two different kinds of glands. The more common eccrine glands (each adult has two to three million of them) are distributed evenly all over the body and give out perspiration that consists of clear water and mineral salts in response to changes in outside temperature or physical exertion. The other glands, called the apocrine glands, are located only in certain areas of the body such as the genitals, underarms, nipples, and buttocks. In addition to water and mineral salts, their secretions contain some protein and certain fatty substances that tend to attract bacteria. This is why the greatest odor problems tend to come from those parts of the body. The apocrine glands respond not to changes in temperature but to changes in emotions. Nervousness, anger, sexual arousal, all turn on their activity.

All-over perspiration can be controlled by daily bathing. You can get extra protection against excess moisture and body odor by using an antiperspirant or deodorant. Deodorants and deodorant soaps work by restricting the action of bacteria on the skin. These products contain antiseptics, which on some people with sensitive skin can cause unpleasant reactions such as blistering or swelling, particularly when skin is exposed to sunlight. Antiperspirants control odor by reducing the volume of perspiration that comes through the skin as well as by combating bacteria. As well as a germicide, a fragrance, and a carrier (lotion or cream to make them easy to apply), these products contain aluminum or zinc salts that penetrate sweat ducts and prevent the delivery of sweat to the surface of the skin, either by blocking the openings or swelling the area around to shrink the size of the ducts. Antiperspirants can cause allergic reactions, although these are relatively rare. The best policy with these products is to use as little as you can get away with and still feel confident. As long as you are healthy, bathe regularly, and wear mostly cotton, silk, or wool clothes instead of mostly man-made fibers, you will probably not need either. If you still tend to perspire excessively, apply a deodorant or antiperspirant once or twice a day when the body is at rest —onto cool, dry skin. (Just after a bath is not the best time, as skin is too damp and perspiration ducts are not fully open.)

If you shun chemicals and prefer do-it-yourself products, chlorophyll is the natural deodorant to try. You can use green leaves, fresh green vegetables (such as spinach or beet tops), and fresh herbs such as mint as natural alternatives to the chemical products. Rub them briskly under the arms a couple of times a day or make the following lavender water and use it instead:

Take six drops of lavender and shake together with a pint of distilled water. Store in a dark bottle or keep in the refrigerator. Apply with a ball of cotton twice a day to parts of the body that perspire easily.

25

Beauty and the Breast

Worry over breasts causes a great deal of anguish to many women. Occasionally it is about their being too large, or about cancer; more often it is about their being too small, or about how to restore a beautiful shape to a neglected bosom. For breasts are funny things—and most women's judgments and perceptions about their own breasts are far from accurate. For a woman, the worry that her breasts are too small or that they are beginning to age can be a manifestation of some other underlying fear or insecurity that is masked behind concern over what is supposed to be the archetypal female sex symbol.

There are a lot of things that can be done to improve the less than perfect bust but it is important before you embark on any of them that you ask yourself if it is really the size, shape, or condition of your breasts that is bothering you, or if it is something else. Otherwise, you can work hard to improve things, find that you succeed in developing an almost perfect bust, and wonder why it hasn't made any difference at all as to how you feel about it. For although many glossy magazines would have us believe otherwise, some of the world's most miserable women are blessed with exquisite breasts.

THE ANATOMY OF THE BREAST

Your breast is over fifty percent adipose tissue (fat) and fibrous connective tissue. These two, which surround the mammary gland itself, give the bosom its shape and firmness, or its lack of them. Each of us is born with a certain genetic inheritance in terms of size and shape and, short of plastic surgery, there is supposed to be little we can do to change it.

This is only partially true. For, although seldom do you find a woman who has markedly changed the size of her breasts, it does happen. After successful psychotherapy some women report that their formerly under-developed breasts have become normal size. Other factors can affect size too—and not always for the better. Hormonal changes such as those brought about by the Pill or estrogen treatment for menopausal difficul-ties sometimes slightly enlarge and improve breast shape—an improve-ment that often lasts after treatment has finished. Weight loss also affects the bosom. If too quick, it can leave you with sagging, flabby breasts that you could have avoided with a less drastic diet. And the quality of what one eats makes an important contribution to breast beauty, too, particu-larly in that you need to ensure that you get enough vitamin C in your diet because of its role in preserving the healthy collagen fibers, which, along with the firmness of your pectoral muscles, helps keep breasts firm and well-shaped.

THE IDEAL BREAST

A so-called ideal bosom rarely occurs, but here is the archetype: breasts well separated with nipples halfway between the level of the elbow and the shoulder when the arm is at the side of the body and at least as far apart as the ears. If this description doesn't fit you and you decide you want to do something about it, then take a look first at your posture. Many a less-than-perfect bosom is simply the result of poor carriage. This is something you can correct, though not by sticking your chest out further in the case of a small bust or adopting a "Twiggy" stance in the case of one that's too large. Instead, try tilting your pelvis slightly up and forward and tucking your bottom under. This will straighten the spine and lift the rib cage at the same time, giving your bust its truest line. Now you can test your breasts for droop by putting a pencil hori-zontally just under each. If it is held in the fold, indicating a true sag, then you can use exercises to improve the muscle tone and other tech-niques to improve the size and shape.

FIRMING UP A BOSOM

Exercise is the only way to lift a sagging bosom—either exercise gotten passively from faradic current equipment such as Slendertone or from simple daily movements in a routine. Swimming, particularly breast stroke, is also good for improving tone of the breast and firming the muscles. Here are some basic movements that, if done daily, will keep your breasts firm and well-shaped and also help restore their beauty where it has been neglected. These exercises are best performed daily before a bath to get results, and then three times a week to keep the sleek new shape.

Small Circles

Stand tall, feet planted firmly on the floor at shoulder width. Stretch arms out to the side at shoulder level and make circles in the air of about eighteen inches in diameter, first in one direction and then in the other. Six times each way.

Large Circles

Stand tall and swing both your arms straight out in front of you with palms down toward the floor. Then fling your arms as far back as they will go as though you were reaching for something behind you, all the while pushing your chest out as far as possible. You will feel a strong pull on the pectoral muscles with each movement. Repeat this twelve times, then go on to the next exercise.

Press-ins, Pull-outs

Standing before a mirror, raise your elbows to shoulder height at the sides of your body. Then bring your palms together and press as hard as you can. (You will be able to see the contraction in the pectorals, and as you practice this movement your breasts will lift with each press.) Keep pressing for five seconds. Then, bending your fingers and making the hands into hooks, lock them together and pull. Hold for five seconds and repeat from the beginning. Do this sequence six times each way.

HYDROTHERAPY AND AROMATHERAPY

In France, where the care of breasts is almost a national institution, they have developed a number of more or less effective salon treatments (some more, some less) that involve exercises to strengthen muscles, hydrotherapy to improve circulation and absorption by skin, and finally the application of creams and oils containing the essential oils of plants and other substances such as embryo and placenta extracts. Although most of the Western world pooh-poohs the idea that such treatment can do any good, there are thousands of French women whose exquisite breasts would belie this skepticism.

Hydrotherapy in the form of a spray of cold water (the colder the better) is directed against each breast for a couple of minutes a day. The combination of the force of the spray and the temperature of the water stimulates the blood supply to the breasts, eliminates any stasis in the tissues, and helps tone muscles at the same time. There is equipment that you can buy specifically designed for giving this treatment at home. It consists of a large cup-shaped cone containing a rotating sprinkler. It is held against a breast and then attached to the cold water tap of your sink with a piece of hose. By turning on the cold water you receive jets of cold water with considerable force on the breast. This treatment should be used daily for two to four minutes on each breast for the best results. But this kind of apparatus has other applications too. It has been used successfully to stimulate the milk supply of nursing mothers.

Creams and oils for use on your breasts should be made from essential oils, with safflower, sesame, almond, or hazelnut (a vegetable oil), used as a carrier in a dilution of 5 percent—that is, one part of essential oil to nineteen parts of the carrier. There are products on the market specifically made to treat the bust using essences that are reported to stimulate circulation, cell growth and reproduction, and to improve the skin in general. Most of the good ones are French. And most of them are expensive. But you can make your own at reasonable cost. Here is a good recipe for a toning oil to use daily:

Mix: five drops lavender oil, 10 drops juniper oil, five drops rosemary, and five drops of ylang-ylang oil in the carrier oil. Apply daily after exercise, a bath, or hydrotherapy, when the skin is warm and most receptive. With the fingers and palms, massage the breasts inwards from the outside and then upward from the space between the breasts in circular motions for three or four minutes until the oil is dispersed.

For the best results in improving the shape and look of your bust, use exercise, hydrotherapy, and oil massage together daily until you get marked improvement—usually a month to six weeks. Then you need only use them once or twice a week to preserve the benefits.

THE QUESTION OF SURGERY

If your breasts are too small, the above kind of treatment can increase their size usually by somewhere between a half to two inches. If they are too large, the same treatment, because of its toning and firming action, will make them appear slightly smaller. But if you want a more drastic reduction, which I think should only be considered in cases of extreme size (a good bra can work wonders for the rest), the only alternative is surgery. Mammaplasty for breast reduction entails making several incisions in the breast area (just where depends on the particular patient) and then removing fat tissue. It usually also means moving the nipple itself, which results in scars around the nipple area and the strong possibility that the patient will be unable to breast-feed a child. But results from this operation are generally good.

Breast augmentation—making them larger—entails a small curved incision made under each breast and then the insertion of prostheses to create greater fullness. Filled with saline solution of silicone gel, the latest prostheses are so good that the shape of the bosom is usually excellent so long as the woman is standing. When she lies down, however, her breasts will not flatten out against her chest as natural breasts do, and of course she will always be left with a very thin crescent scar under each breast. These days modern prostheses never harden as the earlier ones did. They feel natural to the touch if somewhat firmer than most breasts and there is no change in sensitivity. You have to wear a bra for a few weeks after breast surgery while the tissue is healing and then, if you like, you can go without a bra.

The same exercises for firming a natural bosom are useful after breast surgery to strengthen the underlying muscles that give support to your new bosom.

One of the most interesting, useful, and potentially inexpensive (since you can do it yourself) methods of breast augmentation that I've come across has been done by hypnosis. American psychologist James E. Williams conducted a study of women students at North Texas State University who wanted larger busts. The graduate and undergraduate women were aged between eighteen and forty, the average being twenty-four. He hypnotized each woman in sessions of about an hour a week for a period of twelve weeks. Each time he attempted to regress the subject to the age when her breasts were developing and then suggested that she was experiencing the sensations of breast growth. Finally, he asked her to visualize her body image with the large bust size projected into a future date.

The results of the experiment were very successful. Women showed increases in bust size from one to three inches with the average increases being two and an eighth inches. But there is no reason to assume that this kind of size increase in underdeveloped breasts need be dependent on the presence of a hypnotist. The same thing can be brought about through the use of creative imagery. From the deeply relaxed state, visualize yourself in adolescence and imagine your breasts developing and finish off by visualizing yourself as an adult with fuller breasts. Mastering the techniques for deep relaxation and practicing this kind of creative imagery daily should bring similar results.

CAN CANCER BE PREVENTED?

Fear of cancer is widespread. And, unfortunately, the bulk of information about breast cancer disseminated to women concentrates only on the detection aspects—how to examine yourself to check for signs of tumors—rather than on how it might possibly be prevented in the first place.

There is increasing evidence that cancer may be caused by a high fat diet. Deaths from cancer and from coronary heart disease among women are highest of all in areas where the diet is high in fat and low in fresh vegetables and fruits. High consumption of meat may be implicated too. Studies show that groups of people who eat a low meat, low saturated-fat diet tend to have a low incidence of cancer.

SELF-CHECK FOR CANCER

There are certain warning signs that the International Union against Cancer insists should be investigated by your doctor if they occur. The reason for any one of them may well have nothing to do with a malignant growth, but if you experience any it is a good idea to have it checked.

1. Any change in a wart or a mole.

2. Any unexplained loss of weight.

3. Difficulty in swallowing or chronic indigestion.

4. Any change in regular bowel or bladder habits without apparent reason.

5. Unusual discharge or bleeding.

6. Any sore or ulcer that doesn't seem to heal normally.

7. Chronic hoarseness or persistent cough.

8. A lump in the neck, armpit, breast, or anywhere else in the body.

The presence of a possible breast cancer can be detected by self-examination, which is simple to do. The best time for this is just after a period, when your breasts are smallest. If you find any persistent lumps you should see your doctor. Similarly, you need to seek medical advice if you notice any thickening in the breast, any change of shape, swelling in the armpit, retraction of the nipple, or a blood-stained discharge from the nipple.

Here's how: Undressed to the waist and standing in front of a mirror, raise your arms above your head, then lower them again, placing them on your hips. Look for any puckering in the skin, or any bulging or flattening on the surface, or any difference between breasts in two positions. Then lift each breast gently and examine the underneath part. Explore any parts that look different gently with your fingers. If it is sore or there is any discharge you should see a doctor. Now lie down and lift up one arm, with the other folded behind your head, and gently run the fingers of the free hand around in concentric circles toward the nipple looking for any slight thickening or lump, giving special attention to the area between the nipple and the armpit, where tumors are most commonly formed.

Now change arms, putting the other hand behind your head and check your other breast.

If you find any lumps or thickening, go and have a medical examination. Although most lumps are not cancerous, the majority of lumps that are are found by women themselves. This is why self-examination like this is an excellent warning system that you should not ignore. For if a lump does prove to be malignant, early detection may mean that only the tumor itself, and not the whole breast, will have to be removed.

The Face

Introduction

For most people the face is the focus of attention and the most immediate expression of a woman's beauty. It is certainly the area of the body women worry most about. They spend a great deal of money looking after it with creams and lotions, cleansers and toners and masks, and of course the traditional facials, special treatments, and face-lifts. Everything seems to depend on the face. And all of this is done in an attempt to make sure skin stays smooth and young-looking, well colored, and free from blemishes.

Skin is one of the most important criteria for sexual attraction between men and women. Perhaps this is the main reason the face seems so important.

In this section we will be looking at skin and skin care. We will find out what skin is, how it works, and what can be done to care for it well and to prevent it from premature aging. We will also take a look at common skin problems and their solutions.

Finally we will look at the eyes—probably the most expressive feature of the whole body—and investigate how to make them more beautiful and how to look after them well.

26

The Craft of Skin Care

A living, breathing thing, skin is far more than just a superficial covering for your body. It is your largest organ. It covers a surface area of about 17 square feet and weighs between six and eight pounds. So complex is this stuff called skin that a piece of it with only the surface area of your thumbnail boasts a yard of blood vessels, twenty-five nerve endings, one hundred sweat glands, and over three million cells.

Lasting skin beauty is a question of lasting care, not spending lavishly on fancy creams and treatments. It is the everyday way you treat skin that matters year after year. But to know how to look after your skin you must first know something about it—what it is and isn't, what it's meant to do, and the many things that affect it for better or worse. For then you can see that its needs are met from day to day. In return it will give you what you desire: beauty that at the very least is skin deep.

HOW YOUR SKIN WORKS

Your skin is a world all its own: living tissue composed of billions of cells bathed in a lake of liquid with the same salt content as seawater. Each skin cell is separated from its neighbor by a membrane through which nutrients and respiratory gases pass. And all skin tissue is nourished by the myriad of tiny capillaries, which bring fresh oxygen and nutrients to the cell. Cell growth and reproduction go on unceasingly in each of these microcosms. Life is sustained, wastes eliminated to be carried away via the lymph and blood, so that all of these cells can work together to perform the many vital functions that your skin carries out: It protects your body from invasion by bacteria, virus, or fungus. It helps eliminate the waste products of the metabolism directly through its surface. It conveys information about the outside world by way of a vast network of complex sensory nerve endings. It helps guard the inside of your body from the destructive ultraviolet rays of the sun. And it registers pleasure and pain from your environment.

Your skin both depends on the rest of your body for its healthy existence and also offers help to it. And like all live things, in order to function well and look beautiful, it has to be free to carry out all its duties unimpaired by lack of proper nutrients or oxygen, poor circulation, illness, internal pollution, or prolonged stress, all of which threaten its integrity. Real skin care is not just skin deep.

SKIN COMES IN LAYERS

Skin is made up of three layers: the stratified cellular *epidermis* (the part you see when you look into the mirror); an underlying *dermis*, made up of connective tissue, nerves, blood, and lymph systems, which also contain the sebaceous, or oil, glands, and sweat glands with ducts leading to its surface; and finally a fatty layer of *subcutaneous* tissue. The outermost layer, the epidermis, consists of two parts: an inner part of living cells called the stratum Malpighii and an outer part of anucleated (meaning they have lost their nucleus) horny cells, the stratum corneum. The inner part is in direct contact with the dermis, beneath it.

The Outer Skin

Here, at the base of the epidermis, in the stratum Malpighii, a single layer of cells known as the basal layer forms new cells for the rest of the epidermis by continuous cell reproduction. As they are formed, these new cells constantly push outward and upward toward the skin's surface. In the process, they synthesize an insoluble protein called *keratin*, lose their cell nuclei, die, and dry out, becoming mere shells on the skin's surface. Once there, they are forever being sloughed off and replaced by new arrivals from below. Most skin care products concern themselves only with the treatment of this stratum corneum, making sure it does not dry out excessively (moisturizer); that the dead cells are periodically sloughed off (exfoliator, which stimulates the basal layer to produce more fresh cells and leaves the skin looking more translucent); and finally, that it is covered with a chemical or physical sunscreen to guard the deeper layers of the skin from damage as a result of exposure to sunlight.

When the layers of dead cells in the stratum corneum lie flat and smooth against each other, the skin refracts light well, making your skin look beautifully smooth and silky. If, instead, they are turned up at the edges, then the skin looks dry and lacks smoothness. For they are the outermost manifestation of skin beauty and health.

On the stratum corneum, that is on the surface of your skin, there is also a hydrolipidic film composed of water from the sweat glands and oil from the sebaceous glands in a kind of oil-in-water emulsion. This film acts as a natural moisturizer, maintaining acidity (referred to as the pH of skin) to help guard the body against invasion of any kind and to protect it from chemical onslaught. The natural pH of your skin is between 4.5 and 5.5, which means that it is slightly acid. It is important to maintain this acid mantle. It can be disturbed by the use of soaps, most of which are strongly alkaline, and cosmetics which are not acid-balanced. This is particularly true if your skin is sensitive by nature, tends to be either excessively dry or excessively oily, or if it often breaks out in acne.

The Living Skin

Beneath the epidermis, in the dermis, or true skin (which unlike the epidermis is entirely a living thing), are found the nerves. They register pleasure and pain, touch, heat and cold. Here, too, is a rich supply of blood vessels and lymphatics plus all the various skin appendages: the hair follicles, with their sebaceous glands, and the sweat glands. Also important in the dermis is an elaborate network of fibers made by special cells called fibroblasts. These fibers look like the warp and woof of fine cloth. They are collectively known as connective tissues and are made up mostly of protein called collagen together with about 2 percent elastin. This network gives your skin its form and resilience. So long as it remains smooth and ordered, your skin stays young-looking and firm. When its fibers start to bunch up and harden or to cross-link and become disorganized, your skin rapidly begins to sag, to wrinkle, and to age. This aging process has many causes. It can occur as a result of exposure to the sun, internal wear and tear from illness, or an insufficiency of certain vitamins and minerals (particularly vitamin C and the trace element zinc), or exposure to cigarette smoke and pollution. It also appears to be part of your genetic programming.

Much of the beauty and health of your skin depends on the dermal layer. The things it needs to stay strong and healthy come more from the *inside* than from what you apply to skin. This internal aspect of skin care is what is most ignored. Few women even consider it, and yet without ensuring that the dermis gets all it needs through optimum nutrition and regular exercise (not only for the face but also for the body as a whole), there is no way you can prevent or correct the disorganization of connective tissue, its consequent loss of tone, and the resulting deep line formation on the face.

The Subskin

Underneath the dermis, in the subcutaneous tissue, are la
and fatty tissue which act as insulation to the body and which a...
young female skin its characteristic (and very attractive) padding. When
this padding starts to go, either because of hormonal changes that come
with age or because of simple neglect, your skin loses tone and firmness.
Looking after this deepest layer of skin is a *whole body* challenge. Particularly important to it is the health of your endocrine system, in which
constant regular exercise plays a vital part.

Truly effective skin care has to ensure the continuous health and
proper functioning of all three layers, to preserve beauty. This means
treatment and protection from the outside of the epidermis. It also means
treatment of the dermis through first-rate nutrition, vitamins and minerals, rest and exercise, and perhaps, too, the application of specific substances such as essential oils which can be absorbed through the skin's
outer layers into the dermis to stimulate cell metabolism, encourage
waste elimination from cells, and help protect and preserve the collagen
and elastin fibers. Finally, the subcutaneous layer has to be kept intact by
maintaining a firm and well-used, healthy body. In other words, really
good skin care for lasting beauty has to tackle the challenge simultaneously from within and without. And there are no shortcuts.

LET'S BEGIN AT THE INSIDE

It should go without saying (yet this is the most consistently ignored
truth about skin care) that first-rate nutrition is a must. All the nutrients
your body needs for optimum health, your skin needs to keep it young
and beautiful, including the vitamins, minerals, protein, essential fatty
acids, trace elements, and unrefined carbohydrates. So many specific
problems such as brown patches or early wrinkling are mostly the result
of internal neglect, and no amount of expensive stuff rubbed on the outside will stop their formation.

Next time you are in the supermarket, take a look at the skin of the
woman in front of you and note what she has in her shopping basket. Almost invariably, you'll find that people with beautiful skins are buying
lots of fresh fruits and vegetables, while the others have their carts
chock-full of refined foods: white flour, sugar, and other industrially
prepared goodies.

Proper elimination is essential for skin health and beauty. You need a
diet high in natural fiber, or roughage, from raw vegetables and/or whole
grains. If ever you find yourself constipated, take a couple of teaspoons

of bran each morning, with plenty of liquid, either sprinkled on cereals or in yogurt or mixed into a glass of juice (the liquid is vital in providing the bulk necessary for the bran to do its work).

Finally, don't forget to drink plenty of water, an essential nutrient you may never have thought of. It helps detoxify skin, dissolving hard debris that interferes with proper circulation and removal of wastes and which can cause cellulite. If your diet is more than 50 percent raw fruits and vegetables, you don't need to be concerned with drinking too much extra water, for fresh foods themselves contain large quantities of water. If it is not, you should get at least six to eight glasses a day for the sake of your skin.

While all of the nutrients found in the Lifestyle Diet are important for skin, some are particularly vital to its look and health. Vitamin A, for instance. If you do not have enough of it in your diet or if you have some difficulty in assimilating and using the vitamin (many women do), this can bring about dry, scaly, and crinkled skin. For, among its many functions, vitamin A helps regulate the size and functions of the sebaceous glands. A shortage can result in enlarged pores, rough skin, and acne.

Without adequate vitamin C, the collagen fibers in the dermis suffer damage. Vitamin C and the bioflavonoids that are found in natural foods (such as the whitish inner skin of grapefruit) not only keep skin young by helping to protect the collagen fibers and keep them intact, they also ensure the health of the tiny capillaries that supply nutrients to the skin's cells, protecting skin from fragile or broken veins (bruising) and early wrinkling. When capillaries are not strong and working properly, then the skin's cells don't receive all the oxygen and nutrients they need via the bloodstream, and their functioning suffers. Neither are wastes efficiently eliminated. This can lead to stasis in the tissues, and cellulite, as well as contributing to early aging of the skin.

The B-complex vitamins, which help keep nerves healthy and relaxed, also aid circulation in the skin. A lack of one or more of the B group can result in redness, tenderness, or ulcerations around the corners of the mouth. The B group is also useful in controlling excessive oiliness and in avoiding discolorations that often appear on the face and hands in middle age. Some of these blotches will even gradually fade in time when a tablespoon of brewer's yeast, containing the B vitamins, is taken in a glass of juice at mealtimes.

One of the B group, vitamin B_2, or riboflavin, is particularly important in the transport of oxygen to the cells of the skin. Unless cellular oxygen is sufficient, nutrients can't be burnt efficiently for fuel, nor will cellular wastes be completely removed. An insufficiency of riboflavin also causes tiny lines to be etched in the skin around the lips and contributes to the formation of scales and cracks known as cheilosis and stomatitis. When vitamins B$_1$ and B$_2$, niacin, and B$_6$ are added to the diet of women with these symptoms, the symptoms usually disappear.

A professor of dermatology at Japan's Chiba University School of Medicine did some interesting research into skin disorders and the level of certain B-complex vitamins in the skin. In comparing the levels of the B vitamins in people with dermatological problems, with those of normal, healthy skin, he discovered that 27 percent of those with various kinds of dermatosis were deficient in thiamine, 27 percent in riboflavin, and 52 percent in pyridoxine. He also linked a great variety of skin problems, such as eczema, baldness, keratosis, viral infections of the skin, erythema, and various pigmentation disorders, directly with B deficiencies.

Vitamin E, about which there has been such controversy, is vital to skin health and beauty too. Dry, rough, etched, or tired-looking skin often improves when vitamin E is taken in supplementary form. Like vitamin C, vitamin E plays an important role in holding back the skin's aging process, because of its antioxidant properties. It simulates circulation and helps prevent free radicals from causing damage to the DNA—the cell's genetic material. This DNA damage is one of the most important parts of the degenerative process of aging (see chapter on skin aging).

Lecithin, which is such an excellent source of choline, unsaturated fatty acids and anti-stress factors, is one of the most important supplements you can take to look after your skin. It complements all the other anti-stress nutrients and can be taken easily by sprinkling two tablespoons of granular lecithin on your cereals or in yogurt or salads. In some way that is not completely understood, it appears to give support to the skin in a number of ways and to keep it fresh, plump, and smooth-looking.

Minerals for Beauty

Vitamin C and zinc are both essential for the maintenance of resilient collagen and elastin. Human skin contains about 20 percent of the body's zinc. Without enough zinc (and studies show that most women in industrialized countries appear to be deficient in zinc) stretch marks easily appear on the body, and the skin sags and wrinkles easily.

More seriously, zinc deficiency has been shown to cause keratogenesis (a severe skin lesion in rats and mice that resembles psoriasis in people) and also delayed wound healing.

Another mineral, sulfur, is often called the beauty mineral. Although all the body cells contain sulfur, those of the skin, hair, and joints have it in far greater amounts than anywhere else. The keratin of the epidermis is especially rich in sulfur; so are your fingernails and hair. When sulfur in the diet is insufficient (as it is in many women as a result of misguided warnings against egg eating and the widespread cholesterol phobia), the hair and nails become weaker and the skin tends to scale. A few eggs a week can do a great deal to improve these conditions or prevent them from occurring.

Selenium, another antioxidant, like vitamins C and E helps preserve tissue elasticity because of its ability to delay oxidation of polyunsaturated fatty acids, which cause tissue proteins to solidify, so it is also important as a factor in the prevention of premature aging of skin. Selenium is found in eggs, garlic, tuna fish, brewer's yeast, and onions.

Silicon, found in avocados, apples, and honey, is needed to prevent flabbiness in the skin, as it is for producing strong nails and a fine sheen on the hair. And there are more: Iodine helps keep nails and hair strong. Calcium and magnesium are needed to make use of other nutrients in the body. One way or another, every mineral, like every vitamin, has a part to play in ensuring the health of skin and in preserving youth in it. They need to be supplied in good balance from a long-term diet for health and beauty, and if possible any imbalance or deficiency needs to be detected by hair analysis and then corrected by mineral and vitamin supplements where necessary before the beauty potential of your skin and hair will ever be fulfilled.

Skin Destroyers and Helpers

Everyone knows that stress can adversely affect skin, causing lumps and blemishes to appear when you least want them. Long-term stress also contributes greatly to the aging process. But what few women realize is that exercise has also a vital role to play in keeping your skin young as well. This is not only because it stimulates circulation, which improves cell nutrition and firms muscles, but also because when body-muscle mass shrinks as a result of inactivity, the amount of vital hormones, for instance, and the level of steroid hormones from the adrenal glands and the sex glands, decrease in direct proportion to the decrease in the body's muscle mass. Many of these declining hormones play an important part in preserving water balance and youthful appearance of the skin. Vigorous exercise several times a week helps keep this from happening.

Finally, fine skin depends on enough sleep, staying away from such stimulants as coffee, alcohol, and tobacco—all of which are bad news for a complexion—and on making sure your liver is in good order. Since the liver is the organ that has to deal with the neutralizing of toxic elements in our air and food, unless it is functioning well they can back up in the system, resulting not only in early degeneration of skin but chronic illnesses.

SKIN CARE FROM THE OUTSIDE

There are three parts to any good external skin care regimen, regardless of your age or the type of skin you have:

1. Regular, thorough cleansing

2. Protection from moisture loss and external roughness

3. Protection from the ultraviolet rays of the sun

These are the basics. They are simple, and there need be no mumbo jumbo about them. One can include a fourth part to skin care too, and that is *treatment*. This extra can correct problems, help preserve youth, and revitalize the look of skin.

You can give your skin treatments either internally from vitamins, minerals, and diet, or externally in the form of hydrotherapy, or by applying special creams, oils, or herbs, or by using specific exercises to strengthen muscles before they have a chance to sag or to correct neglect. The treatment part of skin care is where the *art* comes into it, and here you need to consider your specific skin conditions and problems. The other three are all parts of the simple *craft* of skin care, and it is very simple indeed.

CLEANSING

The Soap Way

There are two camps when it comes to cleansing: the soap-and-water lovers and the soap-and-water haters. Each feel passionately and dogmatically about their way of doing things and each have a long list of justifications for why they do what they do. Both—within reason—are right. It is true that many grandmothers who have beautiful skin have never used anything on it but old-fashioned soap and water. It is also true that they spent their youth protecting their fair skin from the sun, that they probably had a better diet than we do—a diet mostly of whole foods eaten in their natural state instead of foods that are overprocessed and laced with an increasing number of additives—and that most of their lives their skin was probably not insulted by the vast range of chemical pollutants in the air and water to which ours is subjected.

Soap is an excellent cleanser. Manufactured from caustic alkalies and fats, it removes grease and dirt from the skin's surface easily (although it is usually not as effective at removing makeup as cream or lotion cleanser). Its disadvantage lies in its being extremely alkaline. This means that using soap reduces the natural acidity, or pH, of the skin, which helps protect it from bacterial invasion. Soap is capable of penetrating the skin's outer protective layers and leaching away the hydrolipidic film, making the skin of women who tend toward dryness even drier. Surprisingly, it can also have just the opposite effect on skin that tends to be oily. Because the degreasing action of soap stimulates the already overactive sebaceous glands to produce even more oil, a kind of vicious circle is created: The more you wash with soap, the worse the oiliness becomes, so the more you feel you have to wash with soap to try to control it. On the other hand, soap does give a sense of cleanliness that most women feel they don't get with cream and lotion cleansers.

Thanks to modern technology, there are now many pH-balanced soaps, foaming cleansers, and detergent bars that don't disturb the pH of the skin, so that if you are a soap fancier you can find one to suit you without many of the disadvantages of the conventional type. (It is simple to test the pH of all cosmetic products with litmus papers, which you can buy at a pharmacy. You simply press a strip of the paper against the soap or cleanser and then "read" the color against the chart supplied by the litmus paper manufacturer.)

The Cream or Oil Way

The cream and lotion cleansers, oils, and cleansing milks available now are also good. They will cut through makeup and grime even better than soap, and provided you use enough of one and that you remove it with tonic water or water afterward will do an excellent job of keeping your skin clean. A cleansing milk is an oil-in-water emulsion that cleans by emulsifying water-soluble dirt in its aqueous phase and oil-soluble dirt in its oil phase. Put a lotion or cream cleanser on with your hands as you would soap and then tissue it off, repeating the application until the tissue shows no sign of dirt on it. Then follow with tonic or freshener, preferably one *without* alcohol in it, or simply rinse your face in cool water.

The Double Treatment

Because cleanliness is so important to lasting skin health and beauty, if you live in a city or a highly industrialized area where air pollution is a particular problem, the oil-and-water technique is the most effective means of all. It entails using two types of cleansers, first an oil-based one, which removes makeup and oil-soluble dirt, followed by a water-based one such as a pH-balanced soap or detergent bar to remove the oil and all the rest of the surface grime. Many of the cosmetic industry's most expensive ranges are based on this method of cleansing. But you can put together your own system, which is just as effective, probably from products you own already.

Choose a pure vegetable oil, preferably cold-pressed to preserve all its goodness and vitamin content, such as safflower oil, sunflower oil, corn oil, or one of the more expensive hazelnut or apricot oils. Buy it in small quantities and keep it in a cool place (preferably in the refrigerator), to protect it from oxidation. Pour a tablespoonful of the oil into the palm of your hand and spread it on your face, rubbing it in well. (This is a good opportunity to give yourself a gentle massage to stimulate circulation while the oil is leaching up the makeup and grime on your skin.) Then, using pads of damp absorbent cotton wiped over your face, remove the oil and with it much of the dirt on the skin.

You are ready now for the second stage. Wash your skin in warm water and use a pH-balanced soap, detergent bar, or liquid detergent cleanser, adding plenty of water and rubbing gently with the tips of your fingers and the palms of your hands until the whole face is well covered. Now rinse thoroughly ten times in warm water and then splash with cool.

Whichever cleansing method you choose, follow it twice daily. This is the first step in the craft of skin care.

PRESERVING MOISTURE AND PREVENTING WATER LOSS

Your skin is constantly giving up moisture, not just through the sweat ducts but through a process of transpiration in which water in the cells on its surface evaporates directly into the atmosphere. This is quite different from perspiring, which only happens to any marked degree when the body is warm. Transpiration occurs constantly. The lower the humidity in your environment, the more rapid will be the water loss and the greater the need to protect against it. And what most women don't realize is that the humidity of the average centrally heated home or office is comparable to that of the Sahara Desert. Similarly, chemical pollutants, soaps, makeup, and anything that affects the hydrolipidic film decreases its effectiveness and leads to further dehydration.

I learned the truth of this for myself when I spent a month in a Buddhist monastery in the Himalayas. There was no water to wash with, no air pollution, and no stress, for I was spending most of my days and nights in meditation. Neither was there a mirror. When, at the end of the month, I came down out of the mountains and looked at myself in the mirror, I was amazed to find that my skin had never looked better and without the help of the cleansers, toners, soaps, or creams. Determined to reject all my cosmetics on my return to London, since they obviously weren't doing any good, I was saddened to find after a couple of weeks that back in civilization my skin was looking very poorly indeed. What works in the pure air of the mountains on a superb and very frugal diet with no stress doesn't work at all in the urban world, where one's skin is constantly being bombarded by pollution of one kind or another. I soon went back to the simple craft of skin care.

Another aspect of protecting the skin from becoming dry has nothing to do with moisture or moisture loss. In fact there is some evidence that moisture loss is *not* the most important factor in dry skin. The stratum corneum is composed of flattened cells that have lost their nuclei and overlap in much the same way as tiles on a roof or scales on a fish do. These cells form one of the skin's barriers against water loss. But they are important in another way, too. For much dry skin appears to be the result not of specific moisture depletion but, rather, of changes in these flattened cells on the surface of the skin. When they lie flat and regular against each other, then the skin looks and feels moist and smooth. When, on the other hand, the minute edges of these flattened cells begin to come unstuck from one another, to flake off or to curl up at the edges, you get very dry skin. There is considerable controversy among dermatologists about whether this phenomenon or true moisture loss is at the root of dry skin. The happy news, however, is that a good water-in-oil moisturizer helps solve the problem, either way. It not only protects from excess water loss, it also glues together the edges of these flattened cells, smoothing over the surface and making it look and feel moist.

One partial answer to the problem of dry skin is humidification: the use of a humidifier or simply simmering a pan of water in a room to raise the moisture level of the air to somewhere between 75 percent humidity and 90 percent—the ideal range for preserving the skin's water balance. A humidifier is a worthwhile investment for any woman who values her skin and wants to keep it from rapidly aging. Recent studies show that the use of humidifiers can be helpful in other ways, too: for instance, in helping avoid colds and flu, not to mention preserving antique furniture and keeping plants healthy. But you need surface protection against water loss too.

There are literally hundreds of moisturizers on the market. Some are beautifully cool to the touch and scented, others somewhat greasy. Some come in lotion form and contain humectants—substances such as glycerin, propylene, glycol, sorbitol, sodium pyrrolidone, or carboxylic acid which tend to attract water from the air. The trouble is that when you use them, they tend to attract water from within the outer layers of the skin, too. So moisturizers containing humectants are best avoided.

Other moisturizing products—creams and lotions—contain NMF. This is a catchall term for certain chemical complexes synthesized to resemble the natural moisturizing factor in the skin itself that helps hold water in the cells and in the interstitial spaces. They include such things as urea, free amino acids, sodium lactate, and glucose and fructose in combination. NMFs are a welcome addition to any moisturizer. They do help combat water-loss problems.

But by far the most effective way of moisturizing is simply to *prevent* water in the skin from escaping into the air. This you can do by wearing a water-in-oil-type emulsion on your face every day, winter and summer.

Most moisturizers, particularly the kind that feel so cool and delightful on your skin when you apply them, are oil-in-water emulsions whose fat content is too low to provide the coating on the skin's surface that it needs to be effective in keeping its natural moisture in. Their high water content is what makes the skin feel so lovely when you put them on, since it evaporates quickly from the surface, cooling it and giving a sensation of freshness in the process. But it is just this high water content that makes this kind of moisturizer not very effective—that is unless you want to apply it again and again every few minutes or so throughout the day.

Water-in-oil emulsions contain a great deal more fat than water, which means they are able to cover the stratum corneum with an impermeable film, so that excessive water loss doesn't occur. And they are good for both dry and oily skin. For, unlike so many products specifically designed for oily skin, they are not strongly degreasing. They don't spur the sebaceous glands to produce even more oil in the kind of vicious circle women with oily skin know so well.

Good, pleasant to use, water-in-oil moisturizers are more expensive to manufacture than the oil-in-water variety. First because oil naturally costs a great deal more than water and secondly because there is quite an art to putting them together in a form that is not heavy and greasy but *is* pleasant to the feel and light to the touch. After all, wearing Vaseline—a water-in-oil emulsion—is an excellent way of protecting skin from excessive water loss, but who wants to wear Vaseline? In the past few years, with increased awareness of how to deal with moisture-loss problems, a few new creams of the water-in-oil type have appeared on the market. Find one that you like and wear it every day, applying it twice a day if you can under makeup when you are wearing it or just on its own when you don't. This is the second part of the craft of skin care.

LIGHT CAN BE FOE INSTEAD OF FRIEND

The third part of everyday skin care is simple: Your skin needs to be protected from the sun. This does not just mean when you are lying on the beach, either; it means *all* the time. For ultraviolet light is the worst destroyer and ager of the skin that you are ever likely to encounter.

Long-term exposure to ultraviolet light brings about degenerative changes in the deep layers of the skin that until recently were thought to be an unavoidable part of the aging process: cross-linking and bunching of the collagen fibers and genetic damage to the skin's cells that cause it to lose tone, to wrinkle, to sag, and to discolor. Heavy exposure to the sun's light at the age of eighteen will result in early wrinkling, between twenty-five and forty. This is an unfortunate law of nature that nothing can change—except, of course, wearing some form of adequate sunscreen on the skin. And not just when you are out on the beach lying in the sun, but all the time. For these ultraviolet rays, which are dangerous to the skin and age it, don't come just from being directly exposed to the sun's light. They also come from the sky and from reflections off water and off the earth. In fact, the amount of ultraviolet radiation from the sky is greater than that coming directly from the sun itself. So your skin needs protection all the time.

Which sunscreen product you choose depends on how much light you are exposed to. There is more in Florida or Sydney than in London, Paris, or Dublin. (This is the main reason why the Irishwoman tends to be in such better condition and look much younger than her American sister.) Many makeup products now include a sunscreen in their formation (read labels). There are also a couple of water-resistant sun lotions which themselves make excellent moisturizers-cum-sunscreens for everyday wear, since they happen to be water-in-oil emulsions. By choosing one, you will obtain a dual-purpose product. Wear it all the time, day in day out, winter and summer, so that you never expose your unprotected skin to the light. Twenty years from now, when you compare your face with a friend's of the same age who hasn't used a sunscreen constantly, you will be pleased to find that you look a good ten years younger than she does. I know there is a tendency for women to be particularly negligent in this area of skin care because wearing a sunscreen is entirely preventative and so you feel no immediate benefits from it. But this simple habit will do more to preserve skin youth and beauty than any other external action you can take.

These three things—cleansing, protection from moisture loss, and a sunscreen—are all there is to basic skin care. They are simple, and inexpensive to carry out, and the benefits they bring when used regularly every day cannot be measured in any amount of money.

27

The Art of Treating Skin

When it comes to treating skin, everyone is looking for the fountain of eternal youth. At one time it is thought to be vitamins, at other times plant essences, minerals, fetal or placental extracts. In recent years all of these somewhat exotic substances have been frowned on not only by many dermatologists but also by the so-called hard-hitting journalists who insist that nothing *external* can be done to keep skin looking beautiful and to protect it from premature aging other than to follow the three basic steps in the craft of skin care outlined in the previous chapter: cleansing, protection from moisture loss, and screening from ultraviolet light.

And to a certain extent they are right. These three basics are the most important of all in ensuring that your skin remains intact as long as possible. It is also a fact that most commercial treatments and creams will do nothing more than smooth over cells of the stratum corneum—they will not affect skin at a deeper level. Yet this is only part of the truth. But, armed with this part-truth someone is forever doing some kind of exposé on cosmetics—claiming, for instance, that we have all been hoodwinked into thinking that skin can be fed and will absorb something when, they assure us, everybody knows skin is a complete barrier, between the outer and the inner worlds, through which nothing can pass. Yet while there is not a fountain of eternal youth anywhere in cosmetics, there *are* substances which, when externally applied, can not only be absorbed but will also help improve skin's texture and quality, correct problems, and preserve youth. There are also treatments with masks, exfoliators, massage, exercise, and hydrotherapy which, although the substances used to give them are not taken directly into the skin, will also do a great deal for skin health and beauty. They are all part of the rather esoteric art of skin treatment.

SKIN ABSORPTION—A USEFUL TOOL

In general, your skin is impermeable. Water, for instance, will not go through it. Neither will most oils. However, if it is in prolonged contact with some substances, if it is broken or has a rash, or if it is rubbed with an oil or emulsion whose molecular structure is fine enough to cross the epidermal barrier, then active ingredients in the oil or emulsion can be carried not only through the epidermis but deep into the skin and sometimes even throughout the body via the bloodstream. (The skin's permeability is constantly being exploited by drug companies, which view this percutaneous absorption as a means of getting medication into the body without irritating the gastrointestinal tracts of sick patients.) And the three main routes of skin penetration are through the hair follicles into the sebaceous glands, through the sweat glands, and through the unbroken stratum corneum between skin appendages. Once a substance does get past the stratum corneum by any of these means, its further passage, into the epidermis and dermis, is assured.

Vitamins were first applied this way after the Second World War to treat ex-prisoners with severe vitamin deficiencies who couldn't take them by mouth. Vitamins D, E, and A—the fat-soluble vitamins; vitamin C; and some of the B-complex vitamins have all been used successfully in this way. Hormone absorption is well known. Estrogen creams are often given to postmenopausal women by dermatologists. Many essential oils of plants are also absorbed so readily that they have been shown to appear in the urine of animals half an hour after application.

The important questions are, How do you make positive use of your skin's percutaneous absorption? and How do you protect it from misuse? The second question is easy to answer: Avoid skin contact as much as possible with household chemicals, products containing toxic metals such as aluminum, lead, and mercury, and soaps with cleansers containing hexachlorophene. Also guard your skin from atmospheric chemicals in the air by cleansing it regularly twice a day and wearing a moisturizer/ sunscreen, preferably one that contains the silicones that are particularly useful in protecting from pollution.

Then get to know the substances that can be usefully applied to the skin for treatment purposes, and discover which ones work for you, using them as night treatments or special cures. The French have an excellent idea of treatment in the concept of the cure. A cure consists of a particular product or substance applied daily for a specific period— usually about two weeks at a time—as a kind of shock treatment to stimulate better oxygenation of the tissues. Because this cure is different from what your skin is used to and because your skin doesn't ever get a chance to become accustomed to it and therefore to stop responding positively to it, cures often bring excellent results. A cure can be repeated every couple of months and will be particularly useful when given with the change of the seasons.

Here are some of the commonly applied skin benefactors that can be used on their own or mixed into simple oils and creams. Many of them will be found in some of the world's best manufactured cosmetic products—particularly the European ones and those truly based on plant oils and essences. But there are a lot of so called natural or herbal products that are made of synthetics and have never seen a flower, lemon, or blade of grass—so choose carefully.

The Vitamins

Vitamin A applied to the surface of the skin either from a capsule on its own or mixed into cream and oil preparations has been used successfully in the treatment of dry and aging skin and acne. It appears to work particularly well in combination with vitamin D, which itself has a healing effect on the skin. (This is why vitamin D is often used in diaper-rash remedies and in burn ointments.)

Vitamin E, about which there has been such controversy, and vitamin C are certainly useful in the treatment of skin healing from a cut or burn. There is no conclusive evidence that, applied topically, it will do much for normal skin, although many women who use vitamin E regularly claim good results from it. Both vitamins are natural antioxidants and as such are probably useful in preventing premature aging of the skin (as well as the whole body) but for this purpose should be taken *internally*. In some people, vitamin E used on the skin can cause allergic reactions. So, if you decide to use it, test it out on a small area first.

The B-complex vitamins, applied in the form of a brewer's-yeast mask, are often helpful in correcting skin that is too oily, but even in such cases they are probably of greater use taken internally.

There are two ways of applying vitamins to the skin: You can squeeze the vitamin oils directly from the capsules (which works well with E but tends to smell very strong with vitamins A and D) or you can mix any of the vitamins into a simple carrier oil and then spread it on the face. Good times for doing this are before you take strenuous exercise (the physical exertion improves the skin's absorptive abilities) and after a facial sauna, steaming, or hot bath (when the skin is warm and moist). Leave your preparation on for twenty minutes, then either remove with cleanser or simply tissue off the excess.

The Essential Oils

Plant extracts, or essential oils, are some of the most useful substances for skin treatment that you will find anywhere. The chemical structures of these essences are close to those of the fluids and oils in the skin itself, so that the skin appears to have a natural affinity for them. Essential oils in small quantities mixed with a carrier oil are excellent for general skin treatment as well as for correcting problems such as early aging and excessive dryness or oiliness. Make sure when choosing them that you are buying the pure essential oils of plants, not their synthetic substitutes, which are much cheaper but have no therapeutic action.

Mix your own formulas, using fifteen drops of plant essences (that is, all the various essential oils you may use should total only fifteen drops together) to each ounce of carrier oil. Almond oil and hazelnut oil are particularly good carriers for the face. You can add vitamin E or A, squeezed directly from the capsules (the scents of the plant essences do wonders to mask the unpleasant odors of vitamins). Keep your mixture in a cool place (mix only small quantities each time), preferably in a brown glass bottle to protect them from the light.

Some plant essences such as fennel contain phytohormones, which have an action on the skin resembling that of such animal hormones as estrogen. They have a remarkable ability to firm skin and stimulate cell metabolism in aging skin. Others, such as lavender and orange blossom (neroli) are cytophylactic: They stimulate cell reproduction in the basal layer. Most essential oils used externally encourage the elimination of cellular wastes and help regulate the activity of the capillaries, restoring a look of freshness and glow to the face. Massage them in gently. Here are some of the best essential oils for specific purposes.

For skin that's too oily: lavender, lemon, basil, geranium, juniper, and ylang-ylang.

For skin that's dry: sandalwood, geranium, rose, lavender, jasmine, and camomile.

For aging skin: fenugreek, wheat-germ oil, sandalwood, rose, myrrh, frankincense, lavender, mace, clary.

Placental and Fetal Extracts

Many of the best European skin treatment products contain such things as placental extracts, fetal extracts, or specially preserved plant enzymes. Fetal extracts are taken from unborn animals and placental extracts either from animal or human placentas. They are carefully treated usually by a process of freeze-drying to preserve enzymes and protect their active properties. They are then added to the formulas of some of the best Swiss, German, and French cosmetics on the market. The usefulness of these substances is continually being attacked by the "hard hitters," who insist they are only a lot of nonsense for which you pay an exorbitant price in skin-care preparations. While it is true that simply because a cream or ampoule contains fetal extract or placental extract or enzymes it will not necessarily do good for your particular skin, it is also true that these three categories of skin treaters can be excellent in revitalizing skin, in helping to protect it from premature aging, and even in the treatment of damage from burns, skin disorders, or simple neglect.

Most of the research and development into the use of fetal and placental extracts comes from Germany, where they are regularly used by dermatologists as medical, rather than strictly cosmetic, treatment. One such German preparation, available only on prescription, by the name of Cellcutana, made by Cybila Cytobiological Laboratories, in Heidelberg, is designed to stimulate and regenerate skin that has been either chemically or physically damaged and to prevent abnormal healing, including scars. It is an effective treatment for burns and premature aging. A filtrated extraction of fetal skin, fetal connective tissue, placenta, and suprarenal gland, it comes as a liquid suspension mixed with the supplied dilutant before use. Similar mixtures in diluted form can be found in many of the best French and Swiss treatment creams.

No one is quite sure what makes placental and fetal extracts so effective when used on the skin, but what is known is that they are powerhouses of vital ingredients, including vitamins, amino acids, minerals, and enzymes. Provided they are properly preserved and processed they are also biologically active. Their effects resemble those of enzymes—catalyst-like substances in living things which trigger beneficial reactions in the skin's cells although they themselves don't necessarily take part in the reactions.

The Enzymes

Then there are plant enzymes themselves. Many of the best European skin-treatment products are based entirely on the actions of plant enzymes. These biocatalysts consist of two parts: the protein fraction, or *apoenzyme*, and the *coenzyme*. The smallest particles of enzymes are very large if one takes into account the entire molecule. However, thanks to enzyme splitting, the action of many plant enzymes is not restricted to just the uppermost layer of the skin. They can also produce effects on the deeper layers.

Enzyme splitting is part of the manufacturing process in the production of cosmetics that depend for their effectiveness on the action of those plant biocatalysts. Another part lies in preserving the stability of their actions. For enzymes are delicate substances. All are destroyed at a temperature of 140 degrees Fahrenheit (60 C). Many also lose their activity if they come in contact with oxygen. Traces of iron or heavy metals also render them inactive. Finally, enzymes function best at the same pH as the skin—in a slightly acid medium. So the quality and the activity of vegetable and herbal extracts must always be carefully controlled in order to produce preparations of quality. But plant-based skin-care products that are made with all this in mind are excellent.

Home Treatments

On a do-it-yourself level, raw fruits and vegetables from your own kitchen are rich in enzymes. For instance, the cosmetic effect of the juice of fresh cucumber, which contains ascorbic acid oxidase, has long been known. It is slightly diuretic and astringent and good for all types of skin. Similarly, the juice of fresh lemons, which also contains phosphates and the enzyme esterase, is also beneficial, particularly for oily skins. It is antiseptic and refining. So are fresh carrot juice and fresh papaya, as well as the juice and pulp of many other fruits. The enzymes contained in them help stimulate the life processes in your skin's cells, making it firmer and fresher-looking and giving it a glow of health.

Only infinitesimally small quantities of enzymes—measured in millionths of a gram per liter—are needed for the enzymes to have a beneficial effect on the skin. And the art of using enzymes for cosmetic purposes is an elaborate one. For instance, for dry and tired skin one needs preparations with more proteases in them—enzymes that act on proteins; for blemished skin, or acne, you use more lipases—fat-affecting enzymes. When preparing plant-enzyme treatments at home, you need to make your preparations fresh each time and then put them immediately on the skin. The beneficial results will occur only so long as the living substances from the fresh fruits and vegetables have not yet been oxidized by exposure to air. And this oxidation process takes place rapidly. Here is an easy way of treating skin inside and out. Every day, whenever you prepare raw juices in a juice extractor (see Chapter 4 on the *Rohsäfte-Kur*), spread a couple of tablespoonfuls on your face at the same time. Masks are also particularly beneficial when made with fresh fruit and vegetable juices or pulp plus other ingredients from the kitchen —beaten egg yolk plus a tablespoon of raw, unheated honey for dry skin, two tablespoons of brewer's yeast or two teaspoons of natural yogurt for oily skin. They are best used after a facial sauna, when the skin is highly receptive to whatever is put on it. The following juices can be made with a juice extractor or the fruits and vegetables can be pureed in a blender. Experiment until you find the ones that work best for you, for every woman's skin is unique.

	COMPONENTS BESIDES ENZYMES	GOOD FOR	PROPERTIES AND EFFECTS
Almonds	Oil, natural sugars, calcium, vitamins A and B complex	Dry skin and older skin with underactive sebaceous glands	Lubricating, calming
Apple	Minerals such as copper, calcium, magnesium, iron; natural sugars; vitamin C	Oily skin, blemished skin	Disinfecting, astringent, antiseptic
Apricot	Minerals, vitamin A, essential oil	All skin	Promotes cell reproduction
Banana	Vitamins A, B, C, E; oils; sugars; iron	Dry skin and older skin with underactive sebaceous glands	Good moisturizer; nourishing
Blackberry	Organic acids, iron, lime, vitamin C, tannin	Oily skin with enlarged pores	Astringent, diuretic
Black currant	Vitamin C, citric acid	Good for delicate skin that is blemished	Soothing, healing, decongesting
Cabbage	Minerals such as sulfur, iron, iodine; vitamins A, D	Good for acne and pimples	Disinfectant, good for promoting healing of fresh scars
Camomile flower	Azulene, minerals such as potassium, phosphorus, lime	Healing; good for sensitive or allergic skin, dry skin, sunburn	Healing, soothing, anti-inflammatory
Carrot	Vitamins A, B, C, D, E, K; iron; iodine; magnesium; potassium	Sensitive skin; dehydrated, aging skin; rashes	Stimulates cell reproduction; moisturizer

	COMPONENTS BESIDES ENZYMES	GOOD FOR	PROPERTIES AND EFFECTS
Celery	Potassium, calcium, sodium, phosphorus, vitamins A, B, C	All skin types	Stimulates waste removal from cells, brightens complexion
Comfrey	Allantoin; vitamins A, B_{12}; tannin	Dry skin, acne, inflamed skin, sunburn, blemishes	Soothing and healing; cell proliferant; emollient; moisturizer
Cucumber	Vitamins A, B, C; natural sugars	All skin, especially normal to oily	Helps bleach freckles; soothing, diuretic, anti-wrinkle treatment
Dandelion	Vitamin A, iron, phosphorus, sodium	Cellulite, all skin types, sallow skin	Tonic, soothing; stimulates cell proliferation
Grapefruit	Vitamins A, C; citric acid; natural sugars	Troubled skin, oily skin, enlarged pores	Astringent, mild bleach, brightener
Grapes	Vitamins A, B, C, E	Blackheads, acne-prone skin	Diuretic; encourages cell proliferation
Kelp (*seaweed*)	Vitamins B, C, E; iodine; iron	Aging skin, cellulite	Stimulates circulation, encourages elimination of wastes and water
Lemon	Iron, potassium, tannin, citric acid	Oily skin, particularly skin losing its tone; skin with uneven pigment such as "liver spots"	Mild bleach, antiseptic, disinfectant

Mint	Tannin, essential oil, iron	Oily skin, acne, blemished skin, large pores	Antiseptic, soothing; stimulates circulation
Orange	Vitamins A, C; citric acid; essential oil	Normal to oily skin, enlarged pores, uneven pigmentation	Mild bleach; astringent
Peach	Vitamins A, C; natural sugars; essential oil; citric acid	All skin, particularly dry	Diuretic, soothing, anti-inflammatory
Pear	Vitamins A, B, P	Sensitive skin, inflamed skin	Emollient; encourages elimination of wastes
Potato	Vitamin C; potassium; iron; natural sugars	Aging skin, skin losing tone, waterlogged skin	Tonic and diuretic
Raspberry	Lime, sodium, tannic acid	Large pores, oily skin	Astringent, stimulant, diuretic
Spinach	Vitamins A, B, C; iron	Dehydrated skin, aging skin, troubled skin	Soothing; stimulating circulation
Strawberry	Salicylic acid, lime, iron, sodium, vitamin C, tannin	Oily skin, uneven pigmentation	Astringent, diuretic, toning
Tomato	Vitamins A, B, C; malic acid; natural sugars	Oily skin, blackheads	Rebalances skin acidity; mild emollient

Air—Let Your Skin Breathe

It may surprise you to see such a common thing as air listed among the important treatments for external use on skin, but in many ways it may be the most valuable of all. It is also often the most neglected by women who tend to cover their skin day and night with heavy creams.

Although most of the oxygen your skin needs comes by way of the bloodstream, the skin also helps itself to as much as 2½ percent of the body's total oxygen from the air by direct absorption. Skin also directly eliminates almost 3 percent of the body's carbon dioxide waste. Generally, this direct oxygen intake is used only by the epidermis, where it helps to break down nutrients for cell use at the basal layer and to eliminate wastes. But in an emergency, when the body is short of oxygen, skin respiration can increase in order to partially oxygenate the blood as well. This ability of the skin to take in oxygen directly from the air appears to play an important part in maintaining its health and beauty. In the words of one oxygen researcher, Goldschmidt, "There is no doubt in my mind that skin respiration as such, and all our concern for its perfect function, is vital to health, life, even beauty . . . the retention, holding back of exhaling carbon dioxide must produce a toxic condition in the body which is supposed to be discharged by way of normal respiration through the skin. If such unloading of carbon dioxide is made impossible, the condition of health suffers."

Yet how many women *do* let their skin breathe? We are taught to cover the face day in and day out with cosmetic products, many of which form a heavy, occlusive film on the surface of the skin that severely impedes the natural exchange of gases through the skin's surface. And in some cosmetic products too high a concentration of preservatives can cut down the skin's ability to inhale. On the rest of the body we wear layer upon layer of clothing, much of it made from synthetic materials, which also tend to restrict this skin breathing process. All this, together with the fact that few women breathe deeply and fully even through their lungs, means that they may be severely depriving the skin of vitality both from inside and out.

Recently cosmetic manufacturers have begun to produce products—foundations and water-in-oil moisturizers—that do not interfere with the skin's air absorption. There are also several good treatment creams for older skin that contain ingredients designed to stimulate the skin's use of oxygen, which can be particularly helpful in aging skin. But whatever products you use on your skin, give it time to rest some of each night by cleansing it thoroughly and then leaving it free. For instance, there is no reason to wear a night cream all night long. With any treatment product you put on your skin, the lion's share of what the skin will pick up is taken in during the first twenty minutes after you apply it. Leaving it on longer than that is a waste of time.

A night cream or a treatment oil or a mask can be applied after cleansing, for instance, left on for fifteen minutes to half an hour, and then removed before bedtime, so that your skin will be left free to breathe throughout the night.

On the other hand there are also useful tools for encouraging the skin cells' use of oxygen. As your skin begins to age, its respiration slows down so dramatically that by the time you are sixty your skin may be taking in only half as much oxygen as a teenager's. At that stage it is helpful to take adequate supplies of pantothenic acid and the other B-complex vitamins and to use products containing placental extracts on the skin's surface.

The skin on the rest of your body needs air too. Traditional European naturopathic methods of treatment have for years insisted on "air baths" as a means of increasing resistance to disease and strengthening the whole body. Patients are exposed to air in the nude or near nude for a specific period of time daily and even in cold weather. The treatment is even used with babies and small children, for colds and other infections. Practitioners claim that one of the main reasons women tend to feel so well during the summer months, while they are on the beach, is simply that their skin's surface is exposed to the air for long periods of time and that, although the sun's ultraviolet rays are destructive to skin tissue, the air exposure does it nothing but good: helping to clear up rough patches, lending a youthful glow to skin from improved circulation and better use of oxygen in the cells, and even, they say, revitalizing the whole body. They recommend spending from five to fifteen minutes a day (depending on the temperature) unclothed in the air—preferably outside or if that is not possible at least in a room in which the windows are wide open. They also recommend sleeping in a well-ventilated room. However you do it, find a way to set your skin free in the air for a few hours in every twenty-four.

Herbal Saunas Are Good for All Types of Skin

Every now and then (how often depends on whether your skin tends to be dry or oily and whether you live in the polluted air of cities or the clearer, fresh air of the country) skin needs more than everyday cleaning. It needs *deep* cleansing, and one of the most effective ways of getting it is from a facial sauna. In fact, the only skin condition that doesn't benefit from facial steams, or saunas, is that in which broken capillaries appear in the cheeks and nose, in which case the warm steam could aggravate the condition.

A facial sauna will open the pores, drawing out impurities in them, soften the texture of the face, and tone the skin, all at the same time. If your skin is oily, you can benefit from one a couple of times a week. If your skin is dry, have one only once every two weeks. A facial steam is also an excellent way of preparing skin for treatment with masks, essential oils, creams, and vitamins.

Here's how: Toss a couple of handfuls of mixed herbs (see below) into two quarts of water you have brought to the boil and then removed from the heat. Now cover your whole head with a towel and put it over the steaming pot so the towel forms a tent to catch the steam. Sit in front of the steaming pot (not closer than one foot from the water), and breathe in the scent of the aromatic herbs for five to ten minutes. Finish the treatment by splashing with cool water to remove wastes accumulated on the surface of the skin, and follow either with a treatment cream or mask, or your usual moisturizer.

Here are some of the herbs you can choose from: camomile, elder blossom, mint, basil, rosemary (particularly good for oily skin), sage, slippery-elm bark (good for sensitive skin), comfrey leaf and root (also good for delicate or inflamed or troubled skin), strawberry leaf, raspberry leaf, acacia flower, lavender, and rose petal.

The Mask Effect

Masks are one of the mysteries of the cosmetic world. The manufactured kinds come in many varieties and are designed for several purposes. You have to pick the right one for the right purpose. Many women don't. This is probably why they are often disappointed. Dermatologists disagree about their effectiveness. While some swear by them, others consider them little more than cosmetic security blankets. Chosen carefully, I believe, a mask can be a boon to beauty.

A mask is designed to perform one of the more specific tasks: to deep-cleanse, to tone, to stimulate circulation, to moisturize the skin, or to exfoliate—that is, to remove the outer layers of dead epidermal cells so the skin is refined and left more receptive to whatever treatment product you choose to put on it after. Most commercial masks contain a great amount of water, which makes their evaporation rate rapid and gives the skin a cooling and soothing feel. But this is of little more than psychological help to the user. The deep response to elements in a mask comes through the vascular network in the dermis, where active ingredients coupled with physical tension from the mask drying on the skin bring about increased circulation and help stimulate cellular activity.

1 THE TIGHTENING EFFECT

Putting the skin under a controlled degree of positive stress makes it look good. Most masks are smoothed on and then left to harden. They gently squeeze and pinch the flesh while they are hardening. This constriction of the tissue, coupled with whatever stimulating properties the ingredients have, sets up a kind of temporary tension. When the constricting substance is rinsed away or peeled off, the blood vessels in the inner layer of the skin expand, the skin turns a pink tone, and the inner layer of it swells up somewhat as the fluid escapes from the enlarged blood vessels. This fluid plumps up the skin, making it resemble younger, more hydrated skin and making fine lines temporarily disappear. If the mask's tightening effect is powerful enough (as it is in clay-based masks, used for oily skin), the pores are also constricted, making them look smaller than they are. The whole face appears younger, smoother-textured, and more alive. The only trouble is, this mask effect is very transient. Almost as rapidly as it arrives, it can vanish, for as escaped fluid is reabsorbed, the skin returns to its normal state. But, for many women, this temporary lift, coupled with the fifteen or twenty minutes of enforced relaxation, is a useful beauty treatment.

2 THE EARTH TREATMENT

Some of the most common and useful masks contain a clay base to absorb excess oil and in the process lift out dirt from the skin's pores. They usually also incorporate such ingredients as resorcinol and salicylic acid to slow down the activity of the oil glands themselves. They are designed for oily, combination, and blemished skin ("combination" meaning dry skin that has an oily "T" patch across the forehead and down the nose), and can be a remarkably effective adjunct to your regular skin-care regimen. Most of them dry on the skin. Clay also has a mild bleaching agent in it, which slightly lightens the skin. These masks are definitely *not* for the driest or most sensitive skins and are a kiss of death to any skin with broken capillaries.

3 FACIAL PEEL-OFFS

In recent years, some of the most popular masks have been the peel-offs. Based on rubber, wax, or some kind of plastic, they are applied with a brush or fingertips, left to harden, and then finally peeled off like a piece of cellophane tape, taking surface dirt and some of the old dead cells of the epidermis with them. Because most of the peel-offs are translucent and many even transparent, they can be worn without fear of frightening the postman or the child. They form an occlusive layer on the skin which prevents water from escaping and encourages the tissues to store it up. They also contain specific treatment agents to soften the skin, and they come in formulas for all skin types.

4 CREAMS AND GELS

Other masks are specifically designed for moisturizing as well as treatment. They contain such substances as collagen, NMFs, estrogens, and silicones and are formulated to increase the water retention of the skin and to soften its texture. In the form of a gel or a nondrying cream, they are ideal for dehydrated skin and can be used several times a week if necessary. They do not exfoliate, but they do refine the texture of the skin slightly, leaving it smoother and softer to the touch.

5 EXFOLIATORS

Although usually classified as masks, really these products are simply designed for smoothing out the surface of the skin, much as fine sandpaper does to mahogany. Very young skin doesn't need them. In the process of exfoliation, or skin sloughing, the cells that are dead on the surface are taken off, the pores (which may be blocked by cellular buildup) are opened, and excess pigmentation on the surface of the skin is removed. The texture is improved. Your skin becomes more translucent and a lighter and more uniform color. Exfoliation is particularly helpful to skin after thirty; as skin ages, the reproductive processes in the basal cells slow down. Removing the top layers of dead cells tends to stimulate these cells to reproduce more rapidly. It also makes the skin more receptive to any external treatment given afterward. There are two types of exfoliators on the market. Either will do the job well, so it is a matter of personal choice. One is a chemical exfoliator, which dissolves the cells when it is applied. The other is a pot-scraper physical exfoliator, which comes either as a little pad you wash with; as a mask you put on, let dry, and then rub off like rubber cement; or as a cream containing lots of tiny grains. This kind you put on wet skin and rub gently for two or three minutes while the little particles in it scrape off the surface cells. Your skin can benefit from exfoliation once a week if it is dry, two or three times a week if it is oily.

THE MEDIUM OF MASSAGE

Provided it is done skillfully, massage is a wonderful treatment for the face. But it must be done gently and carefully, for the muscles of the face and neck are made up of fine fibers which, unlike muscles in the rest of the body, are attached not only to bone but also to the skin itself. They are, therefore, delicate and must never be pulled hard, or massage can have a detrimental effect, rather than a helpful one. Always following the direction of the muscle fibers themselves, massage will stimulate blood circulation, which improves the tone of muscles and skin and promotes the use of nutrients in the cells and the elimination of wastes. Massage will also help the skin to absorb active ingredients in creams and essential oils.

Always begin a massage by covering your face with a cream or oil—preferably an essential oil or oils mixed with a carrier (see chapter on aromatherapy). Begin with effleurage, which means moving the palm of your hand and your fingers lightly over the surface of the skin. This has a soothing effect and a relaxing one which encourages blood and lymph flow. Start at the center of the chest with your right hand, sweeping it outward toward the left shoulder and then upward over the left side of your neck. Then do the same for the other side with your left hand. (Actually these movements can be done simultaneously, using both hands at once.) Now massage from the base of the neck at the rear to the hairline. Do each stroke five times. Massage the neck, bringing first one hand and then the other around the curve of the neck from back to front —also five times. Now bring each hand, one at a time, upward over the front and sides of the neck, under the chin, and outward at the jawline (five times each side). Stroke upward from corners of the mouth to temples (five times). Now, using the palms of your hands, stroke upward from the chin, over the jawline to the hairline so that the fingers cover the center portion of the face and the cupped palms go over first jaw and then cheekbones to end at the temples (five times). Stroke around the eyes. Begin at inner corners, at both sides of the nose, and using your middle finger, stroke outward around the eye to the outer corner. Then begin at the same inner corner and stroke upward and outward in a half circle around the top part of the eye, just underneath the bone that forms the eye socket. (Repeat upper and lower semicircle five times each side.) Now stroke across the forehead, using the left hand to move from right to left, followed by the right hand moving from left to right—five times each side. Finally, with the tips of your fingers tap lightly several times all over the chin and jawline, then over the cheekbones, then all across the forehead.

Finish off the massage by removing the excess oil still left on the skin and splashing with cold water several times.

THE ESOTERIC HELPERS

Probably the finest toner you will ever find is simple ice-cold water. This is an excellent shock treatment not only for everyday use but also as part of postoperative care after plastic surgery. It stimulates cells, improves circulation, and brings back life to a neglected face.

Here's how to give yourself a water treatment: Add two dozen ice cubes to a basin of cold water. Tie back your hair and cover your face with a layer of rich cream (oily and thick) or Vaseline or vegetable oil. Put on cotton-lined rubber gloves (I prefer to wear cotton, rather than rubber, gloves). Splash water on your cheeks ten times, under your chin ten times, on your neck ten times, and on your closed eyes five times. By now your face should be tingling and feeling frozen, so you are ready to go to work on the parts that most need firming, such as lines around the eyes, and double chin. Splash each section six to ten times. (You can begin with half the number of splashes everywhere and work up each time you give the treatment.) Finish by patting your skin dry with a soft towel and then applying a little oil or eye cream under the eyes and on the cheeks. You can use this freezing treatment every morning if you like, or only once a week. It is good for all skin types except those with broken capillaries, which should never be put under the strain of temperature extremes.

Another marvelous skin treatment is spring water. Although I cannot say why, the spraying of spring water in microscopically small droplets from an aerosol can can not only hydrate skin but can also help eliminate skin eruptions and alleviate dry skin. I know two French dermatologists and an English one who have found this treatment useful in all kinds of skin inflammation as well. One of them believes that its beneficial results come from its being in such small droplets that the skin will actually take the water into itself. Whether or not this is true I don't know, but I do know it can greatly improve the texture and look of skin when used regularly. It is best to spray your skin after cleansing night and morning, before applying moisturizers or treatment products. I also find treatment products appear to be more effective when used after a skin spray.

Ionization is excellent for improving skin of all types and ages. Ionization is the discharging of negative air ions into the atmosphere and is well known for its ability to speed the healing of severe burns. It has also been shown to be helpful in the treatment of many types of migraine and respiratory ailments and in improving mental clarity. Negative ions, which have often been referred to as "vitamins of the air," are negatively charged air molecules which occur naturally in unpolluted air, particularly by the sea or a river or in the mountains. It is the presence of these molecules, which carry a tiny negative charge, that makes one feel so well standing beside a waterfall in the country. It is also partly their absence in polluted air and in the air of centrally heated or air-conditioned offices and houses that makes some people feel tired or depressed, and which can cause illness and emotional disturbances in weather-sensitive people when the so-called ill winds blow, such as the sharav in the Middle East, the foehn in Germany, the mistral in southern France and the chinook in the Rocky Mountains of the United States.

Scientists still do not know whether the beneficial effects of negative ionization occur as a result of these tiny particles being absorbed by the skin, or taken in through the lungs in breathing, or both. But, besides their other health-promoting properties, negative ions are useful in improving acned and blemished skin and, even more important, in helping protect skin against premature aging.

This particular aspect of ionization is not one that has been proved scientifically yet, for most of the research into the use of air ions has been in the treatment of specific ailments, not as cosmetic treatment, but I can vouch for its effectiveness. I have seen it improve the skin of a number of women with all types of skin and of all ages. An ionizer you can put beside your bed at night will also help you sleep soundly. Ionizers are not cheap, but they are a most worthwhile investment.

28

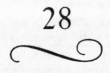

Skin:
When Something Goes Wrong

Theoretically, having beautiful skin is simple: Take one part clear young skin, add the forty or so known nutrients from fresh foods eaten as much as possible in their natural state and whole, and mix together with exercise for overall tone and proper breathing for good oxygenation of cells. Put in a dose of fresh air and a pinch of stimulation now and then. Stir well and you've got a recipe that will last for years. That's the theory. In practice, however, things can go wrong: an early wrinkle, brown spots to mar a perfect complexion, acne, dryness, roughness—that's when you need help from special cosmetics, vitamins, and treatments.

WHEN SKIN DRIES OUT

The Cause

Dried-out, dried-up skin usually comes from underactive sebaceous glands, which, due to a hormone imbalance or vitamin or mineral deficiencies, don't produce enough of this important oily fluid to lubricate the skin and protect it from excessive water loss. It can also be the result of being exposed to excessively drying weather conditions, central heating, or air conditioning. Another, rarer cause is being on a diet too low in essential fatty acids, such as a fat-free slimming regimen. Finally, sometimes dried-out skin is due to an incorrect water balance in the horny cells as a result of their being exposed to water (e.g. in swimming) for so long that they have swollen and burst, or to their having been deprived of water for so long that they gradually desiccate. Excessive dryness of the skin also occurs in people who, unknown to themselves, are suffering from subclinical deficiencies of vitamin A or C or any one of several of the B-complex group or of linoleic acid.

The incidence of dry skin is increasing, probably as a result of air pollution, artificial atmospheric conditions, the use of certain drugs, or the overuse of detergents and soaps on the face. Such skin conditions as neurodermatitis, fungus infections, contact dermatitis, psoriasis and seborrheic dermatitis are often confused with dry skin.

A combination of these factors will result in a skin that can look a dullish gray-white color and boast an ever-increasing number of fine lines. If you look at dry skin very closely, it rather resembles a mosaic. As changes in the hydration of skin take place, the edges of the dead cells in the stratum corneum curl up to form a network of minute "chaps" on the skin's surface. Then, once the keratin in the epidermis dries up, the skin shrinks and becomes brittle.

Prevention and Cure

Use a water-in-oil emulsion on your face night and day to protect against excessive water loss by trapping the water in the outer layer of the skin and preventing it from being given up into the atmosphere. Ensure that you get enough essential fatty acids in your diet by using olive, sunflower, or safflower oil in your salad dressings.

Consider taking supplements of vitamins A and D in the form of fish liver oil, or drinking fresh carrot juice a couple of times a day. Fish liver oil put directly on the skin can help too. Of course it smells foul, but the smell doesn't usually last very long. And you need leave the oil on the skin for only fifteen minutes; then you can remove the excess with a tissue. Vitamin E either taken internally or rubbed on the skin from capsules is often helpful too.

Other helpful things include a humidifier, weekly steaming of the skin followed by an oil massage, and mineral water sprayed from an atomizer before applying your moisturizer or treatment products. Don't wash your skin with soap. Don't use any skin product containing alcohol. Use a mask for dry skin. Use aromatherapy oils you mix yourself to contain the essences most useful for dry skin, such as geranium, camomile, rose, sandalwood, lavender, and ylang-ylang. Always choose an oil-based makeup foundation.

DEALING WITH AN OIL CRISIS

The Cause

Oily skin is the result of overactive sebaceous glands, which usually occurs due to a hormonal imbalance in the body. Occasionally a diet too high in fats and fried foods or refined sugar can contribute to the condition, as can too much stimulation of the sebaceous glands by heat, the sun, or skin-care products containing chemicals such as sulfur, which, although they are designed to dry out the condition, in the long run work in a counterproductive way by removing too much oil and thereby stimulating the glands to produce yet more. Studies show that people on diets slightly deficient in some of the B group of vitamins rapidly develop whiteheads, blackheads, and oily hair and skin.

Prevention and Cure

Treatment for seborrhea is rapidly changing. Dermatologists used to think the way to deal with the condition was literally to dry out the skin. Soaps, lotions, and treatment creams containing sulfur and harsh chemicals specifically designed to degrease the skin were used. Then you were told to wear a heavy, occlusive foundation, which completely covered up the skin and any blemishes, and you hoped for the best. Oily skin was treated roughly.

Dermatologists now realize that oily skin is not the tough and robust stuff they once thought it was. They have found that the use of drying agents in cosmetic products tends in most cases only to treat the problem temporarily by removing excess oil at the expense of worsening the condition in the long run. For these same drying agents that remove the oil also stimulate the sebaceous glands to produce more. Attempts to cover it up and to cover up acne with heavy, drying makeup are generally unsuccessful too. The shine comes through in a few hours and leaves your face a cakey, artificial-looking mess, which, instead of hiding the condition, makes it look worse.

The new approach is different, but it may take time for you to get used to if you are still thinking in the old way. Instead of using harsh, chemical-containing soaps and drying creams on your skin, buy a mild, lotion cleanser without any drying agent (which would degrease the skin) for cleansing and removing makeup. It should be an oil-in-water emulsion, which removes excess oil by emulsifying it in its oily phase while it dissolves other debris in its water phase. Rub it on gently with clean hands, then wipe it off completely with tissues before rinsing with fresh, cool water. It is important to remove it all. You don't need a tonic or a freshener, but if you want one, make sure it contains no alcohol (alcohol is also a drier).

During the day, wear a water-in-oil moisturizer, which will have the effect of stabilizing the flow of sebum from the glands, since it mixes with the natural fats on the face and doesn't degrease the skin. Forget the heavy foundation. Instead, as soon as the moisturizer has had a chance to set, powder your face with double the amount of powder you would usually use, dust off the excess, then spray the face with a fine mist of water (preferably spring water from an aerosol, but you can use ordinary water in a spray bottle so long as the spray is very fine). Now blot with a tissue and then powder again. This will keep your skin looking fresh and matt as well as calming the flow of oil from trigger-happy glands. It will also gradually shrink the size of your pores. Then, throughout the day, every three or four hours or whenever necessary, you can repowder, and you'll never end up with the ugly, cakey mess oily-skinned women usually get.

Also, stay out of the sun. Sunbathing may dry your skin for a while, but when indoors weather comes you will find you're faced with the results of the same situation: overstimulation of the sebaceous glands by ultraviolet light, which results in all the problems you have been trying to get rid of.

From a nutritional point of view, if your skin is too oily, don't eat fatty foods or fried foods and do eat plenty of green vegetables raw and B-complex vitamins from whole-grain breads and cereals, liver, or brewer's yeast supplements. Brewer's yeast both taken internally (a tablespoon stirred into a glass of fruit or vegetable juice three times a day) and also mixed with yogurt and used as a face mask on freshly cleansed skin is very helpful in calming overeager sebaceous glands. Let it dry for fifteen minutes and then wash it off with warm (not hot) water, splashing with cold to finish. Use the mask three times a week until the condition is well under control, and then once a week.

The B vitamins (particularly B_6, niacin, and B_2) in these foods are vital in the treatment of excessively oily skin and the acne that often accompanies it. Vitamin A can also be useful in treating skin that is too oily. It can be taken together with vitamin D as fish liver oil or in higher doses on its own as well. Vitamin C, potassium, and calcium have also been reported helpful. Because vitamin A is an oil-soluble vitamin and excesses tend to remain stored in the body, there is always the danger of taking too much of it. But as most nutritionists who concern themselves with vitamin therapy point out, one would have to take excessively large amounts of the vitamin—probably 150,000 international units a day over a period of many months—for toxicity to develop. And deficiency of vitamin A disturbs the normal activity and size of sebaceous and sweat glands. High-estrogen brands of the Pill sometimes help excessively oily skin, although some birth-control pills seem to aggravate it.

ULTRASENSITIVE AND ALLERGIC SKIN

The Causes

Although allergies and allergic reactions to particular substances are not inherited, a tendency to them can be. If, for instance, both your mother and your father suffered from allergies, you have a 57 percent chance of them too. Approximately 15 percent of all women are said to be highly prone to allergic reactions, 25–30 percent are less easily sensitized (which means they will react adversely only to some substances, sometimes), and 55–60 percent are relatively allergy-free or only rarely prone to allergic reactions. But, on the whole, allergic complaints are on the increase, and cosmetic dermatitis and skin sensitivities are leading the field. For instance, in one study of skin ailments in the mid-seventies it was found that where, four years before, only 3 percent of the patients in Britain seen by dermatologists were suffering from skin reactions, in the space of a very few years it had risen to 14 percent.

The word allergy means "altered response" in Greek. If you are allergic to something, this means that your body has come into contact with it and instead of reacting normally to it or not at all, it has reacted with hostility. This seldom happens the first time you meet the substance (called an allergen), but if for some reason your body takes a dislike to it, it will create an antibody that is a chemical specifically made to repel any future invasion by the same substance. Then, when sufficient antibodies are available, they combine with the allergen, and this combination triggers the release of histamines and histamine-like substances, which by a series of reactions finally results in raised, red, itchy splotches on the skin. This is known as an acute reaction, for it occurs within seconds or minutes after coming in contact with the allergen. You can inhale it, say in the form of a hair spray, or you can take it in through your skin as a face cream or a makeup product.

There are also delayed reactions, which come about only after a few hours or even days after coming into contact with the allergen. This kind of reaction doesn't occur the first time one comes near the substance. In the case of delayed reactions, there is no histamine formation, but, instead, during contact with the allergen the body's white blood cells come to recognize it as foreign and mobilize themselves to attack. Then the capillaries in the area become clogged with waste, and the skin flakes and scales, becoming red and itchy or even very sore.

Prevention and Cure

Antihistamines will alleviate the first sort of allergic reaction, as will special injections to build up tolerance to the allergen. Antihistamines will do nothing for the delayed-reaction-type allergy. And although cortisone and cortisone-like medications are useful in quelling both types of allergic skin reaction, they should be used only in very serious cases and then only for short periods of time. Finally, they should always be used under a doctor's supervision because of the long-term very detrimental side effects that go with cortisone administration. Apart from nutritional therapy to strengthen the whole organism against allergic reactions, the only effective way to deal with skin sensitivities is to locate the allergen —the substance or product causing trouble—and then remove it from your life.

This is not always the easiest of tasks, for an allergen can be almost anything, from a biological detergent to a beautiful-smelling talc. A clue to its identity lies in the area where the red blotches or scaling first appears. If it is on your hands, for instance, check out the detergent you have been washing dishes in, your hand cream, your nail polish, the soap you wash your hands with. If it is around the eyes, it might be an eye cream, an eye-makeup remover, a mascara, or an eye shadow. Test this out by smearing a little of the substance on the gauze of a Band-Aid and then taping it to a newly washed area of your back or underarm. Use a fresh Band-Aid for each substance. Then leave the patches on for twenty-four hours and remove. Any area that shows up as red or blotched indicates that the substance on that patch is one to which you have a sensitivity. After that, avoid it.

Here are the chemical substances that, according to dermatologists, are most often implicated in reactions and skin sensitivities. But remember: The culprit can be almost anything.*

ALLERGEN	COMMON COSMETICS AND HOUSEHOLD PRODUCTS CONTAINING IT
Aluminum salts	Deodorants, antiperspirants, astringents
Ammonia	Bleaches, household chemicals
Ammoniated mercury	Freckle creams, antiseptic ointments
Aniline dyes	Hair colorants, eyebrow pencil
Barium salts	Dipilatories
Beta-naphthol	Freckle creams
Boric acid	Lipsticks, baby skin creams and lotions

* Source: Cutaneous Reactions to Cosmetics; Committee on Cutaneous Health and Cosmetics: AMA, 1965; Lubowe, 1965; Fisher, 1970.

ALLERGEN	COMMON COSMETICS AND HOUSEHOLD PRODUCTS CONTAINING IT
Cresylic compounds	Household antiseptics
Essential oils	Perfumes, deodorants
Formaldehyde	Plastics, preservatives, air fresheners, disinfectants, nail hardeners
Lanolin	Face creams and lotions, hair preparations, skin softeners
Lauryl alcohol sulfates	Water-soluble preparations, cleansing creams, shampoos, body, hand, and skin lotions
Mercuric bichloride	Freckle creams, antiseptic lotions
Para-amino benzoic acid	Sunscreen lotions and creams
Phenylenediamine compounds	Eye shadow, eyelash and eyebrow coloring, other cosmetics, hair colors
Phenyl salicylates	Suntan lotions, creams, sprays
Phthalates	Insect repellents
Propylene glycol	Water-soluble creams, hand creams
Resins	Plastics, drip-dry clothing, balsam of Peru, hair spray, nail polish
Salicylic acid	Face-peeling compounds, dandruff shampoos, acne lotions and soaps, corn removers
Soaps	Cleansing creams and shampoos
Sulfur	Dandruff shampoos, acne preparations
Thioglycolate	Cream rinses, body builders for hair, wave-set lotions, permanent hair-waving lotions, shampoos
Zinc salts	Astringents, deodorants

Avoid contact with any substance or cosmetic product containing a substance to which you suspect you may be allergic. When you cleanse your skin, do it thoroughly with two cleansers: a cream or lotion first, to dissolve makeup and grime, then a specially formulated hypoallergenic soap or detergent cleanser that is pH-balanced. Always dry your skin thoroughly every time it comes in contact with water, and always handle your skin gently, never pushing or pulling it. When you apply creams or oils, use the fleshy parts of your middle or ring fingers, never your index finger, and make sure your hands are scrupulously clean. For applying eye shadow, use cotton-tipped sticks, which can then be tossed away after use. Throw away your powder puff and instead always use a fresh piece of sterilized cotton. Always wear a water-in-oil moisturizer during the day.

Get to know the hypoallergenic cosmetics—skin-care and makeup products made without *known* irritants. Most are inexpensive yet very good and specially formulated with ingredients that have little likelihood of causing problems. The prefix "hypo" means "less." Hypoallergenic products are designed to be less allergy-producing than other cosmetics. They are fragrance-free and leave out such common troublemakers as aluminum salts, wool fat, and phenol.

One of the most common causes of cosmetic dermatitis is nail polish. It is also one of the least-expected offenders, because it seems to cover such a small area. But your hands tend to touch your face and body often, and if you are allergic to the varnish you are wearing, it can wreak havoc with skin elsewhere, so always use a hypoallergenic nail enamel.

From a nutritional point of view, there is a lot to be said about the underlying conditions that appear to make one prone to allergic reactions. Many people who tend toward these reactions have a mineral imbalance: too much copper, for instance, and too little zinc; the presence of excessive quantities of heavy metals in their bodies; or either a subclinical vitamin deficiency or a particularly high requirement of certain nutrients, most often the B group of vitamins. A deficiency of essential fatty acids is also often linked with allergic reactions. Often skin sensitivities can be alleviated by giving vitamin B_6, PABA, and B_2 supplements along with brewer's yeast or another supplement containing the whole of the B range.

Researchers at the University of Uppsala, in Sweden, have linked skin hypersensitivity to the intake of food dyes and preservatives too. It is a good idea, if you have allergy-prone skin, to avoid all overprocessed convenience foods. Often a skin eruption, like simple prickly-heat rashes, will yield itself to supplementation of the diet with vitamin C. Some researchers have had results by giving a mere 1,000 milligrams of vitamin C in two 500-milligram doses each day. Others claim it is necessary to give between six and ten grams per day in doses spread throughout the day. Stress plays an important part in allergic reactions of any kind, so a conscious relaxation or meditation technique practiced regularly can help too.

For immediate relief, skin inflammations usually respond well to calamine lotion, simple witch hazel, and some poultices made with herbs. One of the best to use is comfrey—whose very name denotes healing in Latin. It contains the natural anti-inflammatory substance allantoin, which is often used in skin ointments. Make a comfrey compress by pouring half a cup of boiling water over half a cup of the dried herb. Let it cool to a bearable temperature, near body heat, then put the wet herb on the face. Cover with gauze and lie down for fifteen minutes while it cools. This kind of compress will also reduce the pain and swelling over a bruise or a pulled muscle, as well as calm inflamed skin.

WHEN ACNE STRIKES

The Cause

It is more common among teenagers than among any other age group, although acne, an infection of the sebaceous glands, can occur at any time in life. It shows up as blackheads, whiteheads, pimples, and pustules that occur on the face and neck, back and chest, almost always when levels of testosterone and progesterone—two hormones necessary for growth—are high. Testosterone, known as the male hormone (although women have it in small quantities too), spurs the sebaceous glands to increase their production of sebum. When too much sebum is produced, a keratinous plug can fill the duct, which then becomes infected while the skin around it becomes inflamed. If the problem is severe enough—and luckily most people never get to this stage—the walls of the infected ducts even disintegrate, and cystic lesions may develop in the skin which leave permanent scars after the infection itself has healed.

The cause of acne is still not completely understood, and the recommended treatment tends to vary from dermatologist to dermatologist and even from year to year. Much of the medical profession has tended to ignore the nutritional aspect of treatment, although vitamin and mineral therapy coupled with proper external care has been responsible for many cures. Many people with acne are victims of one or another food allergy —the most common allergens being wheat, milk, or preservatives and colorings. And when the elimination of waste via the alimentary canal is inadequate, often wastes are eliminated through the skin. This is certainly a contributor to acne. Some experts believe that acne is made worse by a diet high in fat and sugar, and there is some evidence linking acne with a disturbance of carbohydrate metabolism. Most doctors agree that iodides and bromides can contribute significantly to acne. Iodides are found in iodized salt, saltwater fish, and shellfish, and some drugs containing iodides or bromides may aggravate the condition; these include cough syrups, sedatives, and cold medications. Finally, stress and emotional upset are often implicated.

Prevention and Cure

Look to your diet first. Eliminate sweets, sugared soft drinks, and fatty foods such as nuts and fried foods. The *Rohsäfte-Kur* followed by a diet in which at least 50 percent of your foods are eaten raw often does wonders for even long-term acne, provided it is used in conjunction with the proper external care and vitamin and mineral supplements where necessary. Vitamin A, taken internally, helps restore and then maintain clear, healthy skin in a daily dose of 10,000 to 25,000 international units. Riboflavin and pyridoxine (B_6) are essential in reducing the secretion of excess sebum and in eliminating the tendency to blackhead formation. Vitamin C in large doses—from 6 to 8 grams a day—can help prevent infection, and vitamin E both taken internally and used on the surface of the skin can be helpful in preventing scarring. The mineral most useful in the treatment of acne appears to be zinc. It can be taken as chelated zinc or zinc gluconate, 15 milligrams twice a day. Finally, some experts in nutritional therapy find that niacin (B_3) taken in doses of 50 to 100 milligrams a day can help because of its dynamic action on circulation and its ability to increase the blood supply to the troubled area. Of course any B vitamin should never be taken alone but be accompanied by the full B group.

Externally, it is essential to keep the skin clean, removing dirt and excess oil or waxy sebum regularly, but this should be done with gentle, pH-balanced soaps or detergent cleansers that do not contain sulfur or bactericidals or other drying chemicals, which in the long run can only make matters worse. Skin should be washed in warm water at least twice a day and steamed twice a week to encourage the release of waste matter. Of course your hands should be immaculate so as not to encourage further infection.

Topical agents are often helpful. Vitamin A acid (available only by prescription) applied to the skin is one of the commonly used and generally effective treatments for acne. It appears to work because by halting the excess growth of cells that clog follicles, it also drastically peels away the layers of dead cells that clog pores. It brings about an intense redness and skin peeling at first, making the acne seem much worse. But after several weeks it reduces oiliness and the number of blackheads and eruptions. It usually takes about six weeks to treat skin with this method, using a 5 percent solution. Another approach to treatment for girls and women is to give conjugated estrogens (1.25 milligrams) just before menstruation, which seems to suppress flare-ups that occur with the monthly period. But there are often complications with this method, as there are with putting women on the Pill for the treatment of acne. It can delay menstruation and of course does affect the endocrine balance in the body as a whole.

Sometimes dermatologists use the antibiotic tetracycline, usually administered in doses of 250 milligrams twice a day. In many cases this has dramatically reduced the acne probably by altering the chemistry of fatty acids in the skin so that the sebaceous glands are rendered less active, as well as acting on the infection itself. But there are disadvantages to antibiotic treatment, too, particularly in growing teenagers, for it does inhibit protein synthesis in mammalian cells. It can also stain the teeth when used over a long period of time and of course disrupts the natural intestinal flora, which produce many of the body's B-complex vitamins.

Sometimes a dermatologist will lance a cyst in order to release the trapped infection in it and help it heal. Resorcinol, a white crystalline antiseptic substance that is soluble in water, alcohol, and oils, is often useful and prescribed along with vitamin A acid. It is antiseptic and antifungal.

An outmoded treatment for acne, X-ray therapy, will slow down the activity of the oil glands by destroying their very active cells, but it is also dangerous since X rays are destructive to skin in general. Indeed, X rays used for acne treatment have been linked with the occurrence of skin cancer later. Like X-ray therapy, sun exposure for acne is also controversial. It does seem to help temporarily in some cases. The trouble is that although it is beneficial while you are in the sun and although tanning makes the appearance of acne less offensive, the condition often becomes much worse after periods of sun exposure. Sunlight, either "sun lamps" or the real thing, should be used only if you have certain proof from past experience that it is helpful to you in the long run. Because of the stress aspects of acne, both regular exercise and meditation or deep relaxation can be helpful too.

Treatment of Scars

The treatment of acne scars is a different matter altogether. It should only be attempted *after* the acne has completely cleared up. There are three methods: dermabrasion, chemical peels, and plastic surgery.

A smoothing operation to minimize the pits and wrinkles on the skin, dermabrasion demands great skill in the hands of the dermatologist, who uses a motor-driven wire brush, rather like a dentist's high-speed drill, to take off the epidermis. The skin is first sprayed with a refrigerant—often ethyl chloride—to eliminate pain. Then the imperfections are abraded using a variety of brushes, or *fraises,* finishing off with a very smooth disk called a diamond *fraise.* Planing away the skin's surface like this makes the acne pits seem shallower. It also makes the follicles shorter and thicker by taking off the top layers, so one can hope the oil secreted by the glands can more easily reach the surface of the skin and they won't become so easily blocked in the future. After dermabrasion, the patient is sent home with pain-killers for a few days while a crusty surface develops on the top of the skin. This is shed in a week or so, leaving the reddish new surface which gradually returns in color to normal.

Chemical peeling aims at much the same thing, but instead of using a physical abrader it relies on a caustic substance such as trichloracetic acid or phenol to do the job. It can be difficult to control the depth to which the burning takes place, but this is terribly important, for if the chemical peeling goes too deep, only scar tissue will grow back all over the face. This is why much peeling that is done nowadays is done with milder chemicals that limit the amount of peeling and drying of the skin. In the case of mild peeling, the edema that develops helps temporarily at least to smooth over irregularities of the skin.

With a deeper peeling, the patient is given an anesthetic; then the chemical peeler is applied. In a few minutes the skin turns grayish white. Then, later, a brown crust appears, which falls off after three to five days. Alternatively the dermatologist can cover your face with occlusive surgical tape to get a deeper penetration. A day or two afterward, the tape is removed to leave an oozy, reddish-brown mask that looks a little like a very bad sunburn; then, in a week to ten days, the crust falls off and the new, pinkish skin appears beneath it.

Chemical peeling for acne scars is expensive and has many possible side effects. It can cause scarring and occasionally serious infection if proper sterilization procedures are not carried out. It makes the skin extremely sensitive to sunlight, so that it often develops brown splotches.

Cosmetic surgery can sometimes help scarred skin simply because the pulling up of the skin smooths it out and lessens the depth of pits and scars. Some surgeons will cut out raised scars and then later treat the flattened scar area that remains by dermabrasion. Often, treatment for acne scars employs a combination of these methods.

One more treatment for acne needs to be mentioned, although it is little known in some countries, particularly the United States. This is the use of pulsed high-frequency (PHF) waves directly on the surface of the skin. Electromagnetic medicine has long been used in the hands of physiotherapists to treat athletic injuries. It can also be an effective treatment for acne, eczema, psoriasis, and other skin problems, probably because of the ability of PHF to stimulate rapid healing of tissue and to minimize scarring. The practitioner directs the pulsed radio waves from a machine to the troubled area for half an hour and then treats the liver and the adrenal area (the pulsed waves enter the body to a depth of 6 inches) to encourage total body healing. PHF treatment is also useful after cosmetic surgery and dermabrasion, to speed healing and minimize scarring.

STRETCH MARKS CAN BE AVOIDED

The Cause

Stretch marks occur frequently on the abdomen and breasts of pregnant women and on the thighs, hips, and buttocks of women who have been overweight—particularly women who are deficient in zinc, vitamin B_6, or both. These two nutrients are necessary for the health of collagen tissue and for the maintenance of a high level of elasticity in the skin. A sudden increase in weight or volume of an area of the body or the swelling of breasts and abdomen in pregnancy results in these unsightly lines, which are difficult to eliminate.

Prevention and Cure

Ensure that you get adequate zinc and vitamin B_6 in your diet—if necessary by supplementing it. Women who are on the Pill are particularly susceptible to subclinical deficiencies of these two nutrients, because oral contraceptives have a marked effect on the body's need for and use of zinc and B_6, along with iron, B_2, folic acid, B_{12}, and vitamin C. If you gain weight or become pregnant, treat your skin from outside with preventative measures by rubbing on an aromatherapy oil for your skin type twice a day or by the use of cocoa butter or one of the products specifically designed for preventing stretch marks.

There is supposed to be no cure for stretch marks once they are formed, for the consistency of the skin itself in that area has changed to resemble scar tissue and therefore remains permanently disfigured. Nutritionist Adelle Davis claimed that when one woman who had developed stretch marks during her first pregnancy took 600 iu of vitamin E and 300 milligrams of pantothenic acid daily during her second pregnancy, she found that the old stretch marks disappeared completely and no others formed. I have no experience of this happening, but it might work. What I have seen is that old stretch marks improve greatly with aromatherapy treatment and connective-tissue massage, which appears to bring life back into the tissue by increasing circulation in the area. But while I have seen them fade greatly—enough for the woman to wear a bikini again without fear of looking ugly—I have never known them to disappear completely.

BANISHING NASTY BROWN SPOTS

The Cause

These so-called liver spots are changes in pigmentation in the skin as a result of the aging process coupled with exposure to the sun's rays. Their proper name is lentigines. They usually mar hands and faces most, and in truth they have little to do with the liver, from which they have borrowed their name. Women deficient in some B vitamins—particularly folic acid and niacin—or women who have a particularly high personal requirement for them thanks to their genetic inheritance or their taking of oral contraceptives, are particularly prone to developing liver spots in areas of the body that are regularly exposed to the sun's light or artificial ultraviolet rays from a sun lamp.

Prevention and Cure

Many dermatologists claim there is nothing internal that one can do either to prevent or to eliminate liver spots. However, some nutritionists—and I have seen personal evidence of this—say that a good B-complex vitamin supplement which is particularly rich in folic acid and niacin (5 milligrams of folic acid and 100 milligrams of nicotinamides taken with each meal) will clear them up—provided of course that the rest of your diet is adequate.

There are also bleaching creams, which, used regularly three times a day, will gradually fade them. But if your skin is particularly sensitive to allergic reaction, you should do a patch test (as one does to test for allergens) before trying any of them, as they contain strong chemicals which may cause irritation.

Professionally, liver spots can be removed by using liquid nitrogen, frozen carbon dioxide, or electrocoagulation, or more simply by skin-peeling with the help of small *fraises* to sand down the epidermis. One thing is certain: At the first sign of any kind of irregular pigmentation like this, you need to shield yourself from the sun at all times on the area where it is developing, using a high-protection sun product. If you are prone to brown spots, stay away from sun products that contain oil of bergamot or any of its derivatives, and never put scent on before going out into the sun.

WHAT IF EVERYTHING GOES RED?

The Cause

A tendency to broken veins and reddish skin is something that is inherited. The veins of some people tend easily to dilate, resulting in congestion under the surface of the skin, which shows itself in red blotches, particularly on the cheeks and nose, where skin is especially thin. It can occur in any type of skin—young or old, dry or oily—but it usually gets worse as you get older. The capillaries in the skin become increasingly fragile and often rupture, which leads to the true broken veins many women are troubled with, particularly on the nose and cheeks. Two things make the condition worse: extremes of temperature on the skin and general inactivity. The more immobile the muscles of the face are, the more the blood tends to collect instead of flowing through the area efficiently.

Prevention and Cure

They are impossible to prevent completely—at least so far as I know—because you can't choose your parents. But once you realize you have the tendency, there is a lot you can do. First make sure you get adequate quantities of zinc and vitamin C plus the bioflavonoids in your diet. Always eat some of the white flesh of grapefruit skins, for instance, as well as the fruit itself. Vitamin B_2 is also helpful sometimes, because it plays an important part in the oxygenation of the cells, and vitamin B_1 is essential for good circulation.

Smoking is about the worst thing you can do for the problem, short of lying for long hours in the sun. Vitamin E is generally helpful in circulation troubles, and some claim that it will help the broken-vein problem when taken internally and also applied to the surface of the skin, although there is no scientific proof to support this. Redness in the skin without broken veins can be treated professionally with frozen carbon dioxide. Once a network of broken veins is visible, they have to be cauterized with an electric needle one by one. The blood in them then coagulates and is gradually reabsorbed, so that they disappear. The face usually has to be treated three or four times before they are completely gone. Preferably treatment should take place with intervals of a couple of weeks between sessions. Always avoid extremes of temperature and always protect your skin from the sun with a high-protection sunscreen if you have a tendency to broken veins.

WHAT IF YOU BRUISE EASILY?

The Cause

Bruises happen when the tiny blood vessels under the skin rupture and blood seeps into the tissue, which is what gives a bruise its bluish color. This gradually fades and changes to a greenish yellow as the blood released is broken down and reabsorbed. They are particularly frequent in women who appear to have a high requirement of vitamin C or who smoke and therefore use up the vitamin, rapidly putting themselves into a mild scorbutic state.

Prevention and Cure

If you tend to bruise easily, increase your intake of zinc and vitamin C, both nutrients essential for the strength and health of capillaries. Carl Pfeiffer, of the Brain Bio Centre, recommends that in addition to natural foods, adults usually need 12 to 30 milligrams of zinc twice a day as well as at least 2 grams of vitamin C. If you bruise very easily, you may even need more vitamin C. It is important to take the bioflavonoids as well, since vitamin C on its own sometimes doesn't clear up the problem, but with the bioflavonoids it does. Immediate treatment for a bruise can be had by applying cold wet compresses.

BLACKHEADS, WHITEHEADS, AND PIMPLES

Blackheads—the Cause

A blackhead—in medical terms, an open comedo—consists of a solid plug of oil that clogs the pore and then blackens due to oxidation on exposure to the air. If it is left alone it will simply stay there in the skin. Blackheads do not cure themselves.

Prevention and Cure

Blackheads on oily areas of the face (such as around the nose and chin) that are not inflamed can be removed easily by steaming the skin first or by applying hot compresses using flannel dipped in hot water and wrung out—hot water to which bicarbonate of soda has been added at a ratio of 1 tablespoon to each pint. This opens the pores and loosens the oily material. Then gently, with scrupulously clean hands and the tips of your fingers wrapped in facial tissue, you can ease out the plugs. Never use your nails. Finish off the treatment with the application of an antiseptic cream.

The occasional appearance of a blackhead or two is nothing to worry about. If, however, you have large quantities, read the advice for the care of skin that is too oily.

Whiteheads—the Cause

A whitehead is exactly the same as a blackhead except that, where the blackhead is open to the air, in the case of a whitehead the comedo remains closed because an accumulation of dead skin cells covers the opening of the duct, making it impossible for the oil blocked up in the follicle to move out of the pore. The oil that is blocked up irritates the cells of the follicle wall so they slough off rapidly and seal up its contents. A whitehead looks like a tiny white lump on the skin. Once formed, it will remain; that is, unless the oil follicle changes the chemistry of the oil-forming free fatty acids, which further stimulates both the increase in sebum production and also the sloughing off of cells, in which case the whitehead turns into a pimple.

Prevention and Cure

It is best to follow nutritional and treatment advice for oily skin if you have many whiteheads. The elimination of a dormant whitehead can be done only by a professional, for the closed comedo has to be opened with a very fine stylet, which leaves no scar. You should never squeeze a whitehead, or you risk forcing its fatty content into the dermis itself, where it can cause inflammation and the formation of raised spots that will take a long time to disappear. Once the whitehead is lanced by a professional, he will carefully remove the entire contents. In such cases of both open and closed comedones, the vitamin-A derivative retinoic acid in a strength of 50 milligrams to each 100 grams of cream is effective applied to the skin.

Pimples—the Cause

When the follicle wall breaks down enough to allow the oil to leak into the surrounding dermis tissue, this irritates the area and inflames it, and a pimple is formed. White blood cells, which are mobilized and sent to the area to fight the inflammation, create pus. When this pus comes to the surface and the skin covering it breaks so that the contents of the pimple are released to the air, it usually heals rapidly—provided, that is, that a secondary infection doesn't take place from the outside. If, however, the follicle break takes place deep in the skin instead, the pimple is more severe and can turn into an acne cyst.

Prevention and Treatment

Besides care in keeping the skin clean and nutritional prevention of excessively oily skin, little should be done with a pimple other than to allow it to take its course. Naturally, it is important that the elimination of waste from the body be efficient and complete, for wastes not eliminated by the bowels can be released through the skin. If you are prone to pimples, it is often a good idea to avoid the use of antiperspirants, as in some cases even this simple discouragement from waste elimination on parts of the body can encourage the formation of pimples on the face.

29

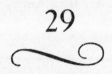

Don't Let Age
Get Under Your Skin

Nothing betrays your age like the state of your skin. When you are young, it is thick, glowing, soft, and elastic. As the years go by, a number of changes take place. The thickness of the skin diminishes by half. It loses its firmness. First, expression lines and minor discolorations form, then these tiny imperfections gradually become wrinkles and blotched skin, which is no longer able to retain water as it once could—skin that has lost its elasticity and turned crepey and old-looking. How fast all this happens depends not only on your genetic inheritance but also on the internal state of your body, your stress levels, and the care and protection you provide for your skin from the outside.

AGING BEGINS ON A CELLULAR LEVEL

The aging process in your skin is really no different from anywhere else in the body, except that it can be faster. This is because, first, the skin's cells tend to divide more often than most other kinds of cells, so genetic mutations are passed on more rapidly, and second, because your skin has to put up with so many external insults from what it is exposed to environmentally.

At the center of the aging process in the skin is a disruption of the genetic material in the cells—the DNA and RNA. This leads to corresponding degenerative changes in the collagen and elastin fibers of the dermis. These changes are brought on by many factors. Two of the most important are the presence of free radicals—highly reactive chemical groups that combine with cell material and cause damage both to the cell membranes and to the genetic material—and ultraviolet radiation from the sun. Both these factors cause the protein in the dermis to harden and thicken so that collagen fibers twist and bind together in a process called cross-linking. Because the firm, wrinkle-free look of skin is dependent on the collagen in it remaining flexible and orderly, when this process takes place the skin begins to sag and wrinkle from habitual expression patterns being etched into skin tissue no longer resilient enough to resist them.

Inadequate nutrition, which leaves the cell membranes particularly vulnerable to free-radical attack—particularly a diet high in unsaturated fats—also plays an important part in aging, as does a diminished blood supply from poor circulation to the tissues as a result of physical inactivity. Finally, some cell loss and damage associated with aging are probably direct results of environmental factors such as air pollution, smoking, and drugs and alcohol in the body. All of these degenerative changes on a cellular level contribute to your skin's losing its elasticity as well as its ability to hold water.

It is firm, healthy collagen and the skin's water-holding ability that give a face its youthful contours and cushiony feel. Eventually the loss of tone and firmness from these internal alterations and a diminishing hydration results in sagging, lines, and wrinkles. Meanwhile metabolism slows down in the cells so that it is increasingly difficult for them to get adequate essential nutrients, while the elimination of cellular wastes also gets less efficient. The rate at which old cells die and new ones are born is also much slower. Gradually the skin becomes sluggish and loses its vital glow, and the epidermis becomes uneven in thickness, discolored, rough, and lined.

To slow down this process and to keep a young, healthy skin as long as possible, you have first to retain a young, healthy body. This is a total, ongoing process depending on good nutrition, stress control, exercise, and protection from the environment. There aren't any shortcuts. But the good news is this: These skin aging changes appear to be not so dependent on the passage of time as they were once believed to be. There is much therefore you can do to retard them.

BEGIN BY STAYING OUT OF THE SUN

To preserve your skin from premature aging, in addition to the constant use of a sunscreen on your face as part of your everyday skin care, you should understand the art of sunbathing—that is if you want to tan at all. Ideally, of course, you would be far better off pale.

As we've already said, the sun is your skin's worst "ager." It has been proved that exposure to ultraviolet light brings about permanent fundamental alterations in the genetic material of skin cells and encourages the process of cross-linking. These changes are cumulative and irreversible. Even when sun-exposed skin from an arm is grafted onto a protected area such as the abdomen and left there for years, it still remains older-looking and darker than the skin surrounding it.

Thanks to an increasing awareness of this ultraviolet damage, sun worship is becoming a highly sophisticated occupation. These days no woman in her right mind would spend hour after hour lying in the sun, developing the deep brown tan which for three generations was considered a sign that one was rich enough and idle enough to spend time lounging around resorts. The fashion in tanning now is to have a lighter skin, just touched with golden light, rather than the previously sought-after, baked look. And for the sake of your skin's future, this change has come none too soon.

Of course in moderate doses, provided your skin is well protected, sunlight can actually be good for you. It stimulates circulation in the skin, makes you feel well, and is deeply relaxing. Also sunlight stimulates the formation of ergosterol, which when drawn into the skin becomes vitamin D. But this happens only if your skin isn't washed for at least twenty-four hours after exposure. Bathing will remove the ergosterol before it can be made use of.

THE WAY YOU TAN

A tan is a protective reaction. It results from the formation of melanin, the skin's natural pigmentation produced by special cells called melanocytes whose action is triggered by exposure to ultraviolet rays. Every woman has a unique capacity for melanin production, depending on her genetic inheritance. Dark, thick, Mediterranean skins produce more. This is why they will turn a darker brown than the "English rose" skin, which produces far less.

Regardless of the claims they make, there is no tanning product on the market that can promise you a tan of any specific depth. The color depends entirely on your skin's ability to produce melanin, and nothing will alter that. The trick to successful and safe tanning is to use a suntan product that will allow the production of the pigment to take place *slowly* by screening out most of the sun's ultraviolet rays, and to expose yourself only gradually to the sun.

Begin with fifteen minutes a day to each side—always between 9 A.M. and 11 A.M. or 3 P.M. and 5 P.M., when the sun's rays are less intense and therefore less likely to cause damage. Then increase your exposure by five or ten minutes a day as you build up a tan.

Provided you have normal skin, a good rule for choosing a sunscreen is to use a moderate filter for your body and a high-protection product on your face. Your body's skin ages much more slowly than the skin on your face, because it is usually protected by clothing. You can allow it to tan more without risk of its aging. Most of the large ranges of suntan products are carefully graded as to the amount of protection a product offers you. You can choose, say, a factor 7, or sun block, which almost completely shields your facial skin from ultraviolet rays, and a factor 4 or 5 for your body.

Although grading is not completely standardized and tends to vary somewhat from one range to another, generally you can gauge the kind of protection you'll get from a product by multiplying the length of time you can safely stay out in the sun without burning, using no protection, say fifteen minutes in midsummer sun if your skin is pale, by the number on the product. This will give you an approximate time that is safe for tanning while using it. For instance fifteen minutes times factor 5 equals an hour and a quarter. Using it, provided you continue every half hour or so to reapply it, you can stay out for an hour and a quarter with safety.

Some suntan products claim to screen out the harmful, burning, UV-B rays while they let through the tanning, UV-A ones. By now technology in tanning preparations has become very sophisticated and there are indeed products on the market that will do just that. The only catch is this: These short, UV-B rays, which are mainly responsible for burning and which these products screen out, penetrate the skin only superficially anyway—mostly to the level of the epidermis. But, according to dermatological research, the longer, so-called beneficial UV-A, tanning rays, which these products allow through, penetrate all the way into the deep layers of the dermis and the underlying tissues. And these UV-A rays are probably most responsible for the degenerative changes in the skin's structure associated with aging. So, whatever product you decide to use on your body, choose a high-protection product for your face that blocks out most of *both* the UV-A and UV-B wave bands. For the sad truth is that there is no way in which you can get yourself a deep tan and still protect your skin from premature aging.

THE TAN ACCELERATORS

There are also products on the market that offer not just protection factors but also tanning factors in them. They usually contain a derivative of the essential oil of bergamot, which has a natural tendency to oxidize certain amino acids in the skin's cells, in particular tyrosine, which accelerates the darkening of the skin when it is exposed to ultraviolet rays even in grayish weather. These products can be useful if you want to begin tanning before the strong, midsummer sun appears. The advantage of tanning this way is that the melanin which is formed and built up gradually is your skin's own protection against burning. But it still won't protect you from aging. Too much ultraviolet is simply too much. Another disadvantage of this kind of product is that bergamot is one of the substances most often responsible for allergic reactions in women with reaction-prone skin.

What about sun lamps? The new artificial tanning equipment is made to block out most or all of the UV-B range. Because of this it makes claims for tanning without burning and without doing damage to the skin. The first claim is valid. The second is highly questionable. For the UV-A rays, on which these machines rely to do their tanning, will still be at work aging skin at deeper levels. Ultimately there is no truly safe way to tan and still preserve young skin. If you are going to tan using this kind of equipment or with a conventional sun lamp that has both UV-A and UV-B wavelengths, you can only hope to minimize damage.

BEWARE OF POLYUNSATURATED FATS

Women are constantly being encouraged by beauty writers to include lots of polyunsaturated fats in their diet for the sake of their skin. Ironically it is probably large amounts of polyunsaturates in the system without sufficient natural antioxidants such as vitamin E to accompany them that is the second-biggest contributor to early-aging skin. As mentioned in the chapter on the Lifestyle Diet, a large dietary survey carried out at the University of California at Irvine showed that people who frequently include polyunsaturates in the diet showed marked clinical signs of premature aging compared with people who did not. Such factors as the degree of wrinkling, crow's-feet, frown lines, loss of elasticity, and discoloration were all evident.

Of course polyunsaturated fats are a necessary part of good nutrition —in *small* quantities. It is only when they are taken in excess, as they are by many people who believe that this will protect them from heart disease, that they may be dangerous. According to age researchers Irwin Fridovitch and Richard Passwater one of the most important things you can do to protect yourself from the possible aging effects of polyunsaturated fats is to increase your intake of vitamin E. This vitamin helps minimize damage done by the free-radical chain reactions triggered by these fats. Because the collagen fibers in skin are prime targets for free-radical attacks, which cause them to bind together and become disorganized, neutralizing these free radicals by increasing one's intake of vitamin E and helping to encourage the production of healthy collagen by taking more vitamin C may be able to slow down the aging process of one's skin. As yet there is no scientific proof of this, for no one has done human experiments; however, animal experiments give a strong indication that this can help.

Just how much of these vitamins in supplementary form one should take for this kind of protection depends on your individual metabolism and age and state of health.

A dermatologist friend who takes a total-body approach to skin care (an unusual approach among dermatologists I have met) recommends daily supplements to all his patients over twenty. Here is his basic list, which he varies to suit each woman's individual condition:

15,000 to 20,000 iu vitamin A
A good, full B-complex vitamin taken at meals, three times a day
100 mg of additional PABA taken once a day
100 mg additional pantothenic acid taken once daily
2,000 mg vitamin C taken twice a day
400 iu vitamin D taken once a day
400 iu vitamin E taken once a day

Expert on vitamin C, Irvin Stone believes that a person may need more C—up to 10 grams daily spread in doses throughout the day—to protect against early aging. Passwater believes that we need extra vitamin C, E, and B complex, and the sulfur amino acids, which occur in eggs, cabbage, muscle meats, and onions, as well as selenium, to help protect the body against free-radical and peroxidation damage.

FORGET THE CIGARETTES

Smoking also makes skin age rapidly. This is probably because of a substance called benzopyrene, which is found in cigarette smoke and which uses up the body's supply of vitamin C rapidly, making it unavailable for the support of healthy collagen. So the skin wrinkles earlier. Dr. Harry Darnell investigated the relationship between wrinkling and cigarette smoking for almost twenty years, looking at eleven hundred patients between the ages of thirty and seventy. He found that the skin of smokers wrinkles and ages up to twenty years sooner than that of nonsmokers. But the problem with cigarette smoke doesn't end there. For it is not only the smoker whose skin can suffer from it. So can the nonsmoker's. She may take in considerable quantities of benzopyrene, tar, carbon monoxide, and other irritating substances just by being in a room with others who are smoking. In a recent study it was shown that in a room of smokers the carbon monoxide level from the leftover cigarette smoke in the air can be as high as twenty to eighty parts per million. The supposedly acceptable level of this poisonous gas in industrial air is only fifty parts per million.

Carbon monoxide in the air is bad for skin in another way, too. It binds together with the red blood cells' hemoglobin, tying up its oxygen-carrying capacity for up to twelve hours. This can lead to oxygen starvation in the skin's cells, much as a high-fat diet can. There are other smoking dangers too of course which, although not directly related to skin aging, probably contribute to allover lowered health—such as the fact that smoking is known to be a contributor to lung cancer, osteoporosis, heart disease, strokes, bronchial diseases, and emphysema. Some dermatologists concerned about the dangerous effects of cigarette smoke on skin recommend that every smoker supplement her diet with additional vitamin C at a rate of 25 milligrams for each cigarette she smokes. But if you are serious about preventing aging, give up smoking altogether—no matter how difficult it seems and no matter how many excuses you can make for yourself about why you think you can't just now.

WATCH THE ALCOHOL

Alcohol is bad for skin too. Each gram of it contains 7 calories—more than any other kind of food except fat. The calories it gives you are empty of nutrition, as they convey no vitamins or minerals or other essential nutrients to the cells of your body. What they do do, however, is stimulate the appetite so that in addition to their calorie-supplying abilities they also tend to make you consume more food. And overeating is one of the worst things you can do to age your skin rapidly. Alcohol also robs the body of its supply of B vitamins, needed for skin health, and depletes resources of vitamin C. As well as all this, alcohol acts directly on the cells of the skin to cause damage.

Freely soluble in water, it attacks the living cell by forcing it to lose its water and to coagulate its protein. This can result not only in cellular damage but also cellular death. And the detrimental effects of alcohol don't stop there. Dr. Melvin Linsely has shown that alcohol also brings about sludging in the capillaries. Instead of the millions of red blood cells circulating freely, they tend to pile up and clog these tiny blood vessels, interfering with circulation so that the cells don't get enough oxygen. As a result of this oxygen starvation, cellular deterioration occurs, and small hemorrhages, or leakages of blood from the capillaries, take place. This sludging phenomenon interferes with skin cell metabolism, as it does with that of cells elsewhere in the body. The tiny ruptures that take place in small blood vessels as a result of the sludging are also a major factor behind the appearance of broken veins on the face. While it is true that the occasional glass of good wine may do nothing but good in relaxing you and improving digestion, more than this is bad for the long-term youth and health of your skin.

SLOUGH OFF THE DEAD CELLS

Men's skin ages less rapidly than women's. One of the reasons for this may be that a man shaves every day and the act of shaving itself removes several layers of the stratum corneum. A slowing down of cell reproduction is one of the things that happens when your skin ages. Many dermatologists believe that exfoliation—the deliberate removal of the old dead cells on the skin's surface—will help keep skin younger-looking. It stimulates cell reproduction in the basal layer and refines the skin's surface, making it look more translucent and smoother, getting rid of the mottled surface that comes with age.

EXTRA CARE FOR OLDER SKIN

Not only does older skin need extra protection from the sun in order to avoid the formation of brown age spots, it needs protection in other ways, too. From excessive stress, for instance, which takes a heavy toll of a woman's face when she is over forty. It is important to get enough sleep.

Both sebum production and the water content of the skin decrease with age, which makes it doubly important to keep your skin guarded from excessive dehydration. Many creams for older skin contain a sebum-like substance to make up for the gradual decline in the natural ability to hold water. Hormone creams, particularly those containing estrogen and estrogen-like substances, can be useful in combating aging too. They plump up skin that is losing much of its padding and form, thanks to their ability to increase the skin's water-holding tendencies. They also soften the surface texture.

The maximum benefits from a hormone cream come about a month after you begin to use it, but they are only truly significant in skin that is genuinely aged. Hormones will do nothing for younger skin, and the benefits from using a hormone cream will only remain so long as you continue to use it. When it is stopped, your skin will gradually return to its previous state. But hormones are powerful substances, which affect the whole endocrine balance of a body. They have to be used with great care and are only available on prescription in the concentration necessary to be effective (10,000 iu of an estrogen-like hormone per ounce of cream).

ON SKIN PEELING, FACE-LIFTS, AND CHEMOSURGERY

Chemosurgery is sometimes recommended for the removal of fine lines on older skin. It involves the destruction of the top layer of the skin with a caustic solution—usually a 10 percent solution of resorcinol spread on and left for a specific length of time. In a week or so the crust formed falls off, revealing firmer, pink skin underneath. This is superficial chemical face peeling. Alternatively, the use of a combination of phenol—a derivative of carbolic acid—and other chemicals, which is applied three or four times to the face to burn away not only the epidermis but part of the dermis as well, is known as deep peeling. They are both supposed to stimulate the formation of fresher, younger-looking skin and also to eliminate many wrinkles.

Both superficial and deep peeling are painful, and the good results they bring in terms of younger-looking skin are short-lived. They usually last no more than a few months. Gradually the new skin loses its plumped-up look and returns to looking much as it did before. I have never seen an older woman who has had the operation and not regretted it later.

Another so-called cure for aging skin is dermabrasion—the planing operation that is supposed to minimize wrinkles much the same way except that it uses a motor-driven brush, rather than chemicals. In my experience, it is even less effective. The one thing both operations will do, though, is eliminate liver spots, freckles, and superficial scars such as some of the scars from acne. Neither can change the condition of the collagen fibers in the dermis, on which depends the long-term look of your skin.

Plastic surgery can be useful, particularly if you are thin—it works far better on underweight women than the rest of us. You must get a good surgeon, for there is a real art to it. It is not just a mechanical job; and you must take good care of your face and the rest of your body both before and afterward. But it is not the cure-all that many women believe it to be. Your diet, level of physical activity, and general lifestyle have to be good in order to maintain the benefit you'll get from it.

MOVE YOUR FACE

One of the most useful things you can do yourself to prevent your face from aging and to correct sags and bags even after they have occurred is to practice face exercises every day.

The bones you were born with give your face its individual shape and structure. Short of plastic surgery or adjustments to your skull through cranial osteopathy, there is nothing you can do to change them. But your muscles are constantly changing either for better or for worse. They are made up of bundles of fibers, each of which works independently to shorten muscle and draw a part of the face into a particular expression. Just like the muscles in the rest of your body, each of these groups of fibers has an antagonistic group. This means that for each muscle that pulls an area of your face into one expression, there is an opposite muscle to pull it the other way.

For instance, one muscle *lifts* the eyebrow and another *lowers* it. So as one muscle lengthens, the other shortens, and vice versa, in a team-like effort. At least that is how it is supposed to work. What often happens, however, is that because of habitual expressions (the polite mask a woman shows to the world, the continual worry that draws the eyebrows together, and so forth) and because of the constant pull of gravity on the face, particular muscles tend to be usually contracted, or shortened, while their partners are just as usually flaccid, or stretched, so that neither get the workout and movement they need to remain firm, full, strong, and in good tone. Then you get muscle tightness and muscle shrinkage, which interferes with proper circulation in that area of the skin and gradually results in distortions of facial contours, such as hollows around the eyes, the valleys that run between the edges of the nose and the outer corners of the mouth, and the sag of the typical double chin.

The only way to maintain the health and firmness of muscles that will preserve youthful contours in a face is exercise. The more you are able to make use of all your muscles in all movements, the stronger they will become. And with it the firmer and more contoured your skin will look. Also your circulation will improve with exercise and you will have a better color. No matter what condition your face is in, whether it is young and smooth, just beginning to lose its firmness, or sagging heavily, exercise will help it. And the worse its condition the greater the improvement you will see. And it is never too late to start. Before long, beginning to work each muscle restores even an aging face to more-youthful contours.

If you are young and have no particular sags or hollows, one of the best ways to stay that way is simply to spend two or three minutes a day in front of a mirror, making the most outrageous faces at yourself. Pull your muscles into all sorts of distortions that in the normal course of your expressions you would never do. Make your lips into an "o" shape hard and open your eyes wide while you raise your forehead. Wrinkle your nose and at the same time open your mouth as wide as possible.

Twist your mouth from one side to the other, then draw down its corners while you tighten the muscles in the side of your neck. Make the face of a fool, or of a monster. The possibilities are endless and the more weird and ugly the faces you can make while going through them, the better a workout you will be giving your muscles.

Face Exercises

After thirty, if lines have begun to form, you have to be more specific about the kind of exercises you do. In effect you have to locate a problem area, say a developing hollow under the cheek, or loose flesh under the jaw and chin, and then work on the specific muscles that will counterbalance it.

This can be done through some simple but specific isotonic-type exercises in front of your mirror, or you can use faradic exercise equipment such as Slendertone to do contractions for you. There are facial electrode attachments, which you can get to go with most passive exercise machines of this type, which when placed at specific points on the face will automatically contract the muscles in that area. There is also a battery-operated face exerciser, which works on the same principles but is small enough to put into a handbag for travel. Faradic exercises are also recommended by many plastic surgeons for use before and after surgery to restore muscle strength and tone.)

Either isotonic movement or passive exercise will work, provided you are conscientious about exercising every day. It is the regular workout you give your face muscles that brings results, and although results can be slow to show themselves—in some cases demanding several weeks' work before you detect significant changes for the better—they can also be astoundingly good. For regular face exercising can transform your face completely, not only making it look ten years younger by eliminating excess and softening expression lines and filling in hollows, but also by enlivening the whole look of the skin.

All exercises have to be done slowly and steadily. The muscles of your face, unlike those of the rest of your body, are attached to the skin itself. When you move them, you naturally move your skin, too. You need never be afraid of the movements, but you should never overtire muscles either—slow and steady is the pace to adopt.

The exercises below are designed to treat the four problem areas of the face: the eyes, the chin and throat, the cheeks (where little smile lines form), and the forehead. The exercises should be done with a well-creamed skin. Moving the face about without this lubrication may deepen any lines already there. The cream you use should be rich—one of the old-fashioned, rather greasy night creams will do nicely, or you can use olive or coconut oil.

EYES

This exercise is excellent for the eye area, which usually goes slack faster than any other part of the face. It is particularly designed to prevent or eliminate crow's-feet. It is in two parts.

Part one   Looking into a mirror, lower your chin to your chest and open your eyes looking straight ahead. Then, slowly and in eight definite steps, close your eyes by bringing the lower lids up to the upper, all the while looking into the mirror until the very last moment. Hold this position with your eyes tightly shut for four counts, then release in the same eight definite steps. Repeat four times. Once you can control these movements in definite steps, you are ready to go on to the toughy that really does the work.

Part two   Place both elbows firmly on your dressing table and, using two small folded pieces of cotton fabric or tissue, place your index fingers over them on the crow's-feet areas and press firmly. Lower your chin to your chest and, looking straight ahead into the mirror, do the same exercise as before but this time working against the pressure of your fingers, which hold the skin in place, as you move lower lids up to eight counts, hold for four, down for eight, rest for four. Do this three times. You will be surprised what it does to tone the eye area and even to brighten the eyes themselves.

CHIN AND NECK

Exercise one   This exercise strengthens and firms the platysma, which covers the neck from jaw to chest and when firm keeps the skin on the neck smooth and free from turning crepey.

Tilt your head slightly backward, placing your hand gently on your throat. Now make your mouth into a hard "o" shape, then pull the muscles around your mouth downward and outward into a turned-down "smile"—a smile in which the corners of the mouth turn down as though you were making the sound "ee." Now push your mouth back to "o" again, then back to "ee," repeating the change a dozen times.

Exercise two   This movement tightens the muscles in the neck and lower jaw while bringing circulation to the skin of the face.

Lying on your back on a firm bed, or better still on a table, let your head and neck hang over the side, bend your knees and place your feet flat on the surface you are lying on. Now you are ready to begin. Slowly, to the count of five, lift your head up so your chin is on your chest. Then, opening your mouth, jut out your lower jaw as far as it will go. Hold for five counts. Finally, keeping your lower jaw thrust forward, let your head flop back over the edge of the table and hold for another five counts. Return your lower jaw to its normal position and repeat. Do this exercise six times.

Exercise three   This exercise strengthens the pterygoids, at the side of the jaw. With your lips together, smile to the sides gently, then push your lower jaw as far forward as possible. Now, maintaining the tension, move your jaw from side to side four times and then return to the starting position. Repeat the full movement twelve times.

CHEEKS

Exercise one   This exercise helps eliminate nose-to-lip creases by strengthening a tiny muscle, just above the side of the mouth, called the canius, as well as the muscles in the cheeks themselves. This will lift the area between nose and mouth corners upward.

   With your lips together, smile upward at the corners of your mouth as hard as you can. At the same time, try to make your lips into an "o" shape so that the muscles are pulling against each other and the whole area is tightened. Hold for five seconds. Repeat twice.

Exercise two   This exercise is designed to remove telltale hollows in the lower cheek area, soften lines, and lift mouth corners. It needs to be done in two parts. The first will train the muscles to your conscious control. It should be followed for a week before beginning the second part. The second part works on the principle of isometric resistance, but it will be effective only after you have trained your muscles in that area to work.

   Facing a mirror, smile to the sides—smile so that there is no movement in the muscles of the eye area—in a series of small definite movements to the count of eight, all the while making sure there is no movement whatever in your eye area; if there is, then you are not using the right muscles. Hold the smile for a count of four. Then, to a count of eight in definite steps, release the smile, returning to the starting position. Rest for a count of four. Do the exercise five times. When you can do this smoothly and with control, then leave it behind and go on to the second part.

   Using a piece of cotton cloth or a folded tissue, left elbow firmly placed on your dressing table, with thumb and middle finger grasp the left cheek area, ensuring that the cloth is centered under the thumb to prevent slipping. Then, holding your cheek firm, smile to the sides just as you did in the first exercise but this time on the left side of the face only, so that your muscles are working against your grasped cheek—again to a count of eight, hold for four, release in eight, and rest for four. Then, using the right hand, do the exercise on the right cheek. Do each side three times.

FOREHEAD

Exercise one This movement strengthens the frontalis muscle, on the forehead, which is the antagonist to the corrugator, which pulls the eyebrows together in a frown. It will help soften frown lines between the brows.

Looking into a mirror, as slowly and gradually as you can, put your brows down, closing your eyes tighter and tighter into a frown. Now open your eyes wider and wider, lifting your forehead as you do. Repeat six times.

Exercise two This is for smoothing out a lined forehead. It also has two parts. Once you have mastered the first, forget about it and go on to the second.

Facing a mirror, raise muscles of your forehead in tiny controlled steps to the count of eight, all the while opening your eyes wider (good for you if you tend to be a squinter) and getting the feel of your muscles in this area. Hold for a count of four, then release slowly in eight steps. Do this five times twice a day.

When you have mastered this completely, do the second part, but *before* you do any of the other exercises, because it needs to be done with a cream-free forehead.

Ensure that your forehead is clean and dry and, taking three pieces of cellophane tape cut to the breadth of your forehead, place them on the brow area, using a small piece to fit between the eyebrows. The tape will act as resistance the way your finger did in the cheek exercise. You work against it for really effective muscle toning. Move your brow up in tiny definite movements, this time to the count of six. Hold for four, opening your eyes wide and looking straight ahead. Release in six. Do this exercise five times.

30

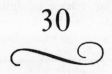

Your Eyes:
The Windows of Your Soul

Not only are your eyes the truest of all physical reflections of who you are, they are also an ageless expression of beauty. For there can be something breathtaking about the eyes of an old woman, as there is about the eyes of a child. Like any other part of your body, to be beautiful your eyes have to be healthy, and to be healthy they need care.

But the care they need is quite different from what we are usually led to believe. For eyes are *not* the delicate, poor, vulnerable things we have been taught they are—overworked, constantly struggling against inadequate light and overstrain, and longing for some well-deserved tinted glasses to rest them. Far from it. Your eyes are tough. They were made for use, and the more you use them, to read and to see with, and the more you exercise the muscles around them, and the more they are exposed to the full spectrum of natural sunlight, the healtheir and more beautiful they will be. And not only will your eyes benefit, so will the rest of your body.

HOW DO YOU SEE?

Sight is a highly complex phenomenon. In fact, it is not your eyes that do the seeing but your brain. Electromagnetic waves in lengths between 0.38 and 0.8 micron (a micron is a millionth of a meter) in the form of light patterns are received by the eye and then pass through it onto the retina, a layer of photosensitive cells at the back of the eyeball. These cells pick up the light and, through a series of photochemical reactions, pass on a nerve impulse by way of the optic nerve to the visual center of the brain, where you can instantaneously "see" the object in front of you. The retina is made up of two sorts of light receptor cells: cones and rods. The cones, in the center are activated when we are in bright light, so we can see fine details and color. The rods, at the periphery, work in dim light. You have about 7 million cones and 120 million rods in each eye.

The part of the eye that allows you to focus (and which is usually at fault when there is a vision problem such as nearsightedness or far-sightedness) is the crystalline lens in the front of the eyeball, which changes from an elliptical shape when you are looking at distant things to a shape more like a sphere when you are examining something close up. This variation takes place thanks to a group of muscles that hold the lens. They are highly elastic when your body is young but become much less so as you get older. This, along with the thickening and hardening of the lens itself, is responsible for presbyopia, the inability to focus on things close to you, which is experienced by the majority of people over the age of forty-five.

A WINDOW TO THE BODY AS WELL AS TO THE SOUL

The eye appears to be a window not only to the soul but also to the internal state of the body. A doctor looking into the eye with the use of a light is able to see if the patient is suffering from many more things than just those ailments affecting the eye itself. Such troubles as diabetes, leukemia, atherosclerosis, and kidney disease can all show up there. Even the presence of 80 percent of all brain tumors is evident from an examination of the shape and color of the optic nerve and the fundus, at the back of the eye.

The light entering your eyes appears to do a great deal more than simply transform electromagnetic wave patterns into nerve impulses for your brain to interpret as images. There is considerable evidence that, acting directly on the pigment granules in the epithelial cells of the retina, it also stimulates the pineal gland, the hypothalamus, and the pituitary gland through neurochemical channels, thereby influencing the health of the whole body.

LET THERE BE LIGHT

Like plants and animals, we *need* light to stay in optimum health. Not only the light available through the tinted windows of the cars we drive and behind our fashionable sunglasses, but the full spectrum of ultraviolet rays one gets only when naked eyes are exposed to the sun in the open air. The work of photobiologists such as Dr. John Ott, author of *Light and Health* (published by Devin-Adair, Old Greenwich, Connecticut) has shown that the type and quality of the light entering our eyes can affect our hormonal balance and body chemistry as a whole, influencing energy levels as well as how we feel emotionally.

If the light reaching the photoreceptor mechanisms in the eyes is the full spectrum of normal, unfiltered sunlight, it helps greatly to keep the functioning of the body normal. Light may even be useful in the treatment of a number of ailments quite unrelated to the eyes. Some physicians have found that exposing patients to the full spectrum of natural sunlight can be helpful in the treatment of many illnesses, from arthritis and diabetes to liver and skin diseases and even depression.

The field of photobiology is a young one and as yet no one understands why light appears to be so important to the healthy functioning of the body, and it may be many years before controlled studies are available to decipher all the mysteries. The most interesting theory to date is that light is necessary to the body because whatever chemical products it helps to produce in the system probably serve as a kind of flame to burn the nutritional fuel that comes from oxygen. If not enough light is visible, then ultimately cell metabolism will suffer. Certain toxic by-products of incomplete oxidation could interfere further with cell functioning and ultimately, therefore, with the functioning of the body as a whole. Many speculate that just as we are now discovering that nutritional deficiencies can bring on a disposition toward many illnesses, in the future we are likely to discover the existence of subclinical *light* deficiencies—something which until recently was never considered even as a remote possibility.

In the meantime, photobiologists are becoming increasingly concerned with three things in modern life which, they say, could prove strongly detrimental to human health in the long run: increasing environmental pollution, which is changing the variety of electromagnetic waves and the intensity of light that now reaches the earth; the increasing use of artificial light, which does not offer the full spectrum of natural sunlight that the body appears to thrive on; and the increasing use of colored glasses as a fashion accessory.

Smithsonian Institution reports show that we have experienced a loss of 14 percent in the intensity of sunlight reaching our eyes in the past half century. Other scientific measurements of light indicate that we have also witnessed a 26 percent reduction in the ultraviolet part of the spectrum reaching our eyes. Living in a modern environment also means that we live increasingly, at home and at work, under artificial lighting, which almost eliminates the important ultraviolet wavelengths. Researchers claim that as a result we are experiencing a kind of "light pollution," which may seriously affect our health and well-being over time. Only a great many more studies will show who are most at risk and how badly they may be affected.

The fashion-conscious woman who wears sunglasses day in and day out may seriously be undermining her health and vitality in the long run. Pink lenses, for instance, worn over a period of time, appear to affect the wearer in a marked psychological way, making one more irritable and disturbed. This phenomenon has been reported again and again from various sources. But *all* tinted lenses filter out specific wavelengths of light and may, say photobiologists, cause adverse effects.

Most women who wear tinted lenses do so because they believe they make them look better, because their eyes feel particularly sensitive to bright light. Much of the sensitivity comes from the practice of wearing the tinted lenses in the first place. When habitual sunglass wearers remove their glasses, they do often experience a few days when their eyes seem bothered by the full spectrum of sunlight, but this apparent sensitivity soon passes.

For the sake of your health and vitality, it is important to spend at least an hour a day out in the open with your eyes exposed to the sunlight—not guarded behind lenses, whether the lenses be glasses or window panes or car windshields. Wear sunglasses when you need them, by all means, but don't wear them incessantly as a fashion accessory. Your eyes and the rest of your body *need* light.

Lighting manufacturers, interested in the reports about the importance of full-spectrum light for health, have begun to develop bulbs that simulate natural sunshine, but they aren't widely available yet.

GOOD GLASSES

This is not to say that sunglasses don't serve a purpose. They do. Wear them when your eyes are exposed to excessive quantities of light to which they are not accustomed—when you are near the sea, for instance, or when you go skiing. A good pair of sunglasses can be a great boon, for your eyes need time to accustom themselves to the increase in light, and wearing sunglasses can make the changeover easier. Also, prolonged exposure of unaccustomed eyes to large doses of ultraviolet light may lead to the inflammation of the cornea known as snow blindness, while too-intense infrared rays can burn the retina. The skin covering the front of your eyes is transparent. It has no melanin cells to produce a protective tan, as does the rest of your skin. This is why, in the past, unprotected workers at glass furnaces who were exposed to high levels of infrared light often lost their sight in middle age. And while Victorian working conditions are a thing of the past, powerful infrared light survives in the tropics. If you are in very intense heat and sunlight, protect your eyes with a pair of glasses that block out not only some of the ultraviolet rays but also much of the infrared band too.

Sunglasses can be useful in another way, too: Worn in moderation, they can help discourage frowning and scowling—two practices that slowly and imperceptibly etch permanent lines around eyes.

When choosing a pair of sunglasses for yourself, look for some that state what percentage of the ultraviolet spectrum they absorb. For wearing in bright sunlight, they need to be dark enough to eliminate 70–85 percent. Also check that the lenses have a scratch-resistant surface. The kind of lenses you choose is determined by the purpose for which you want them. To wear on vacation, in the snow or by the sea, polarized lenses are good. A seven-layered optical sandwich, they cut out glare and are both shatter-proof and shock-resistant. So are some of the new graduated tints, made on the same sandwich principle but without the middle, polarized layer.

Photochromic lenses, which are pale in subdued light and then darken, increasing their filtering capacity when you are exposed to strong ultraviolet rays, are excellent too. But neither polarized nor photochromic lenses are good for driving. The windshield of a car absorbs ultraviolet rays, so the photochromics don't darken as they should and polarized lenses show up the toughening marks in windshields, which can be distracting. Simple glass or plastic lenses are better.

When buying a pair of sunglasses, be sure to test them for optic clarity and quality. Hold them at arm's length, and looking through one lens at a slender vertical image, such as the frame of a door, watch to see if it remains still while you wiggle them up and down. If it does, they are properly made. If not, try a different pair.

EYE HEALTH AND BEAUTY FROM THE INSIDE

Many eye problems, from poor vision and eye watering or itching to premature wrinkles and crow's-feet, can be eliminated and often prevented by improving general nutrition. Japanese expert on eye nutrition Jin Otsuka, professor of ophthalmology at Tokyo University, believes that eating refined sugar is one of the worst things you can do if you want to preserve your vision. He has shown in animal experiments that giving sugar in large quantities will make an animal myopic. This is probably because sugar tends to rob the body of other nutrients essential for the health of the eye and for the nerves which supply it.

Another ophthalmic nutritionist, Stanley Evans, author of *Nutrition, Eye Health and Disease*, claims that much undernutrition that causes eye problems remains undetected, simply because requirements of specific nutrients can vary tremendously from one person to another as a result of genetic differences. Also, there is the fact that your need for various nutrients increases if you are under stress, drink alcohol, smoke, or take drugs. If you have an eye problem or if you find the skin around your eyes sagging or wrinkling rapidly, you might well be someone who needs more of the vitamins particularly important for eyes.

Vitamin A

The ancient Egyptians had no idea that liver is one of our richest sources of vitamin A, but they did know that eating it often improves poor eyesight. Vitamin A is responsible for good vision in poor light. This is why doctors gave extra amounts of the nutrient to pilots and paratroopers during World War II. But vitamin A also plays an important part in ensuring that your eyes' movements remain normal and in protecting the youthful appearance of the skin around your eyes.

Vitamin B Complex

The B-complex vitamins ensure the health of the eyes' nerve pathways and the myelin sheath that surrounds them. As always, the B vitamins all work together and have to be taken together. If you are not getting enough B_1, B_2, pantothenic acid, B_6, and vitamin E to meet your own needs, you risk gradual destruction of the myelin sheath, leading to visual disturbances and the faulty replaying of information to the brain.

Supplements of vitamin B_2 have proved useful in eliminating eye watering and the commonly felt sensation of having sand under the lids, as well as in improving one's ability to adjust to sudden light changes. A deficiency of B_{12} or a lack of folic acid can lead to dim vision, and the entire B complex is important in the preservation of youthful-looking skin around the eyes.

Vitamin C

Vitamin C is important to preserve the strength of the capillaries that feed the eye tissue. It also helps protect collagen fibers in the skin from degeneration and, therefore, helps to avoid wrinkles. If you find the area around your eyes wrinkling, you might consider increasing your daily intake of vitamin C to between six and eight grams a day. Smoking is one of the worst things you can do if you don't want the area around your eyes to wrinkle, since it both robs your system of vitamin C and also tends to make you squint.

Vitamin E

Vitamin E has proved useful in the treatment of a number of inflammatory eye conditions.

Just how much of these nutrients you need for eye health depends on your own, inherited metabolism. But they play such an important part in eye health and beauty that it seems strange that they are so often ignored.

EYE HEALTH AND BEAUTY FROM THE OUTSIDE

How, physically, you handle your eyes has a lot to do with how long the skin around them looks young and how clear and bright they are themselves. Eyes don't need to be favored to stay beautiful and healthy, but they don't need abuse, either. Yet they are faced with it most of the time, in the form of air pollution, smoke, misapplied makeup, and mismanaged makeup removal. The skin surrounding your eyes is thinner and finer than anywhere else on your face. It is also only sparsely supplied with oil glands and therefore highly prone to expression lines. This is where a good eye cream can help. They come in several varieties. Some (usually the more expensive) are designed not only to protect the skin in the area from dehydration but also to plump it up for several hours to minimize the lines there. They are particularly good for women over forty with dry skin, but the plumping action is highly transient: You have to keep using them once you start or your eyes quickly revert to the way they looked before. Others, particularly the herbal gels, are soothing and cooling. Very slightly astringent, this sort of eye cream will help calm swollen lids. Still others are made simply to prevent dehydration and are good for skin of all ages and even the most sensitive skins. If you don't want to spend money on eye cream, a rich oil such as avocado, hazelnut, or apricot dabbed on, in the barest traces, around the eye area will do just as good a job, used mornings before applying makeup and evenings before bed—provided you are not after the tightening effect.

When you put on your oil or eye cream matters. It is important never to use too much of it or you can end up with swollen, irritated eyes, particularly if you are using the plumping-up variety. Apply it gently with your third finger (there is less pressure that way) tapping lightly all around the eye. Never rub or pull the skin. How you apply mascara and how you remove it matters too. Most women open their eyes wide and look directly into the mirror, wrinkling up their forehead in the process. The best way is to hold your mirror at chin level and look down into it; then you don't etch wrinkles into your forehead. This may not seem very important, but when you think that you apply mascara, say twice a day, probably every day of your adult life, the habitual creasing of the forehead becomes a significant force in creating wrinkles there. You will get better coverage, too.

Think twice before you opt for waterproof mascara. It is difficult to remove, so you need a special strong remover to do it and you can end up rubbing and irritating the eye area every time you take off your makeup. Unless you go walking in the rain or swimming with your makeup on, it is better to choose a conventional variety. To take it off, use a non-oily eye-makeup remover if your eyes are sensitive (most are), and saturate a pad of absorbent cotton with it. Then put the pad over the closed eye and hold it there for ten seconds to dissolve the makeup so you can easily stroke it away.

PUT YOUR EYES TO WORK

Like the rest of you, your eyes need exercise. So do the muscles around them, in order for the skin that covers them to remain firm and wrinkle-free. (See Chapter 29.) Here are a few useful toners and refreshers:

Eye Toner

This not only strengthens eyes and helps to keep them healthy, it also improves the musculature that supports the skin and helps prevent sags and bags that belie your age. Hold a pencil in front of your eyes about twelve inches away from them. Focus on it for a couple of seconds, then focus far beyond it. Repeat this fifteen times.

A Victorian Trick

With the thumb and forefinger of one hand, press firmly for thirty sec-onds on the side of your nose at the inside corner of your eye. It hurts. But it is a wonderful way of eliminating tired eyes and getting rid of tension in the face, which usually goes unnoticed and can result in scowl lines. This is something the Victorians used quite successfully to treat hysteria. It *does* calm emotional pressure a lot.

Quick Freshener

Close your eyes tightly, then more tightly, pressing the lids together as hard as you can. Now open them slowly. This is good for when you are stopped at traffic lights and your eyes are tired from driving, or if you have been reading for a long while, or when you wake up and find your vision is not clear.

Palming

Put your elbows on the table in front of you and close your eyes. Then cover them with the palms of your hands. Press gently against the whole eye area for a minute or so. This refreshes the eyes and, provided you breathe deeply and calmly while you are doing it, also revitalizes the rest of you.

Light Relief

Lie for five minutes in the morning or afternoon sun. When closed eyelids get used to the light filtering through them, raise the top lid of one eye at a time, looking downward while the sun's rays shine on the sclera —the membrane that covers the eyeball. Whenever you want to blink, do so. This treatment is one recommended in the Bates method of restoring sight without glasses. It helps relax tense muscles so the circulation of blood to the area is improved.

Special Tricks for Special Problems

Here are some useful treatments for such common troubles as red and irritated eyes, black circles, and puffy lids.

Swollen Eyes

Do the palming exercise and then cover your eyes with cold compresses made from absorbent cotton dipped in ice-cold eyebright tea (1 tablespoon of the dried herb to a cup of water). Or lie down for ten minutes with grated raw potatoes between two pieces of gauze on your lids.

Red and Irritated Eyes

Dip your hands into ice-cold water and then press them against your eyelids, dipping and pressing several times. Put a slice of cucumber on each closed lid while resting for five minutes.

Black Circles

Are you anemic? Retaining wastes? Do you have a low-grade infection? All of these things can cause dark-rimmed eyes. But one of the most common causes is poor elimination or the retention of toxic wastes in the system. The Spring Cleaning Diet can often eliminate dark circles within a week or so. A vitamin B_{12} deficiency should also be suspected.

The Hair

❧

Introduction

Each hair on your head is 97 percent protein in the form of keratin and 3 percent moisture. It also contains traces of metals and mineral substances in about the same proportions as the rest of you. When your body is in homeostasis (that is, all is functioning well) and it is receiving the nutrients it needs and making good use of them, then your hair is strong and beautiful. When something goes wrong *inside*, your hair is one of the first things to show it.

This is one of the many mysteries about hair. In fact, it should not be so. For hair, like fingernails, is *dead*. Only the follicle from which each hair grows is a living thing. And while it is understandable that hair loss can result from a systemic condition since the follicles would naturally be affected by illness as would any other part of the body, there is no apparent reason why dead hair should look so different from one day to the next, depending on how you feel. Yet it is so.

Although there is still a great deal that is not understood about hair, there is a lot more that we do know. In fact, when it comes to external hair care, cosmetic technology is at its very best. In the past fifteen years, excellent products have been developed to deal successfully with hair that is too fine, too greasy, too dry, or damaged. There are also things to protect your hair from the ravages of the sun's ultraviolet rays and some excellent coloring and permanent wave lotions. In this section we look first at what hair is, how it grows, and what you can and can't do to treat it both from inside and out. Then we deal with hair protection and grooming, and finally we look at the most common hair problems and their solutions.

31

What's It All About?

Each hair on your head is made beneath the surface of your skin in a little bulbous structure called a follicle. There, a clump of cells called the papilla, at the base of the follicle, produces the keratinous cells that become a strand of hair. The papillae get good supplies of food and oxygen, since they are well furnished with blood vessels, on which the growth and health of every hair depends. When, for any reason, circulation to your scalp is decreased or interfered with, the papillae get fewer nutrients and less oxygen than they need, and your hair suffers. The function of a follicle is to produce keratin, just as your pancreas produces insulin or your stomach hydrochloric acid. The follicle also contains an oil gland, which produces oil to coat each hair and to protect it from water loss. How efficiently and how well it does this depends on a number of things such as the level of androgenic and estrogenic hormones in your system, your genetic inheritance, and your general health.

You are born with more than 90,000 follicles. This number doesn't change. If the amount of hair on your head changes, it is because some or most of these follicles are not working properly or have shut down, not because they disappear or because you don't have enough.

THE THREE LAYERS OF A HAIR

Each strand of hair, or hair shaft, can be divided into three basic layers: the outside, which is called the cuticle; the medulla, at the center; and the cortex, made up of complicated amino-acid chains, in between. The cuticle serves as your hair's protective coating: It guards against excessive evaporation of water (just as the stratum corneum does for your skin). It is made up of a transparent, hard keratin formation that is itself layered.

These layers overlap, like the tiles on a roof or fish scales. When they lie flat and smooth against the hair shaft, the hair shaft refracts light beautifully and your hair looks shiny. When they are peeling or damaged or raised, each hair doesn't catch the light, so your hair lacks sheen and looks flat and dull. The cuticle provides 35 percent of your hair's elastic strength.

The threadlike cortex, just beneath the cuticle, contains the pigment granules, which give your hair its color. The cortex is softer than the cuticle, yet it provides 65 percent of the hair's elastic strength. It is also the thickest part of the hair. If the amino-acid chains that make up the cortex break up as a result of too harsh treatment from hair dyes, dryers, highly alkaline shampoos, or overprocessing, then you end up with weak and brittle hair that splits easily and breaks off. The most common manifestation of poor cortex condition is the familiar split ends.

The hair shaft's innermost layer, the medulla, is made up of very soft keratin, and in many people there is even a hollow center. It appears to transport nutrients and gases to the other layers of the hair and may be the means by which your hair is so rapidly affected by changes in your body's condition. But as yet not a great deal is understood about the biological functions of the medulla.

THE THREE-STAGE CYCLE OF GROWTH

Hair follicles are the most efficient metabolizers of any organs in the body. This is what makes hair growth possible. They and the hairs they produce function on a three-part growth cycle that lasts from two to seven years. It is important to understand this growth cycle, because understanding it can dispel many of the fears women have that something is wrong when they look at their hairbrush and discover a number of hairs in it. Hair loss is continuous and is a normal part of the cycle. Without it there would be no new hair growth.

During the first part of a hair's growth cycle—called the *anagen* phase —the papilla proliferates keratin at a rapid rate as the follicle expands and imbeds itself deeply in the vascular scalp to provide the oxygen and nourishment needed for growth. During this anagen phase, which lasts between two and six years (depending on your genetic makeup, general health, and the hormone balance in your body), your hair continues to grow from the follicle very much as toothpaste is squeezed out of a tube. The anagen phase is longer when you are young than at the age of fifty or sixty, but no matter what your age, eventually it has to come to an end to make ready for the next phase: the transitional *catagen* stage, which lasts only a few weeks. During catagen, the follicle's metabolism slows down, the follicle contracts, and the papilla's production of keratin stops. This is not a sign that something has gone wrong but, rather, that the growth of that particular hair has run its course.

It is ready to be shed, so soon it enters the last, or *telogen*, phase of the cycle. Now the follicle rests in its contracted state—rather like an animal hibernating—until, in about three months, the hair it contains is physically dislodged from it by normal activity such as combing or washing. The loss of this hair triggers the follicle to enlarge again, and it heads back into the anagen phase, where it produces yet another hair. And so the cycle continues throughout your life.

At any one time, about 85 percent of your hairs will be in the anagen phase and the rest in either telogen or catagen. Luckily, each hair begins life separately, at a different time from the others, or one could end up bald for three months every two to six years. As it is, your hair tends to be shed relatively rapidly in the autumn as more of the follicles head into the telogen stage, and to grow rapidly in the summer.

HAIR LOSS IS NORMAL

Each day, you can expect to lose between 100 and 200 hairs. So you shouldn't be discouraged when you look down at the pillow in the morning and see a few lying there. This only means that new hairs will quickly be growing. That is, provided your hair is not coming out by the handful. Sometimes, as a result of sudden shock, hormonal change, or illness, large numbers of hairs are prematurely pushed into the telogen phase, and lost all at once. This kind of substantial hair loss is called telogen effluvium. But even this is nothing to worry about unduly, so long as whatever triggered the loss is either past (as in the case of childbirth) or being corrected with a relaxation technique and dietary supplements for undue stress or illness. What can be a problem, however, is *stoppage* of the normal growth cycle due to serious hormone imbalance that causes large numbers of follicles simply to shut down permanently. Then baldness ensues. But more about that kind of hair loss later.

WHY YOU HAVE THE HAIR YOU DO

How much hair you have, the color of it, the thickness, curl, and length it will grow before a new hair is begun all depend on your genetic inheritance. There is nothing you can do to change that. The diameter of each hair (its fineness) is determined somewhat by its color. Blondes tend to have more than anyone else (about 150,000 hairs), but the hairs tend to be finer. Brown hair is usually second with about 115,000, followed by black with 110,000 and red at about 90,000. How full your head of hair looks depends on both the number of hairs there and the thickness of the shaft itself. You need a lot of fine hairs, for instance, to give the impression of fullness but considerably fewer thick ones to give the same impression. If your hair is fine, you can make it look thicker by increasing the diameter of each strand with protein shampoos and body-building conditioners or by coloring your hair and giving it a permanent to swell out the shaft.

Your hair's curl or lack of it depends on two things. The first is its shape as it grows out of the follicle. Straight hair tends to be circular, wavy hair oval, and very curly hair more kidney-shaped. The proliferation of keratin in the papillae is also different in straight and in curly hair. Straight hair is formed by a papilla that makes the same number of cells all around the follicle. To grow curly hair, the papilla produces more cells at one side of the papilla for a while, then more at the other side. This causes the hair shaft to bend first in one direction and then the other and results in curly, or kinky, hair.

The color of your hair is determined by the type and amount of melanin pigment granules in the cortex of the hair shafts. But don't think that because you are a blonde you have all yellow pigments. If you examine your hair closely, you will see that the natural color of every head of hair is made up of a number of colors. Pluck ten hairs and if you are blond, for example, the chances are that seven of these will be blond, two red, and one brown, and yet your whole head appears to be blond. Most blond hair is mainly red and yellow pigments; red hair is red and black; and brown hair is red, brown, and black. White hair is white because it is pigment-free. Another thing that contributes to hair color is the number of air bubbles that naturally occur in your hair shafts. All these factors are genetically determined.

So is how *long* your hair gets if you let it grow, although how *fast* it grows appears to be influenced by several things such as diet, how much exercise you get (which improves circulation and overall fitness), and massage—which can be used to stimulate scalp circulation and, therefore, the health and functioning of the hair-producing follicles themselves.

I find there are two things women most worry about: One is wrinkles and the other is their hair. No woman is ever satisfied with it. When it is straight, she wants it curly, and when it is wavy, she wants it straight. The color is either too light, too dark, or too drab, and she either has too much or too little of it. There are a lot of things you can do for your hair and with your hair to make it more attractive, healthier, and more manageable, but it is important to realize from the beginning that you have to work with what you've got. There is no way to change your genetic inheritance, and it is only fruitless and miserable to worry about it.

WHAT TYPE ARE YOU?

Straight hair is often strong and beautiful hair. It can be lank, in which case you should treat it with a thickening product, which will enlarge the shaft of each hair and make it look fuller. It can also be lackluster, which calls for a conditioner to make the scales of the cuticle lie flat and enable hair shafts to reflect light better. Straight hair is often good blunt-cut and worn not too long, or tied up in a twist, or chignon.

Curly hair needs to be carefully cut, for this can make all the difference between its looking fantastic and frizzy. A layered cut is usually best, one in which the direction of each scissor snip goes counter to the direction in which the hair grows, so it makes the most of all your hair's natural curves and idiosyncrasies. It is best not to *impose* a particular style on your hair, but, rather, to go with the natural swing of things. If your hair tends to be wiry, you can correct this by using a softening conditioner.

Thin hair must never be allowed to get greasy, for any excess of oil on it will only make it look limp and lank. It is usually best to have it cut in a short style, and it is useful to shampoo it often. This will give it bounce and fullness. You should also use a body-building conditioner on it each time. Blowing it dry helps increase the fullness too.

Fine hair is delicate hair, but it is usually beautiful hair, too—like a baby's. Unlike thin hair, which is caused by a paucity of hair shafts, fine hair is made up of hair shafts of small diameter. You have to be particularly careful about what you do to it, because fine hair is the easiest of all hair types to damage from chemical treatments such as coloring and permanent waving or by using shampoos that are too alkaline, or by exposing it to the sun. Fine hair does well on protein shampoos and needs to be worn short unless you have a great deal of it.

Thick hair is a blessing, although few women who have it realize this—particularly if their hair is curly. In this case, you should probably not wear it too short, or it can be unmanageable. Thick hair is the easiest to handle and the toughest. It will withstand permanent waving and coloring far better than any of the other hair types and may not even need a conditioner at all when it is washed. If it is straight and you decide to get a permanent, then you should expect the waving process to take a third as long again as it usually does, because the hair shaft is big and tough to break down. But your perm can last you as much as a year, where anyone else's will have to be renewed in a few months.

WHAT STYLE IS RIGHT FOR YOU?

A lot of rubbish is talked about hairstyling. For instance, there is a longstanding convention that the perfect face is the oval face and that every hairstyle should be carefully designed to make every other shape of face, from square to pear-shaped, come as close to looking oval as possible through the clever art of optical illusion—slanted fringe here, some fullness there, and all the rest. Such an idea is old-fashioned and plainly foolish. Whoever said your face should be oval if it happens in reality to be heart- or diamond-shaped? Or even square? By what unwritten convention are you bound never to wear your hair back if you have a large nose, because it will make your nose look larger? The style you choose for yourself should, if anything, *emphasize* your own particular facial shapes and feature idiosyncracies, not try to hide them. A square face, with a wide jaw, often looks great in exactly the hairstyle it is supposed never to be associated with: hair sleeked severely back and close to the head. Forget all the rules.

Find yourself a hairdresser with taste and style (they can be discovered in the most unlikely places, just waiting for an opportunity to do something more interesting than what most women ask for). Take time to get to know him. It is impossible for a hairdresser to design the right style for you the first time he sees you. He needs to get a feel for you and your lifestyle, for how much time you have to spend at the hairdresser and how adept you are at doing your hair yourself. And you need to talk to him at length about how you would like to see yourself— what kind of look you want to emphasize. The whole process can be quite fun and the results pleasing.

The style you choose needs to be one that fits in with the way you live. If you are a businesswoman or young mother, you won't want to be bothered with setting your hair all the time—it is better to choose a style that is simple to look after and perhaps can be blow-dried and then left or, better still, only washed and let dry naturally in the air. Don't hesitate to take advantage of permanent waving, straightening, and coloring— they can do a lot to improve your overall look, provided your hair is in good and healthy condition and gets proper treatments and shampoo before you have any of these hair-processing treatments.

THE CUT IS THE THING

A good cut is more important than any other single factor when it comes to the way a head of hair looks. This is another reason why you must leave enough time to get acquainted with your hairdresser and for him to get to know your hair, how it grows, the way it swings (or doesn't) and all the other little things that make your particular head of hair unique— for it is that. There is no way in which you can take a hairstyle that looks good on one woman, transpose it to another, and expect it to look good. Everyone is an individual, and hairstyling that doesn't take this into account is worse than second-rate.

If your hair is very straight and shiny, a blunt cut often looks great, since it is easy to care for and shows off straight, healthy hair as well. If your hair tends to be thin or lack body, a layered cut can give it shape.

THE NUTRITION OF HAIR

The type, the length of growth, thickness, thinness, straightness, and curl of your hair depend on your inheritance, but the condition of your hair depends on the internal state of your body, which feeds the papillae that produce it. For hair to be beautiful, the cuticle and the cortex have to be strong. It has always amused me when I hear hairdressers arguing about whether or not diet has anything to do with the beauty of hair, because it does, as any farmer knows well. Not only can you change the look of an animal's hair by altering its diet (and that goes for the human animal too), you can also tell a great deal about its internal condition by examining its hair. If you have a sheep that is poorly, its coat shows it. Horses, dogs, and cats are given special vitamin and mineral supplements to improve their coats for shows. But only recently has this aspect of hair care even begun to be looked at for human beings.

What occurs in each hair follicle depends on the current nutritional state of your bloodstream and on adequate oxygen reaching the cells. So true is this that when you put someone on a poor diet, you will detect detrimental changes in the hair bulb even on the second day of the regimen. In a study of people placed on a protein-free diet for fifteen days, researchers have found that hairs plucked from their heads and then analyzed microscopically showed significant changes in color, texture, and structure—damage that took some time to correct.

About the worst thing you can do for your hair is to go on a crash diet or live on typical Western fare, high in refined carbohydrates, processed foods, and white sugar. Both upset the vitamin and mineral balance in your body, and adequate vitamins and minerals are vital to hair.

Iron

Hair's most important mineral is probably iron. If you are anemic, iron-deficient, your hair will tend to be brittle, lusterless, and hard to manage. It may also be thinner than is normal for you. For iron-deficiency anemia is a condition often implicated in excessive hair loss. If you have any of these hair difficulties, it is worthwhile having a serum iron test (which measures the total amount of iron in your bloodstream) and a total iron-binding-capacity test (which gives the ratio of blood iron to the blood's total capacity to hold iron). A normal ratio is about 1 to 4. If yours falls somewhere between 1 to 5 and 1 to 7, then your hair would probably benefit from iron therapy. Your doctor can arrange these tests for you. And it is important to remember, whether or not you take iron supplements, that vitamin C enhances iron absorption by helping ferric iron to be reduced to its ferrous form; also, iron is best absorbed when calcium is present in sufficient quantities.

Sulfur

Another important mineral for hair is the "beauty mineral," sulfur. It keeps your hair glossy and smooth. Sulfur is one of the constituents of keratin. When it is supplied in adequate amounts, your hair is strong. Eggs are particularly rich in the sulfur-containing amino acids and are excellent hair food. Other natural sources include cabbage, dried beans, legumes, fish, nuts, and meat.

Zinc

Research has established that a zinc deficiency is commonly the cause of hair damage in animals. It is probably true of humans as well and is certainly one of the factors contributing to the hair loss that women on the Pill or estrogen therapy experience, since the hormones reduce zinc levels in the body. But the Pill can have other effects detrimental to hair too. It lowers blood levels of vitamins B_{12}, B_6, and B_2, increasing your body's need for these vitamins as well as folic acid, vitamin C, and the trace minerals zinc and iron. If you are an estrogen taker and your hair is giving you trouble, it may be helpful to take supplements of these nutrients.

The B Vitamins

The B-complex vitamins are particularly important to hair health and beauty. Deficiencies of biotin, folic acid, pantothenic acid, and PABA can lead to a loss of color, and there has even been some success in reversing the graying process by giving supplements of these nutrients—particularly megavitamin doses of PABA. One researcher claims to have restored color to graying hair in 70 percent of cases.

A lack of any of the B complex can result in hair troubles and losses. Vitamins B_1, B_2, and B_{12} are particularly important in invigorating lackluster hair, dandruff, scaling, redness of the scalp, and hair loss. Vitamin C is important too, because it maintains the health and strength of the capillaries supplying your hair-producing follicles with nourishment. If your levels of vitamin C are too low, this results in perifollicular hemorrhages, in which these capillaries break and bleed, which results in improper nourishment to the papillae.

How fast your hair can grow depends on adequate, but not too much, protein, since more than adequate amounts can deplete your body of the minerals it needs. The widespread notion propounded by many glossy magazines that if you eat lots of meat and drink milk several times a day, you will have strong and beautiful hair is simply untrue. It is the right *balance* of nutrients that is most important. The condition of your hair is greatly affected by medicines that you take—and I don't just mean antibiotics and sulfa drugs, although these two are common culprits for causing trouble. But aspirin, the Pill, diet pills, tranquilizers, thyroid pills, cortisone, anticancer drugs, and even cold remedies are a common cause of brittleness, dullness, breakage, and loss. Hair follicles are ultrasensitive to hormones. If you are taking a birth-control pill and having trouble with your hair, you might consider asking your doctor to try another brand to see if it improves, as well as taking supplements—or better still, use another form of contraception, such as a diaphragm.

HAIR HEALTH AND BEAUTY FROM THE OUTSIDE

The shine of your hair depends on the condition of the cuticle. Made up of transparent keratin, the cells of your hair's cuticle should form a clear, flat surface that refracts light, making your hair look shiny. But in order for these fish-scale-like plates to lie flat, the cuticle has to be healthy and contracted. This means that the *imbrications*—the natural shingles of the cuticle—need to be *closed*. When they are closed, your hair is protected from much physical and chemical damage and light catches it beautifully. Many things can disrupt the cuticle and lead to the opening of the imbrications: very alkaline shampoos, for instance, which make the hair shaft swell. The swelling pushes out the scaly cells, making them stand away from the shaft. Very strong alkaline substances such as permanent wave solutions and bleaching agents can even *dissolve* some of the cuticle, leaving holes and tears in it, which makes your hair look permanently dull.

Damage to the cuticle can come from physical causes too. For instance, too much heat on the hair from careless blow drying, teasing, or back-combing, and overexposure to the sun. To have shiny hair, you have to be particularly careful not to damage it from the outside. There are some things, however, that help restore a smooth cuticle to hair: mildly acidic substances, for instance, such as vinegar and lemon rinse or one of the proprietary conditioning treatments, all of which shrink the hair shaft and encourage the imbrications to close and the cells to lie flat. These things also strengthen the keratin, which is why if you have fragile, dry, or fine hair or you do not use a pH-balanced shampoo, you should always use an acid rinse (either commercially or at home) after washing your hair. (More about pH later.) The natural oils, secreted from the follicle, which coat the outside shaft also help the hair look shiny. Provided, that is, that you wash your hair often enough. Oil left on hair for too long tends to accumulate dust and dirt on the shaft, which quickly destroys shine.

How much flexibility and bounce your hair has is also something that can be determined by how you look after it from the outside. It depends on the water content of each shaft. Healthy hair has enough water in it to keep the keratin in the hair shaft supple and firm, so that your hair will stretch without breaking, keep a set well, and feel silky. If the hair's water content becomes depleted from exposure to too much heat or the sun or a very alkaline shampoo, then it will become brittle, break easily, and refuse to hold a set. Another dehydrator is chlorine in swimming pools. Conditioners can help coat the outside of each hair shaft to keep it from drying excessively. But the best insurance of all is simply keeping your hair away from too much heat and from chemical desiccators.

Fullness, body, and the overall look of a head of hair are greatly determined by a good cut and by the kind of products and treatments you use on it. We'll look at those in the next chapter.

32

The Craft of Hair Care

To be beautiful, your hair has to be kept clean, well cut, brushed, and protected from external damage. It also needs the benefit of regular massage to ensure that circulation to the follicles in the scalp is good.

SHAMPOOING

There are two types of shampoos: those containing soap and those that are artificial detergents. Most, these days, are detergent-based. The reason for this is that while soap is good for cleansing away old hair spray, dull oil, and epidermal debris, it tends to leave scum, particularly in hard water. Also, modern detergent shampoos do more than just clean. They contain other chemical ingredients, which impart cosmetic properties such as shine and manageability to hair. If your hair is short and you live in a soft-water area, you can probably get away with using soap, provided you use a conditioner afterward. These days they come in many forms: pastes, clear liquids, cloudy lotions, and gels, and also with special ingredients such as herbs, protein, balsam, eggs, and lemon. But whatever their form, most shampoos are put together from the same basic chemicals. First there is the detergent itself to do the cleansing. Then there is a sequestering agent, which is a chemical that traps the minerals in hard water (such as lime) so that the shampoo lathers well and rinses away easily. Most shampoos also contain foam builders to increase their lathering abilities, plus either clarifying or opacifying agents, which do nothing for your hair but render the product either clear or cloudy or creamy depending on what manufacturers think will best appeal to the market. And, of course, all shampoos contain preservatives to keep their ingredients from spoiling.

By far the most important ingredients as far as hair beauty is concerned are the conditioners, which are added to most shampoos nowadays. They vary from one formula to the next, but they include ingredients to eliminate static electricity from the hair when it dries, to coat the hair shaft with protein and thereby enlarge it, making your hair look thicker, and to render the hair shafts slippery so that your hair doesn't tangle when you comb it out. Shampoos become more and more sophisticated every few years in their formulations—a sophistication that is certainly to the benefit of your hair, provided you can find the right one for you. And apart from certain guidelines that depend on your hair type, finding the right one is mostly a matter of trial and error.

THE QUESTION OF pH

There is one more additive—not exactly an additive, rather a group of them—which is important; chemicals are added to shampoos to make them pH-balanced. Your hair, like your skin, has an acid mantle, with a pH from 4.5 to 5.5, made out of the natural oils from the follicle. This acid mantle plays an important protective role keeping the imbrications of the cuticle from opening and the hair from becoming hard to manage, dull-looking, and vulnerable to damage. A shampoo that is pH-balanced, that is, which is slightly acidic so that its pH is about the same as your hair's, helps to maintain the hair's strength and health. If it does not say "pH-balanced" on the label, you can check it with litmus paper. Alkaline shampoos disturb and disrupt the acid mantle, causing the tiny scales of the cuticle to open and the hair shaft to swell. Using a pH-balanced shampoo is particularly important if your hair is fragile, permanent-waved, or colored. If your hair is strong and in good condition, then it does not really matter what kind of shampoo you use on it, provided you put a cream rinse or a homemade vinegar-and-water or lemon-and-water rinse on it afterward. Since conditioners and rinses such as these are acidic, they will close up the imbrications opened by the shampoo, shrink the hair shaft back to its normal size, and leave it looking shiny.

WHAT KIND OF SHAMPOO IS FOR YOU?

Taking into account the things already said, you can choose the cheapest one you like the smell of, since your hair will carry the scent in it of your shampoo for a day or so afterward. But there are certain kinds that are particularly good for certain kinds of hair.

Lemon: These shampoos are especially good for oily hair, because they help remove the oil without leaving the hair lackluster and lank.

Balsam: This is a good ingredient to choose if your hair is very fine or lacks body. Balsam is a resinous substance from the bark of certain trees. In a shampoo, it coats the hair shafts, lending them thickness and strength.

Camomile: This is an excellent ingredient for blond or light brown hair, since this flower has mild bleaching properties. If you use a camomile shampoo regularly, it helps keep light hair bright and shiny.

Herbs: "Herbs" added to a shampoo doesn't mean a great deal, for many herb formulas (unlike camomile) have no real action on the hair and are created only to appeal to women's back-to-nature feelings. Some, however, such as white nettle, can be useful for dandruff.

Protein: Protein shampoos come in two types; both can be useful for hair. The first type contains a simple protein made from eggs, milk, soya, gelatin, beef (or an exotic vegetable called tong bean), which helps to coat the outer layers of the hair, making the hair look thicker. Most protein shampoos are of this type. The second type does far more. Called *substantive protein,* the protein it contains is hydrolized and of the correct molecular weight and size to be absorbed into the cuticle, strengthening it at the same time as aligning its scales and thickening the shaft. This kind of protein shampoo is particularly good for use on treated, damaged, or fine hair. It is not so valuable on strong and healthy hair, for hydrolized polypeptide proteins are absorbed more rapidly by damaged hair than by a relatively compact keratin structure, which does not really need them.

When buying a shampoo, don't worry too much if it does not give much lather, since this is more a measure of the sequestering agent it contains than of its cleaning ability. It should have a good conditioning action, to leave your hair soft and gleaming, and your hair should be easy to comb out afterward. It should also rinse out easily.

How often you shampoo depends on you and on the type of hair you have. If it is dry, not more than a couple of times a week is best. If it is normal or oily you can shampoo every day if you like, provided you use a pH-balanced shampoo. However often you do, you need only lather once, unless your hair is really grimy. More than once strips away too much of the hair's natural oils from the cuticle.

GETTING HAIR INTO CONDITION

A good conditioner can put right a number of hair problems. All cream rinses, conditioners, and treatments are on the acidic side of the pH scale. They are intended to close up the imbrications of the cuticle after shampooing and to shrink it back to normal size. In addition, a cream rinse should contain ingredients such as quaternary aluminum salts to separate the individual hairs and make them easy to comb out and to protect against static electricity. Finally, they should coat hairs with an ingredient such as protein or balsam, which will give more body and protect the cuticle from moisture loss.

Some conditioners contain a large quantity of oil. They are fine for dry hair but will make normal and oily hair into a lank mop that needs to be washed again the next day or so. If you ever have this trouble with a conditioner or cream rinse, then try one of the oil-free ones. They do just as good a job as the others in adding body and protecting hair, but they don't cause lankness.

Protein packs or concentrated treatments left on the hair for from five to twenty minutes (the hair will take up all of a substance it is going to in twenty minutes, so there is never any reason to leave it any longer) are excellent as an occasional treatment for hair of all types (say once a month or every six weeks) and exceptionally good for colored, permanent-waved, and damaged hair, used once a week. They will strengthen and protect the hair and leave it soft and shiny.

STYLING AND SETTING

Because the keratin that makes up hair is a protein, like all proteins it can be treated with heat to change its shape. This makes it possible to curl, uncurl, shape, and mold your hair into a particular style by blow-drying it, by setting it wet and allowing it to dry, or by using heated rollers or a curling iron on dry hair. The protein of hair consists of molecules arranged in organized patterns held together by two kinds of chemical bonds: hydrogen and sulfur. The hydrogen bonds are the weaker of the two. When you set your hair on rollers, or blow it dry while easing it into a particular shape, you break, then re-form, these hydrogen bonds to create a temporary new structure. But it is a tenuous one, for water, heat, lots of brushing, and time can break the hydrogen bonds again so that your hair returns to its former structure and you lose the new shape.

Sulfur bonds are strong. They can be broken only by strong alkaline solutions such as those of permanent waves, straighteners, and coloring products. Sulfur bonds are broken and then re-formed when you have your hair waved, and the new structure formed through these changes lasts far longer.

The problem with breaking either hydrogen or sulfur bonds and then re-forming them is that most of the things used to style a head of hair, such as heat and alkaline solutions, are potentially damaging to it. They have to be used with care.

Blow drying is an excellent way to style straight or curly hair, provided you have patience and strong arms and provided you don't do it too often. Once or twice a week, yes. Every day, no. Hot air can cause progressive, cumulative damage to the cuticle and, finally, to the cortex and medulla, too. Choose a dryer that is not too high in watts (1,000 is enough), as a high wattage may do the job faster but your hair will suffer if you are not extremely careful to keep the dryer far enough from the hair or to use the lowest setting. If your hair is heated above 150 degrees Fahrenheit (66 C), you can do irreversible damage to it, making it brittle, dry, and scorched. There are some protein-based lotions that you can spray on your hair to help protect it from the intense heat—these are specifically designed for blow dryers, and most of them are very good. But you still need to be careful.

Do your hair in two stages: First use the dryer on its own to get the hair almost dry all over, then begin styling with the dryer in one hand and your curved or round brush (made specially for blow drying) in the other. Keep the dryer six inches from your hair and constantly moving. Section your hair into the sides, the back, the side back, and the top front, clipping each section and then letting it down as you need it. Begin on the underneath of one side and then work around the whole head, drying the hair section by section. Do the back first, the front always last, brushing and drying the hair *against* the direction in which it grows. This creates volume. Do the underneath layers first. When they are dry, bring down another layer from above to work on, constantly twirling the brush in the hair to get the curve and the shape you are after. Last of all, do the front or the fringe, brushing it back and then curving it over the forehead and finally brushing it into place. The art of blow-drying your hair yourself is something that takes time and a great deal of practice to learn, and it is important before you begin styling that your hair be almost dry or you will exhaust yourself in the process.

Setting your hair can be done wet on rollers or dry on heated rollers or the hair can be curled dry on a curling iron. A wet set will last you longest, provided you dry it thoroughly under a dryer or in the air. Heated rollers, like blow drying, are something you should not use every day, for they tend to damage the ends of the hair, making them dry and brittle. This can be avoided somewhat by wrapping each roller with a piece of tissue paper or toilet paper before putting it into your hair. Never use heated rollers on wet hair—they won't work. And never use a curling iron on wet hair, or you may damage it badly. Always section your hair carefully when you are putting rollers in—the more rollers you use and the less hair on each the better and longer-lasting will be the set you get. A useful technique is to blow-dry the hair and then put in a couple of heated rollers at the front to give it extra swing and shape. However you style your hair, always let it cool before brushing out, or you will ruin the new structure of it.

BRUSHING AND COMBING

Brushing is good for hair, provided you have a good brush and you do not overdo it. It stimulates circulation of the scalp, removes loose scales from the skin on the head, and distributes your hair's natural oils well, which means it helps protect the cuticles and create shine. The brush you choose should have evenly spaced bristles with *rounded* ends. The best brushes for your hair are still made from animal bristles.

Nylon bristles have blunt ends, which can cause splits and cracks to the hair. Some brushes have bristles set in rubber. They are particularly good, for they give a massage to the scalp while you brush. About thirty to fifty strokes a day is good—more than that is too much, and with less you are not really doing anything. When you brush, you need to bend at the waist and brush your hair from underneath as well as back from the crown. The more positions you can brush from (leaning to the side, with head hanging down, etc.) the better job you will do. Lowering your head while you brush back the side does something else, too. It brings circulation to the scalp in the way that the yoga headstand does. If your hair is long, don't pull the brush through the full length of it. Instead, brush to the shoulder and then, taking hold of the rest of the hair with your other hand, pull the brush down the rest of the way to the ends. You should always brush firmly, but never drag. And you should never brush wet hair, for the disruption of the hydrogen bonds that comes with wetting makes your hair a great deal more susceptible to breakage and damage than when it is dry. Some women fear that brushing is going to take out too much hair. This is unfounded. You will only lose the telogen hairs, which are ready to be lost anyway, and their loss will simply stimulate new growth.

When choosing a comb, pick one with the largest teeth you can find that are blunt at the ends so they don't scratch the scalp. Hard rubber, nylon, or bone are the best. Always comb your hair gently, never yanking or pulling at a tangle.

MASSAGE CAN BE WONDERFUL

Anything that increases circulation to the scalp and activates the papillae and follicles tends to make for sturdier hair shafts and to improve hair growth. Besides daily brushing, the best thing you can do for the hair is to massage the scalp. Many people have a genetic tendency to restricted circulation in the scalp, which shows itself in slow hair growth and poor-quality hair. Each hair root is fed by the complex vascular network in the scalp that brings nutrients and oxygen through the blood and carries away carbon dioxide and other metabolic wastes. When circulation there is poor, the hair root suffers. Waste products build up in the tissues, so that the hair cells grow only slowly and may even die, resulting in thinning hair. This can be avoided (and often corrected, too) by scalp massage.

People with a tendency to oily hair can also benefit from massage. A healthy scalp is loose, rich in vascularity, and thick. The scalp of someone who produces excessive oil is usually just the opposite of this: tight, with poor circulation, and thin. Daily massage can do a great deal to correct this. The idea that massaging your head will make an oily condition even worse because it stimulates the follicles to produce even more oil is just not true. It is far more likely to help normalize trigger-happy oil glands than to stimulate them to further production. Many a too oily head of hair is put right by massage.

Here's How to Massage

Using your fingertips and the palm of your hand just below the thumb, push them firmly into your scalp at the sides and, keeping them in the same place, rotate them in small circles. You will be moving the scalp, not your fingers—it is important that fingers stay in the same place to stimulate circulation well and so that you never pull your hair. After you have worked in one position for about thirty seconds, remove both hands from your head and take up a new position, rotating fingertips again firmly for thirty seconds there and so on until you have done your whole scalp. The massage shouldn't take more than three minutes, and it will leave you feeling fresher as well as doing something good for your hair.

If you suffer from tension in your neck and shoulders, this, too, can interfere with proper circulation to your scalp and create hair problems. Use the neck exercises in the chapter on posture to correct this. An electric vibrator is also a good investment for hair: Use it both on your scalp and on your neck and shoulders.

THE COSMETIC TREATMENTS

Permanent Waves

Waving and straightening hair involve pretty much the same process. First you break down the sulfur bonds connecting the protein molecules by using a highly alkaline solution containing a chemical such as ammonium thioglycolate. Then you rearrange the softened hair into the structure you want it to have. Finally, you use a peroxide neutralizer to halt the chemical action of the bond-breaking chemical and to encourage the new shape to set. Since the neutralizer is acidic, it also helps close up the imbrications in the cuticle and encourages the hair shaft to become strong again. Finally, your hair is treated with some kind of conditioner to restore some of the damage done by the process.

In the case of the permanent, the reshaping of hair takes place while it is wound tightly on curlers. With straightening, the reshaping takes place while it is being combed, stretched, and encouraged to give up its natural tendency to curve. The secret of successful permanent waving is twofold: First, the hair must be wound carefully in *small* sections on the curlers in order for the right curl to "take." Second, the timing has to be right. The thioglycolate has to be allowed to stay in the hair long enough to disrupt its chemical bonds and give it new ones, but not so long that it softens the hair too much, or your hair will suffer real damage. The neutralizers, which chemically reverse the action of the thioglycolate and reharden the hair, need to be put on at just the right time. And the right time varies greatly from one head of hair to another. Fine or damaged hair will need very little time (neither will it hold a permanent very long, once it is given). Coarse, thick hair will take much longer, but it will also keep its curl for months.

Caring for Processed Hair

Once your hair is waved, it is more vulnerable to damage than ever before, so there are a few special precautions you need to take in order to preserve its health and sheen. For instance, instead of brushing 50 strokes a day, cut it down to only 20. Use scalp massage or an electric vibrator instead, to give scalp circulation the stimulation it needs. Also, only use acid-balanced shampoos when you wash your hair, and always apply a conditioning rinse. Protein conditioners are particularly good for permanent-waved and colored hair. They keep the cracks in the cuticle closed and make your hair smoother and shinier.

How often you get a permanent depends on the condition and length of your hair. If it is long, you should only need one every six months—shorter hair perhaps every two or three. If you have only a body wave—

a soft wave in which the hair is wound on larger rollers—then you will need to have it redone more often than a regular permanent, which is much tighter. If your hair has been bleached or tinted, it is a good idea to have one of the new permanents especially designed for bleached or damaged hair. They don't last so long, but they do ensure that the hair remains in good condition, and you don't run the risk of a permanent's not "taking" because the cuticle has already been broken down so much that there is not enough elasticity left in it to remold the hair's shape.

Provided your hair is healthy and you look after it well after the permanent, there is no reason to worry about its condition being spoiled by the waving. A permanent will add a lot of body to lank hair and can often improve a too oily condition as well.

It is a good idea when having your first perm to go to a hairdresser. That way, you can learn about how the curl winding is done properly and also get to know the characteristics of your hair, such as how much time it needs for the wave to take. After that, there is no reason why you can't give yourself later perms at home if you prefer. It is a lot cheaper.

Straightening Hair

Besides the thioglycolate straighteners, which are put on hair still damp from having been washed, left on for about fifteen minutes, and then combed through for another fifteen minutes before neutralizing, there are two other types of chemical straighteners commercially available. The first are the ammonium bisulfate or sodium bisulfate straighteners, which are not as effective on very curly hair as the thioglycolates but are much safer. You put them on wet hair, tuck it under a plastic covering for fifteen minutes, and then comb it out for twenty minutes. They are ideal for hair that is not excessively curly.

The other type, the sodium hydroxide straighteners, are highly alkaline and have to be carefully applied or they may irritate the skin. They can also be very dangerous if you get any in your eyes. They are the fastest-acting of all the straighteners and demand only about half the combing time to do their work before you apply the neutralizer. But they are not good for hair that is in less than perfect condition.

There are also some short-term but simple ways to straighten hair. It can be done by blow-drying with a brush to smooth it out or by washing your hair and then wrapping it wet around your head in a circle, like a cap, fastening it with clips and letting it dry. Then, when it is dry, you simply comb it out straighter. Finally, the old-fashioned and very efficient method for long, curly hair is simply ironing it with an electric iron. Spread the hair out on a board, keep the iron on the lowest setting, and go over it gently from roots to ends. But the same advice given for blow drying and heated rollers stands here: Be careful not to put too much heat on it. Burnt hair is irretrievably lost.

A CHANGE OF COLOR

One of the simplest and most effective ways of changing your appearance is to change the color of your hair. As we get older, the color of hair tends either to fade or to go darker, so that a once shimmery golden mane or deep mahogany tresses can become lackluster and dull. One of the best ways of remedying the situation is with a color boost. Hair coloring these days is effective and reasonably priced and can look even better than most natural hair—provided, of course, it is done correctly. Otherwise it can end up looking like a burnished haystack.

There are two categories of hair colorants: *permanent* colorants, which enter the cortex and cannot be washed out, and the *temporary* and the *semipermanent*, which can be used to highlight and intensify your own hair color but won't alter the cortex.

The Temporary Colorants

These are the easiest to use. They coat the cuticle of the hair with color that washes away with the next shampoo. You can get temporary highlighting shampoos and color rinses in a great variety of colors that don't disturb the cuticle imbrications. Most of them have a shine-promoting pH, too. But what you can do with them is limited, for while they will darken the hair—say from blond to red or to black—they are really designed for minor color changes only. If you try to go too many shades away from your natural color, they tend to streak and give uneven coverage. They also cannot make your hair lighter than it is, because they have no action on the cortex, where the melanin granules are —they merely coat the outside of the hair shaft.

The Semipermanents

Like the temporaries, these contain no peroxide. Instead, they are a combination of the same vegetable dyes with other chemicals such as a thioglycolate or sulfur, which suspend minute molecules of color for deeper penetration of the hair shaft and make them longer-lasting. They, too, coat the outside of the hair shaft and so are not good for drastically changing hair color. Nor will they lighten. What they are good for is touching up hair that has just started to go gray, highlighting your own natural coloring, and making gray hair look shinier and more attractive without really changing its shade. The "semis" are more alkaline than the "temporaries," and so may do some damage to the hair cuticle. If you use one, be sure to use a pH-balanced shampoo afterward.

The Permanents

There are three kinds of permanent hair colorants: vegetable dyes such as henna, metallic dyes such as those used to gradually cover gray hair, and the aniline dyes or oxidation tints, which include most of the colorants used professionally in salons.

THE VEGETABLE DYES

Henna is the best-known, since its use dates back thousands of years. Taken from the *Lawsonia* plant, which is indigenous to Africa and Asia, henna varies in color depending on which country it comes from. It can be strong orange in color, as Moroccan henna, or a deep red, as the henna that comes from Iran—the most sought-after in the world. The plant is harvested, dried in the sun, and then crushed into a greenish powder, which is what one puts on the hair. It coats the hair shaft's cuticle a reddish color.

The standard way of using henna is to add hot water to make a creamy paste and then put this on the hair and leave it for up to one hour. Daniel Galvin, Britain's top colorist, who is an expert in the use of herbal hair colorings, uses a different method and gets beautiful results. He adds hot black coffee to the powder, mixes it into a paste, and then adds the juice of a fresh lemon and the yolk of an egg. The coffee brings out the depth and richness of the hair color, the acid in the lemon accelerates the reddening, and the egg yolk keeps the mixture moist and easy to maneuver through the hair. Sometimes he also adds some 10 percent peroxide to lighten the whole effect.

Henna will give brunette and black hair a lovely reddish glow—the darker your hair the more chestnut is the effect. Lighter hair goes Titian. Henna does not do well on mousy hair, as the resulting tone is usually an unattractive orange. It should never be used over a tint, is no good on gray hair, and can be very drying to any hair, so it is better to avoid it if your hair is already dry. Many of the henna products now on the market claim to have henna of many colors: brown, black, blond, etc. They contain metallic chemicals, which coat the hair and are troublemakers if later you want to tint or wave it. Avoid them. The only color of henna you should use is *red*, which in its natural, powder form is a pale green.

Camomile, another herbal colorant, has a gentle lightening effect on hair and is wonderful for "sun-streaking" blond and light brown hair.

But you must be patient, for it takes several applications and plenty of time to work. Its advantage over other bleaching methods is that, like the sun, it never brings a brassy or yellow tone to hair. Camomile-bleached hair looks exactly like natural hair with sun streaks. Even a professional colorist can't tell the difference. It is not useful for brown hair or dark hair, but it will gently lighten red and works beautifully on all shades of natural blond. The herb also adds shine to the hair. There are two methods of using it: You can make a camomile rinse to use after each shampoo as the last rinse by taking 2 tablespoons of dried camomile flowers and tossing them into a pint of boiling water. Simmer for fifteen minutes, strain, cool, and use as a final rinse (you can make more at once and refrigerate it for up to ten days). You leave the rinse in your hair and towel it dry. The alternative way is faster in its effect. I devised it as a way of making use of the very delicate British sunlight to lighten hair. I do it about three times each summer to keep my naturally blond hair bright. Add one cup of dried camomile flowers to half a pint of boiling water for fifteen minutes. Cool. Simmer and strain. Add the juice of a fresh lemon to the infusion plus two tablespoons of a rich cream conditioner. Put it on dry hair, comb through, and then go and sit in the sun (with a sunscreen on your face, of course) until it dries. Finally, shampoo and condition as usual. You can use this method whenever you are going to be out in the sun for a few hours, and simply let the mixture dry on the hair. Your hair will be in beautiful condition by the time you shampoo it, at the end of the day.

Daniel has several other herbal tricks he often uses (in fact, he even mixes herbs with proprietary hair colorants for special effects, something no woman should ever do at home). For instance, he boils saffron root in water for thirty minutes and then dilutes his solution to whatever strength is required for use as a water rinse on blond hair. It gives a vibrant, canary-yellow tone. He uses an infusion of marigolds as a final rinse to give blond hair delicate yellow tones, and he relies on sage to darken graying hair by adding herbs to a pint of water (the amount of sage depends on the darkening effect required), boiling for fifteen minutes, straining, and using as a final rinse.

All herb treatments except perhaps henna are gentle and not intended for drastic changes in color.

THE METALLIC DYES

These you have no doubt heard about—they are supposed to be the magical cure for graying hair and are often called *color restorers*. They deposit metallic dyes and salts of various metals such as manganese, cobalt, silver, and copper on your hair shaft, which gradually darkens the hair. But hair dyed this way does not permanent-wave well, nor is its condition very good, as this kind of dye tends to make the hair look a dull, flat color. Metallic dyes have to be removed completely, with the use of a special preparation, several days before waving or tinting with a permanent colorant. Because of their many disadvantages, I think they are best avoided.

BLEACHING

Hair bleaching is done with hydrogen peroxide, which affects the hair shaft both physically and chemically. Combined with an alkaline compound such as ammonia, it opens the imbrications of the cuticle so that it can penetrate the hair shaft, and then inside the cortex it chemically oxidizes the melanin pigments, fading their color, thus bleaching out the hair in the process. There are products on the market that are simple bleachers—they are called lighteners, and they consist of peroxide together with ammonia. Sometimes a "drabber" is added in order to remove the red highlights that come from bleaching darker hair. Bleaching forms an important part of the other permanent tints, which also rely on oxidation processes to work.

THE ANILINE OR OXIDATION COLORANTS

The most permanent (and the most successful), these dyes are included in a number of products for coloring hair such as tinting shampoos, highlighting shampoos, and the single-step and double-step permanent colorants you can buy in packages at the drugstore. They are permanent dyes, because the artificial pigment is made to penetrate into the cortex of the hair shaft. There it stays. How this happens is most interesting.

Tiny molecules of colorless dye are mixed with a "developer" such as hydrogen peroxide and then put on the hair. The hydrogen peroxide opens up the imbrications of the cuticle, and the molecules enter through them into the cortex. Once inside, they react with the oxygen from the peroxide (a very unstable substance), which spurs the molecules of the dye to oxidize and combine, forming larger molecules. In the process, these new and larger molecules develop the desired color, but they have now become so large that they can no longer pass through the cuticle, so they get *stuck* on the inside. There are more than 50,000 aniline dyes, each different in shade, thanks to slight changes in the arrangements of their molecules.

They are potent and effective. They are also potential allergens, since about one woman in ten cannot tolerate an aniline dye without reacting adversely to it. This is why it is important, whenever using a permanent colorant on your hair either at home or at the hairdresser, that a patch test be done first. The anilines can even cause blindness, so they should never be used to tint your eyelashes or eyebrows. If you have your hair dyed with an aniline dye, you must wait at least a week before having it permanent-waved or straightened, and you must use a pH-balanced shampoo and conditioner every time you wash it. One of the advantages of the anilines is that tinting limp, straight hair that won't hold a set can often make it more manageable, since the peroxide in the dye disturbs the cuticle just enough to give the hair some body and eliminate its lankness.

In this category of hair colorant you will find shampoo tints and high-light shampoos, which can be used at home to cover gray if there is too much of it, to lighten hair a couple of shades, to add depth, or to high-light hair that is drab and dull. You put the products on as you would an ordinary shampoo and then leave them in the hair for a few minutes while the peroxide and dye does its work, and then rinse off. They are simple to use.

The single- and double-step tints also fall into this category. They are the dyes most frequently used by hairdressers. If you want to change the color of your hair dramatically, you should have it done professionally. There is quite an art to color mixing and application (I know women who literally fly 5,000 miles to have their color done by someone who is a real master at it). Although there are some excellent products available for home use, if it were my hair, I would still shun them and head for a salon that specializes in color.

The single-step tints are a mixture of aniline dyes, peroxide, and ammonia in an oil base. They are applied carefully to sectioned hair, starting an inch or so away from the roots to the end. The hair is left to sit for a few minutes and then the root area is done. The hair is rested for another half hour or so. These dyes can change the color of your hair to almost any other color, but they are not successful in changing very dark shades to blond. For that, you need a *two-step tint*, which bleaches out the existing pigment in the hair shafts in the first step and then adds dye separately in the second. All aniline dyes and bleaching procedures have to be touched up often as the roots grow out, particularly if you change the color drastically from your normal hair shade. They also cause considerable damage to the hair shaft. If you have your hair tinted with them, you must look after it using a pH-balanced shampoo and conditioner and having a protein treatment every couple of weeks.

FROSTING AND STREAKING

One of the best and most easily manageable ways of changing your hair color is to have it streaked or frosted. This involves the same procedures as the single- and double-step tinting, but instead of being done all over your head, they are done only on some strands or areas. Streaking and frosting are particularly useful for older hair that has darkened or faded. They can bring new life to a head of hair by lightening some of the strands, but they create no harsh lines between the tinted and natural hair at the scalp, as total dyeing does. This means that you don't need touch-ups more frequently than every two or three months. There are an enormous number of techniques used in frosting and tinting. Some of the most interesting involve three or more colors put into the hair to give a remarkably natural look.

SPECIAL CARE FOR BLEACHED OR TINTED HAIR

The golden rule for processed hair is to stay out of the sun. The sun does harm in two ways: It dries out the hair, and it alters the color. Keratin needs water to stay soft and flexible. When too much water is lost as a result of sun or of using heated rollers or of blow-drying too often, then its fibers crack and split and the hair becomes so dry and brittle that it breaks off. It also loses its shine. Sunlight does strange things to hair color. It can turn it greenish or very brassy, or simply make the tint go flat and gray. If you are going into the sun and your hair is bleached or tinted, wear a hat or a towel wrapped around it. Even virgin—that is, un-treated—hair needs protection from sunlight. You can use one of the sunscreen products especially made for hair or simply rub in some high-protection suntan lotion you use on your body—shampooing it out at the end of the day.

WHAT ABOUT CANCER RISKS?

There is some indication that about 1 percent of the chemical hair dyes used on hair will penetrate through the skin and be absorbed into the bloodstream. The question is, What damage will they do? Professor Bruce Ames, at the University of California, has tested 169 hair dyes on bacterial cells to find out if they cause mutations to the cells. Of these, 89 percent were found to be mutagenic. Although all carcinogens (cancer-causing substances) are mutagenic, not all mutagens are car-cinogens, nor do we know if the same results will occur on human cells. The people most at risk from exposure to hair tints are those hair colorists in salons who use them daily without wearing gloves (something you should never do). It is unlikely that cancer risks are very great for the average woman who has her hair tinted. If you are uneasy about it, use one of the semipermanents or herbal dyes instead.

Now let's take a look at some of the most common hair problems and their solutions.

33

Problem Solving

WHAT CAN BE DONE FOR DRY HAIR?

That depends on the cause of the dryness. If your hair is naturally dry due to there being fewer than normal oil glands in the scalp, then it will still be strong and healthy hair—not at all the same thing as a head of hair that is dry from overprocessing (permanent waving and coloring), overexposure to the sun, or overuse of hot-air dryers and heated rollers. Then the individual hairs are weak and fragile. Naturally-dry hair needs an occasional oil treatment to coat the cuticle and help protect it from further moisture loss—in other words, to replace the hair's natural oils, which should be doing the job themselves.

Here's how to give an oil treatment: Place 2 ounces of olive oil in a blender and add to it the same amount of boiling water. Turn on high for a few seconds, until all the oil has been broken up into little droplets, and then immediately put it on your *dry* hair, massaging it in well all over. Wrap a hot towel around your head and leave it for twenty minutes, changing the towel for another hot one whenever it cools. Then remove the towel, and shampoo with your regular shampoo, finishing off with a cream rinse that contains a hair-softening chemical such as quaternary ammonium salts. Silicone and balsam are also useful ingredients in conditioners and cream rinses for dry hair, since, like the oil, they coat the cuticle and help protect it from excess water loss. You should also stay out of the sun, be careful about blow-drying your hair, and use heated rollers only when absolutely necessary. Make sure you get enough B-complex vitamins—dry hair is often a symptom of insufficiency. Try taking brewer's yeast three times a day.

If your hair is dry from overprocessing, then an oil treatment will do nothing for it, because the hair itself has already been damaged. It is *weak* hair. A cream rinse with a softener in it is also out, since that will only exacerbate the weakness. You need something to help repair damage to the hair's keratin instead: a protein treatment pack, which is left on for twenty minutes after washing with a pH-balanced shampoo. The more often you can give yourself this treatment, the better the results will be. Two or three times a week is ideal for severely dried out and overprocessed hair. It will gradually restore flexibility and strength.

If your hair is in damaged condition, it should go without saying that you need to steer clear of further processing until the dryness has cleared completely. This may take several weeks or even months, depending on how bad the problem is. You should always protect your hair from sunlight and not brush it too much until it is better (no more than twenty strokes a day).

HOW DO YOU TREAT OILY HAIR?

You wash and brush it often and well to distribute the oil evenly throughout the hair shaft and make it shine. You also massage your scalp daily. The scalp of someone with oily hair needs a lot of stimulation, for when the circulation is poor, the follicles don't get the nutrients and oxygen they need to function efficiently and you risk hair loss. The common notion that brushing, washing frequently, and massaging oily hair will stimulate the oil glands to produce more oil is simply untrue. A head of hair that is too oily is that way either because of the hormone balance in your body or simply because you have larger or more oil glands in your follicles than most people. Occasionally, a diet that is too rich in fat can contribute to excessive oiliness.

Lemon shampoos and a fresh lemon (the juice of a lemon in a pint of warm water) as the final rinse after washing is good for controlling too much oil in hair. Lemons are slightly astringent, so they not only clear away excess oil but also close the follicles. There are some good shampoos on the market especially formulated for oily hair. The trouble with them is that they work for a while, but then your scalp and hair seem to become accustomed to them and they become less effective. One way of getting around this is to buy three different shampoos for oily hair and to alternate them each time you wash your hair. You can also leave the shampoo in your hair for five minutes before rinsing it away, which helps dry out the hair shafts. When choosing a conditioner, look for an oil-free one. It will give your hair body and never leave it looking lank, as oily hair tends to look. Don't be afraid of washing your hair every day if you want to. It won't do any harm.

WHEN HAIR IS TOO FRAGILE

You need to stop any processing you have been doing to it (such as coloring with permanent tints or permanent waving) for several weeks and go on to a pH-balanced protein shampoo plus a protein conditioner. You can use a heavy protein pack on the hair for twenty minutes twice a week. This will close the imbrications of the cuticle and help heal whatever damage you have done to the cortex, which is the cause of fragility. You should have split ends cut off and steer clear of very hot blow drying, overbrushing, and heated rollers. Wear your hair in a simple, easy-to-care-for style until it has responded to the treatment and healthy hair is showing at the roots (usually about three months). Then you can consider having a gentle permanent (but it should be professionally done). Stay out of the sun.

IF YOUR HAIR IS DULL, WHAT ARE THE REMEDIES?

This depends on the cause. Some hair has become dull as a result of pigment changes associated with age or illness. Some is dull because of raised cells in the cuticle, which poorly reflect light. Usually dull hair is dry hair, so much of the problem and advice for dryness goes for you, too. If the dullness is a color problem, it is best to seek professional advice, since correcting it is usually easy, provided you know how. The hot oil treatment can help dull hair, as can an intense protein treatment every two weeks.

ARE SPLIT ENDS INEVITABLE?

Yes, everybody has them to some extent although on a normal head of hair they are few and far between and so go unnoticed. Split ends in large numbers are almost always the result of poor hair care such as blow drying with too hot a setting, sun damage, washing with a highly alkaline shampoo, too much brushing with a sharp-bristled brush, or overprocessing. If you have split ends, you are probably doing some of the wrong things to your hair. Don't wash your hair more than once or twice a week, keep it away from heat and sunlight, don't tease it or brush it with nylon bristles, and avoid chlorinated swimming pools. Have the ends cut.

WHEN HAIR TURNS GRAY

Gray hair is the result of loss of or changes in the melanin granules in the cortex. This can be the result of age—when the body is gradually losing its ability to produce melanin from enzymes and proteins—pernicious anemia, a vitamin or mineral deficiency (see section on nutrition), a thyroid condition, or prolonged stress. Sometimes graying hair can be halted or restored to its natural color by giving supplements of PABA, biotin, and pantothenic acid plus the other B-complex vitamins and zinc.

When hair turns gray, there are several things you can do for it. You can use a semipermanent rinse or highlighting shampoo to cover graying, provided no more than 30 percent of your hair is affected. You can have your hair tinted with an aniline dye, in which case you will want to opt for a color two or three shades lighter than was your original color, because as the hair ages and loses pigment, so does the skin. Too dark a tint will make it look artificial. Or you can leave it gray, and should you have any yellowing in it, simply treat it with a blue rinse to tone it down and turn it silvery. The natural beautiful silvery quality that some gray hair has depends on how the light hits it and on the condition of the cuticle. If your hair is not in the best of condition, put it through a series of protein treatments to improve the way the scales of the cuticle lie. If it seems coarser, it is probably the result of its being drier than it used to be. Use a hot oil treatment on it.

TWO KINDS OF DANDRUFF

Simple dandruff, which affects 60 percent of the population, is nothing more than a dry flaking of the scalp. A form of *hyperkeratinization*, it is the result of the scalp's most superficial layer of cells drying out too fast as they move up from the reproductive layer to the skin's surface. When they finally get there, they are so desiccated that they are rapidly shed, creating the flakes of skin we call dandruff. In most cases, the presence of dandruff indicates too little brushing (which will remove the offending flakes before they fall, unwanted, on their own); poor circulation of the scalp, which can be improved by daily massage; or the use of too many alkaline products, which have irritated the scalp and encouraged it to scale. If your scalp is dry, use a mild dandruff shampoo once a week to keep it under control—one containing zinc pyrithione or selenium sulfide, which will remove the scales. Brush your hair well every day with a natural-bristle brush, and use pH-balanced products to condition hair and for "in between" washes.

If your dandruff is the other variety, which is far rarer, it will look like thick, rather greasy or crusty scales on your scalp. It is the result of the same hyperkeratinization but with the added ingredient of scalp irritation caused by a large amount of excess sebum. In the long run, the zinc pyrithione shampoos tend only to exacerbate the oily type of dandruff, by encouraging the head to become even oilier. Shampoos containing coal tars or selenium sulfide are usually better for this. Sulfur tends to quell the oil-producing effect of the glands, while it helps remove and eliminate the scales. Regular brushing and massage are important here, too. Sometimes dandruff can be the result of microorganisms, allergens, hormonal imbalances, and diet deficiencies, so if self-treatment doesn't clear up the condition, it is a good idea to see your doctor about it. Dandruff shampoos are useful only in bringing the condition under control. If you use them every time you wash your hair, you can make matters worse. Sometimes it is helpful to own three different dandruff shampoos and alternate them, using a regular shampoo after each application of dandruff shampoo.

WHAT IS THE CAUSE OF HAIR LOSS?

There are many causes. The most simple is that of poor circulation in the scalp, hair breakage from poor treatment or overprocessing, and temporary illness or stress. Other reasons include hormonal imbalance, underactive thyroid, drugs, and poor diet (specifically too little B vitamins, vitamin C, zinc, sulfur, and iron). If you find you are losing your hair at a rapid rate, don't panic. There is a strong link between anxiety and hair loss, and a temporary excess shedding of hair at the telogen stage can be made much worse by worry about it. Instead, go through the process of elimination to discover possible causes and then seek whatever treatment is necessary to help correct the excess shedding. Start by asking yourself the following questions.

Are you taking any medication? The Pill or estrogen in hormone-replacement therapy is a common cause for thinning hair—thinning that is usually corrected in a few weeks after stopping it. Anti-coagulants, cortisone, and diet pills such as amphetamines are other offenders, as is boric acid, which occurs in many common proprietary products, from ointments for cuts and burns to eye baths. Thyroid medication can also be the culprit. So can simple aspirin, if you take as many as one or two a day.

Have you had any major traumas in your life or illnesses recently? Shock, illness, and emotional worry are among the most common causes of heavy shedding of telogen hairs—called telogen effluvium. Help can be had from vitamin supplements—particularly a good vitamin B stress formula including vitamin C, eating liver frequently, and taking brewer's yeast eight to twelve tablets after each meal). In addition, get plenty of physical activity, to help deal with stress, and practice meditation or deep relaxation techniques twice a day.

Is your scalp tight? Poor circulation, particularly in a scalp that tends to be oily, can result in hair loss. Give yourself a daily scalp massage. Try brewer's yeast. Brush fifty strokes a day.

Are you anemic? Women, who suffer from anemia far more often than men do, frequently find their hair has thinned greatly. Have a serum iron test and a total iron-binding-capacity test done to find out.

Is your hair breaking off near the roots from overprocessing, sun bleaching, or too much heat on it? This is fairly easy to detect, for if you sit in front of a mirror with the light coming from behind, you will be able to see a myriad of tiny hairs standing up out of the scalp no longer than a half to three quarters of an inch. If you examine them carefully, you will find that even these short hairs are damaged, with split ends. See the section on overprocessed hair for help, and consider cutting your hair short until the damaged hair has grown out and healthy hair shafts replace it.

Have you recently been pregnant? Women commonly lose hair during pregnancy. It may be the result of hormonal changes or some kind of subclinical vitamin or mineral deficiency—perhaps zinc, which is very low in most women just after childbirth. Happily this condition usually disappears a few weeks after the baby is born, provided the diet is adequate and you are generally well.

Do you wear your hair pulled back too tightly, or have you been putting rollers in too tightly? Another common cause of hair loss in specific areas of the scalp is simple traction caused by a tightly wrapped rubber band around a ponytail, or curlers that are too tight. The pull on the hair interferes with proper circulation there and results in damage to the hair follicles, which shed their hairs. If this is the case, you need to change your hairstyle, stop rolling curlers tightly, and give yourself daily massage or treatment with an electric vibrator. If you are using a nylon-bristled brush or rollers with brushes in them or too fine-toothed a comb, you should replace them, as they can also cause hair loss.

Is the hair coming out in patches? Then you might be suffering from *alopecia areata*, which looks like bald patches the size of a quarter sprinkled here and there in a normal head of hair. Its exact cause is unknown, although it often occurs when people are under severe stress. Some dermatologists think it may be linked to a vitamin B_{12} deficiency, others that it is a freak reaction of the body's immune system, like an allergic reaction in which one begins to reject one's own hair. In most cases the condition cures itself and the hair grows back into the bald patches until no evidence remains of this most distressing condition. You can seek medical help, although there is no standard treatment established for the condition.

WHAT IS MALE-PATTERN BALDNESS?

It is a hair-loss condition that occurs as a result of the follicles' sensitivity to a high level of certain hormones in the system—primarily the androgenic, or male, hormones. When these hormones are present in the bloodstream in raised concentration, they tend to shut down the functioning of the hair follicle. This results in either temporary or permanent hair loss. The condition is more common in men than women, because their bodies produce far higher levels of androgen—the hormone usually responsible. It does occur in women, too, however, probably as a result of the androgenlike hormone progesterone, which is made in the female sex glands and adrenals. Hair loss from hormonal causes is particularly likely to occur around the time of menopause, when estrogen levels fall dramatically in a woman's body, for estrogen is the antagonistic hormone to progesterone and tends to keep it in control. The tendency to this kind of hair loss is genetically determined, although there appear to be dietary factors which influence its onset—particularly insufficiencies of some of the B-complex vitamins. It occurs in a specific pattern, thinning at the crown and at the hairline. Sometimes estrogen therapy in postmenopausal women helps the condition. There is no adequate treatment for it in men.

OTHER HAIR COMPLAINTS

There are a number of other conditions of the hair and scalp that demand medical help, such as impetigo, fungus infections, psoriasis, sebaceous cysts, mites, and ringworm. They are all the province of the dermatological profession—your doctor's office is the place to seek help. Don't go to a hairdresser or a trichologist.

The best news of all about hair health and hair care is that with proper treatment even the most severe damage to hair or scalp can usually be completely repaired. But it takes time. Your hair grows at the rate of about $\frac{1}{72}$ of an inch a day. Be patient, keep caring for it, and in nine months to a year it can look absolutely fabulous, no matter how it looks now.

The Fun of It All

Introduction

The chores of facts and treatments over, we come to the part of beauty that is pure delight: makeup and scent. They are fanciful icing on the cake that, no matter how stoic and disciplined an approach you take to health and beauty, are just too good to leave out.

Making up your face can be enormously creative—like working on a canvas to paint a picture of mood and intent that reflects whatever you want to project at that particular moment. The colors and textures themselves are wonderful. There is great variety in them, and short of completely changing your face, there is almost nothing you can't do with them.

When it comes to scent, the fun and frivolity of change and indulgence can take on even deeper meanings. For perfumes affect us subliminally and can be exquisite not only on their own but also in the wide variety of moods and images they can convey for us.

Both makeup and scent are far too alive for their power or their delights to be conveyed adequately in cold words on a page. The only way one can experience them is by immersing oneself in their world and *playing*—much as a child would play with colored paints or build a castle out of various-shaped blocks. For both have tactile, sensual qualities that are missed if you approach them too logically or coldly.

Still, perhaps it is useful to have some guidelines about how to use makeup and what kinds of things to buy, and a little knowledge about the various families all the scents fall into, so one can get to know them better and appreciate their subtle messages. That is what this section is all about.

34

The Magic of Makeup

When you use makeup, you are practicing the age-old art of illusion. But the illusions makeup offers you are subtle ones, not complete changes of character, age, and coloring. Try to achieve that, and you carry the use of makeup too far; then, instead of being your friend, it will suddenly become an enemy and make you look foolish, too old, or simply less well than you could look. So the first rule of good makeup is simple: Never try to *change* your face with it.

After that has been said and after you have come to terms with the fact that whether or not you like it, your jaw is square or your eyes small or your skin a different color from what you ideally would like, then there is a lot you *can* do with color to make you look better. And that, after all, is what making up your face is all about. Whether you are after a freshly scrubbed, natural look (which incidentally takes a lot more artifice to achieve than you might imagine) or a more elaborate-looking, sophisticated face, the makeup you choose and the way you apply it should make you look more attractive, more interesting, healthier, and simply more yourself.

THE NAKED FACE

What about going without makeup? Great—provided you are healthy and your skin is good and provided you wear a moisturizer and sunscreen day in, day out for protection. Half of my life is spent without even the faintest touch of makeup. There is something I like about the "honesty" of an un-made-up face. When you blush, it shows. When you are tired, it shows. When you are really well and vital, there is no mask to cover up the translucence of your skin. A naked face can be beautiful.

Indeed, why should any woman feel she has to wear makeup simply because most do?

THE MAGIC THEATER

On the other hand, makeup is great fun. It can be a real pleasure to apply and to wear, because there is so much you can do with it. That is why the other half of my life is full of it. I find it somehow exciting to begin each morning by deciding what colors I want to wear that day and how I want to wear them—according to my mood or my imagination. You can also vary your makeup colors according to what clothes you are wearing or to go with the feeling of fashion of the time. The one essential thing about wearing makeup, however, is that you don't get into a rut with the same old lipstick all the time year after year. Nothing dates a face like wearing the same colors applied the same way over and over again.

NO EXCUSE FOR NEGLECTED SKIN

Long ago, makeup was worn to cover up defects in the skin. Like a mask, it covered over everything in a world where women still wore "falsies" in their bras to make their bosoms bigger, boned waist cinchers to make their middles smaller, and lots of hair pieces to give them the look of a Hollywood extravaganza. No longer. Makeup, like everything else in fashion and beauty today, is not something obviously artificial. Product textures are lighter and smoother, and the modern look in makeup is one of natural clear skin, no matter how much color you choose to put on your eyes and cheeks. If your skin is less than perfect, spend your time and money on getting it into shape before indulging in makeup products and colors.

INVEST IN GOOD TOOLS

The brushes you use, the sponges and absorbent cotton, and even your mirror and lighting are all-important in getting good results from your makeup products. You need to acquire a collection of them, keeping your tools immaculately clean and using them every time you put on your makeup. It is always tempting to put on an eye shadow with your finger or to apply powder with a dirty puff, but the results are never good, and the makeup you put on that way doesn't last as long as it should. Also, many of the little padded wands and brushes supplied with eye shadows and cheek colors look great in their compacts but won't really do the job of applying colors properly. And once any applicator wand or brush is dirty, you will never get good, smooth application from it.

Here is a suggested list of makeup tools as a general guideline. You need not buy all the things at once. The more expensive ranges of blushers, compact powders, and eye shadows sometimes contain sable or real-hair brushes, which are good enough to keep and will last for years. The other things you need you can buy from a shop that specializes in makeup products. Stage-makeup sellers usually have particularly good brushes, or you can sometimes get them from a good druggist. Buy brushes of real hair or sable. They are more expensive than other kinds, but the investment is worth it, since with the use most women give their makeup brushes, they will literally last a lifetime. You can find good brushes in an art supply shop, too. Their handles tend to be long, but these brushes look quite lovely in a jar on a dressing table.

2 large brushes for powder
3 slightly smaller brushes for blusher, highlighter, and shader
4 small brushes for eye shadows and for highlighting small areas
1 stiff toothbrush-like brush for brows
1 circular hard tiny brush for clearing excess mascara from lashes (this can be saved from a used mascara wand and then washed thoroughly)
1 fine-line lip brush
In addition, you will want some sponges for applying foundation and liquid blushers. They can be either natural sponges (the tiny ones used for cosmetics) or white rubber sponges. I think the natural ones are best.
Absorbent-cotton balls or pads
Cotton-tipped sticks (the kind used for cleaning babies' ears) for clearing away mascara accidentally smeared on your face and lipstick that has gone where it shouldn't have
Facial tissues
A spray bottle, used for misting plants, filled with pure spring water. The spray should be very fine so that using it will cover your skin with a delicate mist, not drops of water.
Good light—either natural light (which is best for applying any kind of makeup, because it gives a true picture of what colors are doing on your face) or ordinary incandescent lighting, which is second best.

Get as much light as possible—certainly on both sides of the mirror you are using. Fluorescent lighting is bad for makeup: It grossly distorts colors.
A scarf to tie back your hair while you are working is also useful.

It is important to keep your tools and brushes for makeup immaculate. The brushes can be washed in warm water with a little detergent shampoo or simple soap and then left to dry naturally in the air. The cotton of course is simply tossed out as you use it, as are the tipped sticks. Your makeup sponges will also come clean by washing them in soap or in shampoo—which is better at removing grease, especially in hard water, on which soap tends to form a scum. Wash them at least once a week and keep them well aired and ready for use.

THE PRODUCTS

Makeup products offer you two things: coverage, which to some extent will conceal minor flaws and blemishes in your skin, and most important, color. There are literally hundreds of different makeup products on the market. From the amount of advertising that accompanies the launch of each of them—the new wand-lipstick or foam cheek color or moisture-encapsulated powder—you would assume that to do a good job of making up her face a woman needs all of them. You don't. In fact you need very few.

Neither do colors change a great deal from season to season, in spite of the fact that each cosmetic house brings out new autumn or spring collections. If you gather together a simple range of shades for eyes, cheeks, and lips that you know look good on you, there is no reason to replace half of them with each new season's arrivals. Yes, there might be the new shade of fuchsia lipstick which you fancy or a new-formula foundation (foundations seem to get better and better each couple of years), but the quality of a makeup product is not dependent on its price, although the package—including the little compacts, mirrors, and applicators—is usually better the more you pay. More-expensive compacts are less likely to break in your handbag. But the texture and quality of colors for cheeks, eyes, and lips and even the foundations can be just as good in very inexpensive ranges as they are in the high-priced ones. Textures, however, do vary a lot from cosmetic house to cosmetic house, as does a product's staying power, so it is a good idea to shop around even among the expensive ranges to find products that offer long-lasting good colors.

THE COLORS

The idea that makeup color—say an eye shadow—is only to be used on the eyes, or a blusher only on cheeks, is absurd. Color is color, and it doesn't matter what you call a product, provided it serves the purposes you want it to. For instance, a touch of shimmery gold or silver eye shadow in the middle of your bottom lip after applying lipstick can give a mouth a full-lipped, pouty look that's very sexy. Or a little blusher in a burnished copper shade brushed just below your brow at the inside of the eye can give a tired face a lift. When you have a set of brushes, you can dip into any product you like to get the effect you are after, and you shouldn't hesitate to play around with them all. You will discover some remarkable effects when you do.

The colors that you use on your face should go together. It just doesn't work (unless you are very skilled and after a most unusual effect) to wear a bright red lipstick with a brown-toned blusher and vivid green eye shadow. The colors you choose should all give *support* to each other so they work together to create an overall effect that is pleasing.

There are two basic possibilities: warm color schemes and cool ones. The effect of a warm color scheme on the face—which includes the earth colors such as browns, greens, beiges, golds, apricots, coppers, or-anges, and peaches—is to enliven it, making your face look healthier and stronger and more glowing. Warm colors look wonderful on older women, too, because they accentuate youth. A little peach or apricot blusher can make almost any face look younger, whereas bluish-pink blusher applied to a face over forty can age it drastically.

The cool colors—the blues, purples, pale ivories, silvers, fuchsias, ber-ries, magentas, blued pinks, and whites give a look of delicate vulnera-bility to a face, especially when they are applied, as they should be, over a very pale foundation. They can be exciting because they are almost electric in their boldness. But to wear them you have to have perfect skin and you have to be young; otherwise they will make you look tired, older, and even unwell.

A warmer color scheme is also better in a climate such as ours, in Brit-ain, where there is relatively little sun, because it adds brightness to the habitually gray days and the dull colors that most British women wear. In a warm, bright country such as Australia, southern Italy, or the United States, a cool color scheme, particularly worn in summer, can bring welcome relief from so much strong light.

This is not to say that you cannot occasionally mix a warm makeup color with a cool makeup scheme, or vice versa. You can. A brilliant blue-pink lipstick can look superb on a face that is wearing peach and pale green eye shadow and a gentle rose blusher. But then the theme is still predominantly warm—only a single brilliant lipstick has been added to give surprise to the look.

PRACTICE IS THE ROAD TO PERFECTION

The only way to learn about using makeup is by experimenting with it over and over again until using it well becomes second nature. Books can give you guidelines, and a professional can teach you a trick or two, but only you can create the skill needed to make the very most of your face. This is why top models often prefer to do their own photographic makeup, in spite of the fact that there may be a very expensive and skilled makeup artist hired to do it for them. It is *their* face, after all, and through the years of applying color to it they have gotten to know each little part, each flaw, each particularly good feature, and how to work with them. If you want to get the best from makeup, you need to do the same.

Set aside some time to yourself—about forty-five minutes a month, say, in which you simply sit in front of your mirror and experiment with makeup colors and textures, to see the kind of effects you can get. If you don't have many colors of lipstick and eye shadow, then buy some inexpensive ones (the kind aimed at the teenage market, which are very cheap), including several basic shades of lipstick (true red, rose, orangy brown, beige-pink, fuchsia, etc.) and the four basic shades of blusher (rose, red, bronze-gold, and russet). The best basic eye-shadow colors are a flat neutral brown or gray for contouring, a softened blue (not too bright), a beige for highlighting (either with or without frosting), a cinnamon or pink, and a dull green. You can always add brilliant colors to your collection—the vivid yellows, deep violets, golds, silvers, and so on —but these are a good basic set of colors to begin with. You will also need two shades of foundation: a flat beige nearest the color of your skin and a shade in the same tone but slightly darker.

One of the mistakes most women make when working with color is that they tend to use the same colors all the time. You know the kind of thing: the standard baby-blue eye shadow or the same pink lipstick. They feel safe with them, and so they stick to them. While it is good to have some colors you know look good on you and to wear them often, it is a shame to limit yourself to these alone. For one of the most wonderful things about colors is how much they can do to express your various moods. For instance, a brilliant red lipstick can be fun to wear occasionally, particularly if you consider yourself not at all the type for red lipstick. So can wonderful soft, muted shades on eyes, lips, and cheeks, which, blended together on your face, will give you the look of someone standing in the light of a morning mist. Every woman has many faces and many moods. Makeup can help you explore and express them all.

One of the most important parts of experimenting with makeup is simply getting to know your face well without any makeup on it at all. Few women do. There seems to be a kind of fear about really looking at one's own naked face. It is something most of us avoid. Sit down and spend fifteen minutes simply looking at your clean, naked face. What do you see? If you look long enough, you will begin to see beauty, regardless of what previous ideas you may have had about yourself. Everyone has something about her face that is truly remarkable. It may be the way your upper lip seems to curve out that gives a sense of emotional sensitivity to your face; your eyes, which are particularly clear or large; or your lashes, which are very heavy. It can also be your bone structure, which makes lovely planes on a face that catch the light. Or it can be your skin itself.

Whatever your particular virtues, get to know them, and then by experimenting with colors, light and shade, and highlighters you will learn to accentuate your best characteristics. And don't just let it go at that. Every few months, take another long look at yourself. Forget what you saw last time and see how your face has changed. Faces do change remarkably—and I don't just mean with age, either. They change as women change and grow. Your makeup needs to change with you.

35

Makeup:
Putting It into Practice

Every good makeup begins with a water-in-oil moisturizer and a sunscreen lavishly applied over clean skin and then given a chance to settle in. It is rather like making a mayonnaise. You can't rush things. You need to wait for your skin to take to the moisturizer before you put on your foundation; otherwise you will end up with a flawed finish and your makeup will not last. "Taking" time is usually about two minutes.

MANY MOISTURIZERS

In addition to the ordinary moisturizers, there are also tinted ones on the market. These products are halfway between moisturizers and foundations. They impart some color and also provide you with some measure of protection from water loss. In France they are often called *crème sport*, because they can be worn, by women who ordinarily would not want to cover their skin with a foundation, for instance during a tennis match. They give a very light cover but can be a nice way of simply adding a healthy glow to your skin. Some of them also contain sunscreens.

When choosing a tinted moisturizer, look for one that is not too far away from your own skin tone, or you will find it doesn't blend in and cover well. Some of them give little color, and others are much stronger —even *too* strong. You need to experiment.

Among the tinted moisturizers are the "color correctives"—products tinted a specific hue in order to change the look of your own, natural coloring. They are worn under your ordinary foundation. A green moisturizer will soften a florid skin, toning it down and making it look more neutral, so that your naturally high color doesn't interfere with whatever eye shadows, blushers, and lipsticks you are going to use. Green will also help conceal red blotches and spots on your skin. A mauve-colored moisturizer will improve a dull complexion and brighten the face of someone who is too pale. An apricot-colored corrective should be used only by the very few women who are really sallow and then only sparingly, on areas of the face that would naturally be expected to blush, such as the cheeks, the chin, and the upper part of the forehead, just beneath the hairline.

When you use a corrective, put it on with a sponge that has been dampened and then had all the excess water removed from it by wiping it against a towel.

THE FOUNDATION

Once your moisturizer has set, you are ready for the foundation. But why all over? Instead you can wear it only on parts of your face such as around the eyes, where it gives a good base for eye shadows, on your chin, and on your cheeks. The advantage to this is that you still get the wonderful, delicate shading of natural skin, rather than that all-over deadness that can come from covering your whole face with one opaque color. Or you can wear two shades of foundation: a lighter one in the center of your face (on the nose, forehead, cheeks, and chin) and the slightly darker one of the same tone around the outside (near the hairline and along the jawline). This has the effect of preserving a natural-looking gradation of color and still lending the finished look of a well-made-up face.

Another alternative is to go without foundation altogether, applying your colors (best to use cream and liquid eye shadows rather than powders in this case) directly to well-moisturized skin. For evening, however, or a very sophisticated look, an even, single-colored foundation lightly covering your whole face is best.

Foundations (sometimes called makeup bases) come in all colors and textures. Finding the right one for you is a matter of trial and error, and unfortunately in the process there often seems to be more error than anything else.

There are far too many colors on the market. About 80 percent of Caucasian skin should wear one foundation color: a flat true beige with neither pink nor peach overtones to it. It will look good on all ages of "northern European" skin, because it gives a neutral canvas on which to put your eye and lip colors. Many women—particularly Americans—make the mistake of opting for a peachy or golden foundation color in the belief either that their skin is too dull or that the extra brightness in their foundation will make them look younger. Neither notion is true.

A foundation is not *meant* to give strong color to a face. It is supposed to be flat and neutral. Blushers and shaders, and eye and lip colors, provide the color interest to a face. If your foundation is too bright already, you only end up looking overdone and in bad taste. You also won't get the mileage you should out of your lip, cheek, and eye colors, for there will be too much skin color for them to compete with.

If your skin is olive or yellowish or very dark, then choose a foundation as close to its natural color as possible but slightly flatter. When testing out color, put it on your naked face, and then go out into the daylight to look at the results, before buying anything. Cosmetics counters, with all their lavish atmospheres and artificial lights, can greatly distort colors. And the skin on your hand (which is where most consultants try to put a sample of makeup) is very different in shade and texture from facial skin. It just won't do.

The kind of foundation you choose depends on what kind of skin you have as well as on personal preference. Dry or aging skin does best with a cream or oil-based-liquid foundation that contains powder and gives a matt finish with any degree of cover you want. Oily skin demands a water-based liquid or cream or a cake or block-type makeup. But beware here. Many women make the mistake of wearing a foundation that is too heavy and end up with a greasy mess at the end of the day. For daytime wear, most oily skin is better off without foundation at all, simply covered with two layers of light, translucent powder to give it a matt finish which can be renewed periodically by applying more powder if necessary. This will avoid stimulating the sebaceous glands, as drying makeups can, to produce yet more oil. It also makes it possible to renew your matt finish easily so your face never becomes discolored or cakey-looking. The best way to apply foundation is with a sponge. Of course you can apply it with your fingertips, but you will never get the same perfect light coverage that you can with a sponge that has been dipped in cool water and then thoroughly wrung out until it is almost dry.

Put a little foundation in the palm of your left hand (if you are right-handed), and then dip the sponge into it and apply it to your face, brushing it lightly over your skin again and again until everything is well blended into your skin. If you want a heavy cover and a very matt look, instead of applying a thick coat of foundation, apply two thin coats, allowing a couple of minutes for the first one to dry before applying the second.

COVERING THE BLEMISHES

Now is the time to deal with any problems you want to conceal, such as black circles under your eyes or discolorations here and there. Concealer creams and sticks are good here, although some of them are greasy and, particularly under the eyes, tend to sink into tiny lines and make matters worse. If you use a concealer, buy one that is not too light-colored. Many brands are far too pale and, used under the eyes, make you look ghoulish.

Put your concealer on and pat it into the skin with your little finger until it blends perfectly with the surrounding area. If you add a little powder here—particularly under the eyes—even if you don't wear it on the rest of your face, you will get just the finish you need to make the undesirable area fade into the surrounding skin tones.

THE MAGIC OF LIGHT AND SHADE

The whole secret of successful makeup, no matter what look you are after (the natural, clean face or pure glamour), lies in using light and shade well. The rules are simple. Whatever part of your face you want to bring out or emphasize, you apply a light color to, and whatever part you want to minimize, you cover with a darker shade. In practice it becomes a little more complicated. Shaders and highlighters come in several forms: creams or lotions you put on a naked face or just after applying your foundation, powders you brush on after applying translucent powder, and simple light and dark shades of foundation you put on various areas of the face for effect.

In the fifties and sixties the well-made-up face boasted great exaggerations. Brown shaders swept under cheekbones (either real or imaginary cheekbones) gave the face a sculptured look, while brilliant white highlighter smeared under the brow was supposed to "lift" it and make the face more interesting. In truth it all looked very artificial, which in itself would have been all right except that the skill with which the photographic model applied her light and shade was considerable, while the average woman copying her tended to make a great mess of it all and ended up looking slightly ridiculous.

Now, thanks to changing styles in the seventies and eighties, things are different. You can still use a darker shade of foundation to minimize a large jaw or soften a big nose or give a bit more shape to the under-cheekbone area of too round a face, but the difference between the two colors is less exaggerated and the whole effect far more subtle.

The secret of making light and shade work for you is simply to apply both sparingly and only where it matters to your face, and always to blend well into the surrounding area. Don't get involved in complex theories that may work well when a makeup artist has three or four hours to prepare a face for one color photo with a particular kind of lighting. They are simply not for everyone, nor for everyday wear. Above all, make sure, when you have applied highlight and shading, that there is no dividing line between the darker and lighter areas of your face.

Here are some of the things you can do with shading:

To minimize a jaw that is too large or too square, apply darker shade along the jawline, blending it under the jaw and fading into nothing at the sides of the face.

To shorten a pointed chin, apply shader to chin only, blending underneath into the neck and fading to nothing at the sides.

To fade a double chin, put shader on the double chin and blend it skillfully. This will make it recede into the background and look less prominent.

To give more interesting shape to a square face, apply shader in the temple area and all around the jawline, carefully blending.

To add cheek hollows when there aren't any, use a *small* amount of shader in a gentle curve just under where the cheekbone finishes (you can feel it with your finger even if your natural cheekbones don't show through the skin). Then blend carefully down to nothing just above the jawline at the sides.

To minimize a nose that is too large, apply shader (preferably liquid or cream) in a single stripe down the center of the nose, carefully blending into the color at the sides so that no definite line appears.

To slim a broad nose, apply a shader—preferably a slightly darker foundation or cream—in a stripe down each side of the nose and blend it carefully into the skin to make the nose look narrower.

LIGHT DRAWS THE EYE

Highlighter is a powerful tool when it is used wisely. When carelessly or wrongly applied, it can make a face look positively absurd. The best highlighters are not white. Bone white is too harsh. Instead choose a pale ivory foundation to use as a lightener on the areas of the face you wish to make prominent or draw attention to. Or you can use a peach or beige eye shadow.

When, during the makeup process, you apply the highlighter depends on what kind you are using: creams and liquids just after foundation, powders after using face powder. It also depends on what you are using it for. If you are adding a strip of highlight down the center of a perfect, slim nose to show it off, then apply the highlighter just after your foundation. If you are using it to exaggerate the bow in your lips, then apply a powder highlighter—perhaps a frosted one—after powdering your face but before applying lipstick.

Here are some of the things you can do with highlighter. But don't do more than two of them at any one time, or the effect will be counterproductive and you'll lose all of the wonderful impact highlighter can give:

Add a thin edge of matt lightener just under the brows to make the eyes look wider.

Brush shimmery highlighter down the two ridges between the center of the bottom of the nose and the bow of the upper lip, to draw interest there.

Brush shimmery highlighter on the bow of the upper lip at the center.

Brush a touch of highlight in the center of the upper eyelid to add brightness to the eyes and more shape to the eyelids.

Stroke a little highlighter across the cheekbone, just under the outer corner of the eye, to exaggerate the bone's prominence.

A carefully blended line of light down the center of a beautiful nose will draw attention to it.

A little, very light foundation used in the hollows that run from the edge of the nose to the corners of the mouth will minimize the age hollows there.

Put a little highlighter on collarbones when you are wearing a décolleté dress.

THE EYES HAVE IT

For most women, one of their best features is the eyes. Perhaps this is because eyes reveal so much of what goes on inside one. Makeup for eyes should emphasize this and show off the eyes' beauty and color. It should never be applied gratuitously, as it often is.

There are lots of ways to use eye makeup to improve eyes: to make deep-set eyes more prominent, to give more interesting shape to eyes that have little, to improve the look of an overhanging upper lid, and so forth. But all of them begin with the same principles: Use neutral tones such as flat browns (without red tones in them), grays, and grayed greens for establishing the shape of the eyes (the darker shades to define the sockets and the lighter beiges on the lids and under the brows), and then, after you have done that, add other colors for effect, if you wish.

All eye shadows are best applied with a brush, whether they are liquid, cream, or powder. Brushes give you good control over color application and make it possible, by brushing over and over the area, to blend colors masterfully so that there is perfect light coverage, with no demarcation lines. Of course there is no reason why you have to add other colors after doing the basic contouring. Indeed many faces look best without bright colors near the eyes, which can not only draw attention away from the natural shimmer of the eye itself but also detract from a particularly lovely shade of lipstick you may be wearing or the good bone structure of your face.

All eye shadows are best applied to skin that has a foundation on it—even if you don't put foundation on the rest of your face. You will get a better, longer-lasting finish from them this way. And when using eye shadows, the same rules apply as on the rest of the face: A light color will make the part of the eye it's on look more prominent, and a dark color will make it recede. Beware of frosted shadows if you are over thirty-five or have crepey eyelids. They can be very aging, and you will get better results from matt finishes.

THE EYEBROWS

The natural shape of an eyebrow usually goes with the face it is on. That is why it is usually a bad idea to alter yours greatly just because the kind of brow you particularly like looks good on somebody else's face. What you can do to improve a shape is to pluck the extraneous hairs from your brows, giving them a cleaner line and making it possible to wear eye shadow successfully—eye shadow looks awful smeared over skin with tiny hairs sticking out of it. Another thing you can do is exaggerate the natural shape of your eyebrows slightly. An angular shape adds a feeling of planes to a round face; a sweeping shape looks good on narrow faces and also balances a very large mouth; and a rounded shape makes the eye look more open and young and is particularly good on a face with large eyes and a wide forehead.

If you have heavy brows, then pluck them to keep them tame, and let them be. If your brows are short and thick, don't try to change them by elongating them on the sides, until you have taken a long, hard look at them and decided that that is really what you want to do. This shortened brow is a favorite of many models, because it gives surprise and a youthful look to a face.

HOW TO PLUCK YOUR EYEBROWS

Before you begin, brush them first one way and then the other to remove any loose hairs or makeup, and clean the skin around the eyes thoroughly. Now put moisturizer in the area, before you reach for the tweezers. Brush your brows into shape and take a good look at them. Start by removing stray hairs between the brows and the stragglers that have nothing to do with the main body of the eyebrow. But never pluck from above the eyebrow. And always remove only one hair at a time, pulling it in the direction in which it grows. Work carefully, from the lowest hairs upward, clearing away the unnecessary ones. When you have finished with one brow, apply antiseptic or a simple toner to it before going on to the next one. This will help soothe the irritated skin. Don't try to apply makeup for an hour after plucking ends.

The shape of a brow then can be accentuated or the density filled in, using a sharp eye pencil in a light shade—even if you have black brows you should choose an eyebrow pencil lighter than the natural hair color or you will make your face look older. If your brows are brown, choose a light brown color. The strokes from the pencil should be feathery and put on in the opposite direction to that in which the hairs grow. Then, when you've finished with the pencil, brush your eyebrows back in their natural shape to soften the strokes and make them look like natural hairs.

THE EYELIDS

Apply the lighter neutral shade or the lighter shade of colored shadow you have chosen to the section of the lid nearest the lashes, and then brush it out, fading it away to nothing toward the eyebrows. Now you can add the darker neutral in the socket to define the shape. There are lots of tricks you can play here with colors and light and dark to enhance the look of your eyes, make them look bigger, and so on.

EYELINERS

Finally put on your eyeliner. A good way of emphasizing eye shape without looking too obviously made up is to use a pencil in the same tone you are using for your eye shadow, dotting it all along the upper lashes and then just under the lower ones so the two lines meet at the outer corners and form a little triangle. This kind of liner looks good when it is gently smeared with a brush or fingertip to blend it into the surrounding area and keep it from looking too heavy. You can also use another color line drawn on the *inside* of the lower lid if you like. If you use a light color there, such as off-white, it will make your eyes look bigger. If you use a bright color such as electric blue or brilliant green, it can look great for evening.

The other way of applying eyeliner is with a brush, in which case you use liquid or cake liner and get a more definite line—a real line instead of an intensified eye-shadow color near the lashes. It is drawn just above the roots of the upper lashes and just below the roots of the lower ones, again meeting at the corner. Many women use black eyeliner, but usually a gentle gray or slate or muted brown is better. If you are over thirty-five black can be very aging.

MASCARA

Mascara makes eyes look more glamorous. It seems to create an aura of mystery about the eyes when lashes are darkened and thickened. Unless you are planning to walk in the rain or to go swimming with your makeup on, you are better off using a mascara that is not waterproof. Waterproof mascara is very hard to remove, and you often have to do a lot of rubbing in the process, which can stretch the delicate skin around the eyes and slacken it.

Some mascaras contain fibers to lengthen the lashes and make them look even thicker. They are fine so long as you don't have particularly sensitive eyes; otherwise you are better off with a simple, fiberless one.

Apply your mascara by looking down into a mirror held next to your chin and you will not etch lines into your forehead, the way most women do by crinkling it up. You will also get better application this way, since the brush or wand strokes the lashes easily from their origins to tips from underneath and slightly curls them to make them look even longer.

CHEEKS

The single most important makeup product to help a face look younger is a little cheek color applied in a sweeping line over the cheekbone and fading to nothing at the temples. You can also use cheek color on your chin and forehead and even on the upper part of your eye socket, just below the brow, for a healthy glow. The best colors for everyday wear for most women are warm burnished copper or dusky peach, because they make the skin look particularly healthy. When you wear a warm cheek color, your lipstick should be warm as well, and vice versa. Where you apply blusher depends on the shape of your face and the effect you want from it. Use it high on the cheekbones and it accentuates a well-sculpted face. Use it across the cheeks and it gives a simple warm glow. Never use it in the way we did in the fifties and sixties, to make hollows under the cheeks. This is far too obvious for today's natural-looking face.

LIPS

Balance your eyes and lips, making one or the other more prominent. If both are strong or in very bright colors, it tends to make a face plastic-looking, and there is little in the way of contrasts to create interest. Most women tend to pick lipsticks that are too bright or too pink to flatter their coloring. There is certainly a place for fire-engine reds and vivid fuchsias, but for everyday wear you are probably better off with a muted brownish pink or a softened melon or salmon. Shop around until you find four or five lipsticks in differing tones that look good on you. They will go with almost everything you wear normally and will work with most makeup looks you are after.

When applying lipstick, use a pencil or a lipbrush to outline your mouth first, so you get a good, sharply defined edge. Then apply your lipstick and blot it and apply again if you want it to stay.

Fashions for lip gloss come and go. If you want to wear it, it's usually best to apply it only on the bottom lip, so it catches the light, and not to carry it all the way to the edge of the mouth, or it tends to blur the lips' outline. Some lipsticks are translucent and impart a kind of see-through color. They look great on younger women. So can the frosted lipsticks. Older women are usually better off with cream lipsticks, since frosting shows up wrinkles on the lips and the see-through ones don't give enough definition.

POWDER

Recently powder has been making a comeback although for years younger women have insisted that powder could be aging and that they wanted shiny, freshly scrubbed-looking faces. In fact just the opposite is true. A little translucent powder that imparts no color but gives a smooth, matt finish can actually make a face look younger. It is also an interesting effect to powder only parts of your face, such as the sides below the cheekbones, the nose, and the forehead, and then leave a sheen on cheeks and chin. Just as one can mix light and shade to make a face more interesting, so one can mix finishes.

The best way to apply powder is either with clean absorbent cotton, dabbing it lavishly all over and then brushing off the excess with a new piece of cotton, or with a brush. I prefer the brush method, because it always seems to stay better that way. Always use a powder that gives no color, just a matt, smooth finish, and always brush away every speck of excess once you have applied it.

THE FINISHING TOUCHES

Last of all, after you have applied your makeup completely, you need to set it with water. This step is very useful, for it will make a face last far longer than it otherwise would. Spray your face with spring water from an aerosol can or with a fine mist from a plant-misting bottle. Then blot gently once with a tissue.

The whole process of making up may sound complicated, but with practice it should take very little time—no more than ten minutes from start to finish.

36

~~~

Scentsational Beauty

Scent is a passion. For me it is an irresistible one. And like a beautiful painting or a well-written novel, a fine perfume is a work of art. Wearing one can be a vivid expression of a woman's feeling and intention. For scent is not only a delight to indulge in, it also carries one of the most potent beauty messages you will ever send out. Change the scent you wear and you can change the way you feel, the image you project, the mood you want to set. If I had little money to spend on beauty products, I could do without makeup altogether and would buy only the simplest creams and lotions, but I would never stop buying scent—bottles and sprays of it, sachets to put into drawers and cupboards, oils to drop on pads laid on heated surfaces which waft their perfumes into the air. Scent has always had magic to it.

Even the multimillion-dollar perfume industry is a fascination, mysterious and paradoxical—none the less so for all the mechanization of the past twenty years. For in spite of advanced market-research techniques, manufacturing technology, and selling methods, perfumers still do not understand some of the most basic things about their raw materials and why they affect people as they do. How does the human sense of smell work, anyway? What makes it impossible to reconstruct perfectly even one essential oil from a plant or flower that goes into making a fragrance? Why does the simple act of smelling involve such a vast range of primitive emotional responses in the human being? And how can these responses be calculated? Nobody knows for sure.

Psychologists and biologists working with the sense of smell only know that they do. For we respond to perfumes unconsciously. Various odors can even bring about abreactions, in which specific events are relived, releasing pent-up psychic energy, much as Proust reacted to the madeleine. The smell of vanilla, for instance, often brings out tender memories from childhood. Other smells, such as lavender, are calming to a disturbed mind. Still others, such as carnation, mint, rose, and tobacco, act as mental stimulants. Even mass hysteria and fear are being linked with our sense of smell; the hormonal changes accompanying violent feelings of fear appear to cause the body to give off odors that are then subconsciously recognized by others. These kinds of smells may be as important to human behavior as they are in the behavior of animals, even though we are entirely unaware that we are smelling anything. In the future, scent may well be made using ingredients as much for their physical and psychological effect as for their pleasant smell.

Meanwhile scientists are looking at the far-reaching effects and implications that various odors have in human life. A German neurologist, Dr. Edinger, has experimented and found, for instance, that work rates in factories can be significantly improved simply by supplying workers who get dirty from their jobs with large quantities of strongly perfumed soap instead of the plain carbolic variety. Similarly, in France during World War II, researchers reported that people remained markedly calmer and more easily organized in air-raid shelters that were well aired and scented than their counterparts in ordinary shelters. So far, no large perfumer has explained this kind of information, but it is there just waiting for the adventurous marketing man to find a way to use it.

THE MYSTERY OF SMELL

Scientists have been working for generations trying to understand how our noses distinguish one smell from another, to find a classification for scents, and perhaps to develop some kind of notation system for their description. So far without much success. One of the most interesting theories about the sense of smell comes from J. E. Moore, a British chemist. He claims that there are seven primary odors, under which all smells can be classified. Each of these, he says, has a distinctive molecular shape, which the olfactory cells in our nose recognize and react to. And this reaction is not only chemical, as you might expect. According to Moore (and several American researchers agree with him) these special-shaped molecules slot into submicroscopic pores of differing sizes and shapes in the receptor cells. The researchers claim that any change in odor is the result of a change in the *overall* shape of the molecule. But just *how* a fragrance affects the nervous system and brings about many-layered emotional responses remains yet another unsolved mystery.

THE MAKING OF A PERFUME

Each good perfume is like a carefully gathered bouquet of flowers or a Bach fugue. It is intricately and exquisitely constructed from a number of components: the essential oils of plants, notes from animal ingredients, and synthetic chemicals in alcohol or perhaps in one of the newer emollient bases. And a fine scent, like a piece of fine music, is far greater than the sum of its parts.

There are several thousand natural and man-made odorous materials that can be used to make a perfume. Most perfumers (in the business they are called "noses") work with about two thousand of them, of which, by smell alone, they can recognize between six and eight hundred. A fine perfume is a blend of between twenty and a hundred and fifty ingredients. Until fifty years ago, the ingredients were almost entirely taken from plants and flowers, with the exception of a few remarkable animal notes such as musk from a Tibetan deer, civet from the glands of the civet cat, and ambergris from the sperm whale. This century, chemists have developed a wide variety of synthetic materials called aromatics, which have new smells. Some of the best scents rely heavily on them. The beautiful Chanel No. 5, for instance, takes its special character from a group of aromatics called the aldehydes. Just because a perfume contains a large number of synthetic chemicals doesn't mean that it is second-rate or "cheap" compared to one that is predominantly essential oils. But it is also true that there is something special about the true plant essences in perfumes too. They seem to give a depth and richness that most of the man-mades lack. Ideally, a good perfume should make use of both: the natural plant and animal notes for character and body, and some of the synthetics for a special unique individuality and modernness which the naturals cannot offer.

Grasse, in southern France, is still the world's capital of fine scent. It has been since the beginning of the fourteenth century, when scent as an industry was born, although the raw materials of perfume now come from all over the world. There and nearby the ground is covered with small fields of all kinds of odorous plants and flowers: roses and jasmine, tuberose, violet, lavender, narcissus, and carnations. In the factories the flowers, herbs, and woods are each carefully processed by distillation, enfleurage, or extraction to trap and preserve the valuable essences that will eventually be treated and mixed to make fragrances. Each flower is handled differently, and each essential oil produced from it has its own individual smell. Some sell for as little as a few dollars a pound. Others, like rose and jasmine, require hundreds of pounds of flowers to make even a few ounces of the precious essential oil, which may then sell on the open market for thousands of dollars a pint.

It is far more than a figure of speech when one likens a fine scent to a piece of fine music. So close to music in composition is the art of creating perfumes that perfumes and composers use many of the same words to speak about the two processes. For as musical notes and chords are the raw materials for music, so these essential oils, along with the aromatic chemicals and animal substances, make up the individual notes of scent.

And each good scent is composed like a piece of orchestral music, a blend of various ingredients striking various notes and eliciting various emotional responses from the nose smelling them.

The base notes of a fragrance are profound and long-lasting. They are made up of the heavier-smelling substances, many of which are even unpleasant alone. They form the foundation of the scent, giving it richness and lasting ability. The base notes make a scent reverberate hour after hour. Many animal substances are used in constructing a base, as are oak, moss, patchouli, and vetiver.

A perfume's middle notes don't last quite as long as the base, but they give the scent breadth and variety. Common middle notes come from Bulgarian rose, iris, jasmine, thyme, and ylang-ylang. The middle notes give a perfume its warming, diffuse glow as it develops on the skin.

The top notes of a perfume are the most immediately apparent when you first put it on. They produce scent's first impression. They also add brilliance to the blend, giving it clarity of statement, much as a flute adds simple purity to an orchestra. These top notes are highly volatile substances, often drawn from citrus or spicy materials: neroli, lemon, coriander, bergamot. The perfumer carefully blends and reblends base, middle, and top notes in a kind of harmonious composition that not only smells complete when it is first encountered but has depth and dimensions that continue to speak as it changes on your skin. The difference between a fine scent and a poor one is unmistakable to a discerning nose. And anyone's nose can be made discerning simply by being exposed to good perfumes.

THE FAMILIES OF SCENT

Roughly speaking, there are four families of scent. First the florals, which include both the simple single and multiple flowery perfumes and the more complex aldehyde florals with their sharp elegance. Second the chypres, which are mossy in character with either fruity or leathery tinges. Third the modern "liberated greens," which give a sense of cleanliness and the great outdoors. Fourth the sultry, powerful orientals. Every scent will fit into one of these families, although most will have faint overtones of another as well. For instance, Caron's Bellodgia, with its strong carnation character, is a single floral, yet it belongs in the same family as Elizabeth Arden's multifloral Blue Grass, which is flowery with an oriental tinge to it. And in the green family you will find the lovely Aliage, by Estée Lauder, with unmistakable chypre overtones, right next to the striking Weil de Weil, another green scent but with strong floral tinges to it. The possibilities, like variations on a theme, are endless.

Each family has its own charm and will tend to appeal to a particular biological and psychic makeup in a woman or to her particular mood. And every woman, like every scent, is different, although most of us, without knowing anything about the families of scents, tend to choose our perfumes from the same family over and over again. It is useful to get to know and understand the families: what they "say" and which perfumes are related to one another. Then you can avoid getting into a rut by using the same scent all the time. It can also help you steer clear of costly mistakes at perfume counters. For instance, if you like Cabochard, by Grès, a leathery chypre with floral overtones, you might also try Balmain's Jolie Madame, which is similar in character. Or if you want a more decisive change in the same genre, you could sample Courrèges Empreinte, another leathery chypre but with rather a woody than floral overtone. Another way of using knowledge of scent families is to choose a couple of scents from each of two or three families and then use them to express your mood changes.

Finally, it is simply interesting to trace the development of fine perfumes from the early-twentieth century, when François Coty first launched his exquisite L'Origan—a spicy, single flowery carnation from which a whole family of floral scents was born—right up to the eighties, when we are witnessing a kind of floral jubilee right across the market— from Guerlain's exquisite Parure to Revlon's inexpensive but excellent Jontue and the bright and tuberosy Adolfo, by Frances Denney. That perfume is as much an art form as painting or literature or music is something few people appreciate, partly because there is no adequate language for describing something as ephemeral as scent and partly because in the area of perfume most of what is written in women's magazines and advertisements is not only inaccurate but simply silly. The advertising copy for new scents, for instance, year by year becomes more fantastic. The power of advertising in the selling of scent is one of the reasons so many women are dissatisfied with the perfumes they buy. They see the image of the woman who supposedly epitomizes the new perfume and decide they like the way she looks and, therefore, that the perfume is just right for them. Then, when they buy it and wear it a little, they find they simply don't like it. This is how dressing tables become littered with half-used, expensive bottles and how women become disillusioned with perfume.

Charles Revson turned his good but, I believe, not exceptional scent Charlie into one of the world's biggest money-makers through brilliant advertising. He created the image of the trouser-suited, straight-haired young woman who symbolized the liberated girl of the moment in her walk and the way she tossed her head. He was able to take the social temperature of the time and cash in on it. But that doesn't necessarily mean that the scent Charlie is right for you, even if you do wear trouser suits and toss your head. The only way to buy scents is by *feeling*—sensing, smelling, and trying them on you. If you buy perfumes any other way, like most women, you will find yourself dissatisfied. If you don't respond to a particular scent instinctively, who cares how beautifully it is packaged, who else wears it, or how exciting an image of womanhood the advertisements for it communicate? It is simply not for you.

Let's take a closer look at perfume families, what they have to say, and what kind of woman or mood they will appeal to. And let's begin with the florals, since that is where it all began.

Fabulous Flowers

The floral family is the most important of all the scent families. It is composed of simple florals created to give off one predominant floral note, such as Diorissimo (lily of the valley) or Chloé (tuberose) or the multiple floral bouquets which are harmonious mixtures of several flowers' fragrances without any particular one predominating. Jasmine and rose often form the major part of these blends, for example the rich and elegant Joy, by Patou, with its clear woody overtones, the spicy L'Air du Temps, of Nina Ricci, or Guy Laroche's lovely Fidji, a floral spiked with green.

In the early twenties Coco Chanel's talented perfumer produced a wonderfully flowery scent with a remarkable difference. He added large quantities of some new chemicals called aldehydes to it. The story goes that it was an accident, in that he added several times the quantity of aldehydes called for in the original formula. But when Chanel smelled it, she loved it. It was a truly original blend, and so Chanel No. 5 was launched—a scent that was literally to revolutionize the perfumery world. He had created a new branch of the floral family, a floral with a clear, sharp chemical statement of elegance which gave inspiration to other modern perfumes—from Lanvin's Arpège to Madame Rochas in 1960, Calèche, by Hermès, in 1961, and many more.

The floral aldehydes have a kind of stamp of acceptability about them. They are cool and elegant, and the woman who wears them wants to project that kind of image: collected, in control, yet richly feminine and warm. The simple florals are pure fantasy and charming and each has its own nature and personality. They are never heavy, always womanly, can be worn anywhere at any time and are the hallmark of women who like the idea of being feminine and have no wish to hide it. Some of the more important florals include Estée Lauder's Estée, Halston, Chloé, and Chanel No. 22.

The Dark, Mysterious Chypres

These scents, which make up the second-most-important family of perfumes, have tremendous tenacity and are said to have originated in Cyprus centuries ago from "eau de Chypre," although that particular chypre differs tremendously from the modern chypres and hybrids. Chypres have rich, mossy undertones that are reminiscent of dark green woods after rain, luxurious ferns, and luscious fruits. Women who prefer scents in the chypre family and wear them often are attracted to their warm, sensuous aura, which lasts for hours. The chypres are subtle and seem continuously to unfold their secret loveliness as you wear them.

The chypre family is a large one, with many branches: The two most important are the fruity scents, which include those chypres with green and citrus overtones and the leathery chypres, which often also contain either patchouli or vetiver.

The common denominator of both branches is the unmistakable mousse de chêne, or oak moss. Fruity chypres tend to be delicate yet full-bodied. Perhaps the best example is Guerlain's haunting Mitsouko, which has inspired many others in the same family, from Femme de Rochas to the more recent Azzaro. Some fruity chypres such as Miss Dior, Revlon's Intimate, and Givenchy III have aldehydic green tinges to sharpen their warmth; others, such as Diorella and Chanel's Cristalle boast pure green overtones. Matchabelli's Cachet is a chypre made even richer by the addition of amber, and recently three lovely chypres with floral tinges have appeared: Dior Dior, Tamango, and If, by Lenthéric.

The leathery chypres are the warmest of all and the most long-lasting. The tone for leathers was set back in 1944 with the appearance of Piguet's striking Bandit, which for the first time used a leatherlike chemical to help form the main character of a scent. Jolie Madame followed the theme in the fifties, and the elegant Cabochard appeared in 1960. Since then it has influenced many successful perfumes, from Estée Lauder's Azurée to Courrèges Empreinte, as well as the men's fragrances Aramis and Revlon's Braggi.

The Bold Greens: A Bid for Freedom

Sharper and clearer in character than the chypres, the green scents seem to get more and more popular every year. Their notes are reminiscent of nature's foliage as well but this time of leaves and stems and cut grasses, often blended with budding hyacinth or jonquil. Many of the "lifestyle" fragrances of the seventies, such as Revlon's Charlie, have incorporated a green note as a variation on their own family themes. Others, such as Lauder's Aliage and her Private Collection, use green notes as their main theme. These scents appeal to the woman who prizes independence and freedom, who likes to think of herself as moving swiftly and thinking clearly. The greens are dynamic, clear, never cloying, as some of the heavier perfumes can be. They are also particularly popular with men, who are attracted by their fresh-air quality.

Balmain's Vent Vert was the first composition to carry this accentuated green-foliage note. When it first appeared, in 1945, it was considered very bold. It had a following, but it didn't become the trend setter that some of its contemporaries, such as Miss Dior, Bandit, and L'Air du Temps did. At least not until Pucci launched Vivara, a spicy, flowery variation on the theme, some twenty years later, in the sixties. Then, in 1971, Weil de Weil, the green floral aldehyde composition, appeared, to be followed by the richer and more tenacious, as well as more successful, Aliage, in 1972. Soon after, Estée Lauder launched her Private Collection. It was a bolder interpretation of the green theme, with a wider variety of green chemicals in its makeup, combined with tenacious musks.

The Sultry Orientals

Women who wear them like to be seen and heard. These perfumes are strong, full-bodied, often overtly seductive fragrances, which many women choose to wear only in the evening. They are based mostly on nature's raw materials, including many culinary components such as cloves, cardamom, coriander, and ginger, which accord with oils of lemon and orange, patchouli, olibanum (frankincense), myrrh, and many balsamic resins, which, like the oak moss of the chypres, give these perfumes exceptional tenacity. Many also incorporate herbaceous oils, lavender, and rosemary for breadth and body.

Of the oriental family, the semiorientals such as Youth Dew, by Lauder, and Yves Saint Laurent's Opium are lighter variations on the same theme. Other true orientals include the more aldehydic Shocking, by Schiaparelli, and Dana's Tabu, with its animal tones.

Many women find the semiorientals the most beautiful of all scents, because they seem to be a kind of bridge between the florals and the sultry orientals. Youth Dew sets the tone of this branch and has inspired many others, such as Germaine Monteil's Royal Secret and Revlon's lovely Ultima, as well as Saint Laurent's Opium and Lauder's Cinnabar. One of the most beautiful of all the florals, Guerlain's Chamade, which appeared in 1969, is closely related to this semioriental group, although it properly belongs to the floral family.

Just as there are families of scent, so there are trends in scent that have closely followed social changes and new fashions in the past seventy years. Each decade appears to have its own particular character and qualities. New chemicals in the future mean we will probably have new branches and even new families. But fine scents from any decade will never grow old. And the same floral, chypre, green, and oriental themes will be around to haunt and delight us as long as there are fine perfumers to create new scents, and noses to appreciate their artistry.

THE WORLD OF PERFUME NOW

By the seventies, fragrances had invaded every area of our lives, from the smell on the paper tissue or kitchen towel to the myriad of perfumes we can choose from for bath products, shampoos, colognes, laundry detergents, and fine scents at almost any price. Now we are also witnessing the development of new psycho-scents—essential oils used for their effect on mind and body, and carefully chosen incense that smells the way it does to clear the mind for meditation or to soften the edges of reality more gently than the mind-bending drugs of the sixties did. Whether we are aware of it or not, we live in a world of scent that affects us on almost every level of response.

Fine perfumes used to be the province of the French. If someone wanted a good perfume, he went to France to have it made. It had to have a French name and French quality, and the advertising used to promote it showed a particularly French flavor. Then the Americans got in on the act. They began to use advancing technology to produce good new scents (sometimes at remarkably low prices) that hit you between the eyes. What they lacked in subtlety they made up for in overt sexiness and power.

Following Estée Lauder's lead with the successful Youth Dew which appeared way back in 1952, a great gamut of strong, unmistakable "American" fragrances appeared, from the phenomenally successful Charlie to Lauder's Private Collection. These newer scents had some important things in common: They were stronger and more tenacious than any before; they were usually associated with a particular image or lifestyle (remember Babe, Blasé, Smitty, Jontue, and so on); and many of them were "super perfumes"—made so by increasing the levels of aromatics and by adding an emollient to the alcohol. This helped control the evaporation rate of the perfume on the skin. It also gave the perfume an oily, velvety texture when it was spread on the skin. Thanks to clever advertising, this new silky feeling of perfume became associated in the consumer's mind with tenacity and quality—so much so that many women now believe, quite wrongly, that if a perfume doesn't have this velvety feel it is not really good quality and won't last.

But the trend was set and it has remained. Even the finest French scents that have appeared in the past few years bow to American technology and style.

FORGET THE TRENDS

Trends in scent are all very well, but no woman selecting scent for herself should give too much consideration to them. When choosing a scent, remember that it should be an extension of your own personality. Select it as you would a piece of music to complement how you feel or what you want to do while wearing it. Here are a few basic guidelines for choosing.

1. Go shopping alone; friends can influence you wrongly either by telling you what you want to hear or by giving an opinion about what they like for themselves. Your scent is the most personal of all your purchases.

2. Shop for scent only when you are in a good mood. One's judgment about the subtleties of fragrances can be severely clouded by fatigue or by being in a bad mood.

3. Don't wear scent when you are going to buy some. It will only distort your judgment.

4. Give yourself enough time. Choosing scent is not something to sandwich between buying bedspreads and meeting friends for lunch.

5. Ask for help from the expert behind the counter. She knows her products—or she *should*. Tell her about your lifestyle. For instance, if you're an active sportswoman or a busy mother with small children, you may not want a heady, sensual fragrance.

6. Get to know the families of scent; go to perfume counters and sample various fragrances from each with no intention of buying. Give yourself a chance to just get the *feel* of the types of scent and the individual perfumes. How does each make you feel? What does it make you think of? Is it a feeling you would like to have more often?

7. When testing scent, put it directly on your wrist and then wait a few moments before smelling it so that the alcohol has evaporated, or you will not get the true odor of it. Some scents such as Aromatics, by Clinique, can seem unremarkable or even unpleasant when first smelled, but after you have been wearing them for half an hour or so their fullness and beauty emerge. Others such as Nina Ricci's Farouche are wonderful when you first smell them but quickly seem to fade, since their middle and base notes are not good enough to support the lovely

first impression. So when getting to know a scent give it time on your skin. Never be in a hurry to buy.

8. Limit yourself to testing six scents at a time, no more. The nose becomes fatigued and is no longer discerning after that.

9. If you are a "one-scent woman," you might try some of the other products scented with the same fragrance—a cologne, sachets, or bath powder, for instance. But consider, too, that many women like you have eventually found it is better and more fun to use various scents for various occasions: a crisp, sharp green for outdoor sport, a light floral for day wear, a rich sensual oriental for evening. Don't be afraid to experiment. When you find a scent you like, buy it rather than the cologne or toilet water—it is stronger, more concentrated; it will last longer and give the richest representation of its particular personality. The cologne or toilet water can come later.

Epilogue

Perfumes, exercise, nutrition, aromatherapy, meditation, and hair care—
how do you make use of it all? By doing everything at once? By putting
yourself on some new regimen and spending every waking hour concerned with whether you are taking the right vitamins and just how
stressed (or unstressed!) you feel? Certainly that would be a mistake,
although it is a mistake a lot of women make. There is little more boring
than sitting across the table from such a person while he or she lectures
you about the food you eat and what kind of life you should be living.
This is a person who has become so obsessed with exercise or weight
watching or personal appearance that he or she has lost touch with what
being beautiful is all about. For these things—the exercises, the wholesome foods, the face creams and body lotions—are not ends in themselves.
They are simply tools for you to use if and when you need them. And,
like all tools, they are not very interesting on their own.

Michelangelo insisted that he never set out with an image that he was
going to carve into a piece of marble. Instead, he used his tools to chisel
away the inessential parts of a block to reveal the beautiful form hidden
within the stone. That is just the way the tools in *The Joy of Beauty* are
meant to be used. Pick one up here when you need it—a meditation
technique or the raw food diet—use it to center yourself so you feel
stronger and clearer about who you are and what you want. If it works
for you, hang on to it and integrate it gradually into your lifestyle so
that it becomes not something external, which you are imposing on yourself with self-righteous vigor, but an integral part of day-to-day living
and enjoyment. Meanwhile, it and whatever other useful tools you've
picked up along the way (such as particular ways of treating your skin
or hair, or an exercise program) will gradually shape themselves into a
transformed (and transforming!) new lifestyle that will help gradually
clear away the inessential and reveal the beauty you have been hiding

beneath the "stone" of excess fat, long-term tension, physical neglect, inappropriate makeup, or any number of other things which obscure the essential form beneath.

I have always found the biblical expression "Become what thou art" full of meaning. And becoming beautiful is like that. But it is not a static state of perfection, as the glossy magazines would have us believe—one fleeting moment on a well-made-up, well-lit face, captured for eternity by the camera. It is a living process, an unfolding of your uniqueness no matter what your age or where you start from—a kind of journey which, for me, is one of the two most exciting things in life. The other, I believe, is creativity itself, whether it is expressed in painting a picture, cooking a meal, running a business, loving a man, or caring for a child. And the wonderful thing about the whole process of becoming more beautiful— becoming what you really are—is that it inevitably leads to greater creativity and satisfaction in what you do. What could be more re- warding?

Bibliography

Book One: The Foundation

The Self

Assagioli, R. *Psychosynthesis*. New York: Viking, 1965.

Beecher, H. K. "The Powerful Placebo," *Journal of the American Medical Association*, Vol. 159 (1955), pp. 1602–6.

Bugental, J.F.T., ed. *Challenges of Humanistic Psychology*. New York: McGraw-Hill, 1967.

Cannon, W. *The Wisdom of the Body*. New York: Norton, 1942.

Dunbar, F. *Emotions and Bodily Changes*. New York: Columbia University Press, 1954.

Dunn, H. L. *High Level Wellness*. Boston: Mount Vernon Press, 1961.

Howard, B. *Dance of the Self*. New York: Simon & Schuster, 1974.

Huxley, L. *Between Heaven and Earth*. London: Chatto & Windus, 1975.

Jourard, S. *The Transparent Self*. Princeton, N.J.: Van Nostrand, 1964.

Jourard, S. M. *Disclosing Man to Himself*. Princeton, N.J.: Van Nostrand, 1968.

LeShan, L. *The Medium, the Mystic, and the Physicist*. New York: Viking, 1974.

Lewis, H. R. and M. E. *Psychosomatics*. New York: Viking, 1972.

Lewis, H. R., and Streitfield, H. S. *Growth Games*. London: Souvenir Press, 1970.

Lowen, A. *The Language of the Body*. New York: Collier, 1971.

Maslow, A. *Farther Reaches of Human Nature*. New York: Viking, 1971.

———. *Toward a Psychology of Being*. New York: Van Nostrand, 1968.

Miller, J. B. *Toward a New Psychology of Women*. London: Allen Lane, 1978.

Otto, H. A. *Guide to Developing Your Potential*. New York: Scribner, 1967.

Oyle, I. *Time Space and the Mind*. Milbrae, Cal.: Celestial Arts, 1976.

Pearce, J. C. *The Crack in the Cosmic Egg*. New York: Julian, 1971.

Pelletier, K. R. *Towards a Science of Consciousness*. New York: Delacorte Press, 1978.

——. *Holistic Medicine.* New York: Delacorte Press, 1979.

Penfield, W. *The Mystery of the Mind.* Princeton, N.J.: Princeton University Press, 1972.

Phillips, A., and Rakusen, J., eds. *Our Bodies, Ourselves.* London: Penguin Books, 1978.

Reich, W. *Selected Writings.* London: Vision Press, 1960.

Rush, A. K. *Getting Clear.* London: Wildwood House, 1974.

Rogers, C. R. *On Becoming a Person.* London: Constable, 1977.

Salk, J. *Man Unfolding.* New York: Harper & Row, 1972.

Shuttle, P., and Redgrove, P. *The Wise Wound.* London: Victor Gollancz, 1978.

Simonton, O. C., and Matthews-Simonton, S. "Belief Systems and Management of the Emotional Aspects of Malignancy," *Journal of Transpersonal Psychology,* Vol. 7 (1975), pp. 29–47.

Smith. M. *When I Say No, I Feel Guilty.* New York: Bantam, 1975.

Tart, C. T. *Altered States of Consciousness.* New York: Wiley, 1969.

Weinberg, G. *Self Creation.* London: Macdonald & Janes, 1978.

Fuel for Health and Beauty

Agradi, E., et al. "Diet, Lipids, and Lippoproteins in Patients with Peripheral Vascular Disease," *American Journal of the Medical Sciences,* Vol. 268 (1974), pp. 325–32.

Altschule, M. D. "Is It True What They Say About Cholesterol?" *Executive Health,* August 1976.

Anderson, T. W. "Magnesium, Soft Water, and Heart Disease," Second International Symposium on Magnesium, Montreal, 1976.

Andrews, Sheila. *The No-cooking Fruitarian Recipe Book.* Wellingborough, England: Thorsons, 1975.

Ashley, R., & Duggal, H. *Dictionary of Nutrition.* New York: St. Martin's Press, 1975.

Beedell, S. *Herbs for Health and Beauty.* London: Sphere, 1972.

Bircher, Max E., and Bircher-Benner, M. *Fruit Dishes and Raw Vegetables.* London: C. W. Daniel, 1974.

Bircher-Benner, M., and Bircher, Max E. *The Bircher-Benner Raw Fruits and Vegetable Book.* New Canaan: Keats Publishing, 1977.

Charmine, Susan E. *The Complete Raw Juice Therapy.* Wellingborough, England: Thorsons, 1977.

Cheraskin, E., Ringsdorf, W. M., and Brecher, A. *Psychodietetics.* New York: Bantam, 1976.

Courtier, G. *The Beansprout Book.* New York: Simon & Schuster, 1973.

Crawford, Michael and Sheilagh. *What We Eat Today.* London: Neville Spearman, 1972.

Cott, Allan. *Fasting As a Way of Life.* London: Bantam, 1977.

Davis, Adelle. *Let's Get Well.* London: Unwin, 1979.

——. *Let's Eat Right to Keep Fit.* London: Unwin Paperbacks, 1979.

De Vries, Arnold. *Therapeutic Fasting.* Los Angeles: Chandler, 1963.

Donsbach, Kurt W. *Nutritional Approach to Superhealth.* Huntington Beach, Cal.: International Institute of Natural Health Sciences, Inc., 1980.

Ehret, Arnold. *Rational Fasting.* New York: Benedict Lust Publications, 1971.

Fernstrom, J. D., and Wurtman, R. J. "Nutrition and the Brain," *Scientific American*, February 1974, pp. 84–91.

"Food and Fibre." A symposium held at Marabou, Sundbyberg, Sweden, September 4, 1976.

Greden, J. F. "The Caffeine Crazies," *Human Behavior*, April 1975.

Hardinge, M. G., and Stare, F. J. "Nutritional Studies of Vegetarians: Nutritional, Physical and Laboratory Findings," *American Journal of Clinical Nutrition*, Vol. 2 (1954), p. 73.

Hoffer, Abram, and Walker, Morton. *Orthomolecular Nutrition*. New Canaan, Conn.: Keats Publishing, 1978.

Hovannessian, A. T. *Raw Eating*. Tehran: Aterhov, 1967.

Hunt, Janet. *The Raw Food Way to Health*. Wellingborough, England: Thorsons, 1978.

Hunter, B. T. *Yogurt Kefir and Other Milk Cultures*. New Canaan, Conn.: Keats Publishing, 1973.

Jensen, Bernard. *Health Magic Through Chlorophyll from Living Plant Life*. Provo, Utah: Provo BiWorld Publishers Inc., 1973.

Kirschmann, John D., ed. *Nutrition Almanac*. New York: McGraw-Hill, 1979.

Kolata, G. B. "Brain Biochemistry: Effects of Diet," *Science*, April 2, 1976, pp. 41–42.

Kunz-Bircher, Ruth. *The Bircher-Benner Health Guide*. London: George Allen & Unwin, 1981.

Lappe, F. M. *Diet for a Small Planet*, rev. ed. New York: Ballantine Books, 1975.

Leonard, J. N., Hover, J. L., and Pritikin, N. *Live Longer Now*. New York: Grosset & Dunlap, 1976.

Longgood, W. *The Poisons in Your Food*. New York: Simon & Schuster, 1960.

Lust, John. *Drink Your Troubles Away*. New York: Benedict Lust Publications, 1976.

McGovern, G. *Dietary Goals for the United States*. A report of the Select Committee on Nutrition and Human Needs, U. S. Senate, Washington, D.C. GPO Stock No. 052-070-04376-8, February 1977, and the Second Edition of the above document in expanded form, Stock No. 052-070-04376-8, December 1977.

Passwater, Richard A. *Supernutrition*. New York: Dial, 1977.

Pfeiffer, Carl C. *Mental and Elemental Nutrients*. New Canaan, Conn.: Keats Publishing, 1975.

———. *Zinc and the Micronutrients*. New Canaan: Keats Publishing, 1978.

Prevention Magazine, ed. *Vitamin A, Everyone's Basic Bodyguard*. Emmaus, Pa.: Rodale Press, 1973.

Roberts, Sam E. *Exhaustion, Causes and Treatment*. Emmaus, Pa.: Rodale Press, 1977.

Rodale, J. I. *The Complete Book of Vitamins*. Emmaus, Pa.: Rodale Press, 1977.

Schwartz, George. *Food Power*. New York: McGraw-Hill, 1979.

Scientific American. *Human Nutrition*. San Francisco: W. H. Freeman, 1978.

Shears, Curtis C. *Nutritional Science and Health Education*. Berkeley, Cal.: Castle Press, 1974.

Shelton, Herbert M. *The Science and Fine Art of Fasting*. Chicago: Natural Hygiene Press, 1978.

Simons, P. *Lecithin—The Fat Fighter*. Wellingborough, England: Thorsons, 1977.

——. *Garlic*. Wellingborough, England: Thorsons, 1980.

Szekely, Edmond Bordeaux. *Guide to the Essene Way of Biogenic Living*. Cartago, Costa Rica: International Biogenic Society, 1977.

Tudge, Colin. *Future Cook*. London: Mitchell Beazley, 1980.

Volen, M., and Bresler, D. *A Guide to Good Nutrition*. Los Angeles: Center for Integral Medicine, 1979.

Walker, N. W. *Become Younger*. Phoenix, Ariz.: Norwalk Press, 1949.

Watson, George. *Nutrition and Your Mind*. New York: Harper & Row, 1972.

Williams, Roger J. *Nutrition in a Nutshell*. Garden City, N.Y.: Dolphin Books/Doubleday & Co., 1962.

——. *Nutrition Against Disease*. New York: Bantam, 1973.

——. *You Are Extraordinary*. New York: Pyramid, 1974.

——. *Physicians Handbook of Nutritional Science*. Springfield, Ill.: Charles C. Thomas, 1978.

——. ed. *A Physician's Handbook on Orthomolecular Medicine*. New Canaan: Keats Publishing, 1979.

Wilson, F. *Successful Sprouting*. Wellingborough, England: Thorsons, 1978.

Zorn, J. *Seaweed and Vitality*. New York: Popular Library, 1974.

Movement

Astrand, P. O., and Rodahl, K. *Textbook of Work Physiology*. New York: McGraw-Hill, 1970.

Astrand, P. O. *Health and Fitness*. Canada: Minister of Health and Welfare, 1979.

Balaskas, A. *Bodylife*. London: Sedgwick & Jackson, 1977.

Barlow, W. *The Alexander Principle*. London: Hutchinson, 1979.

Brannin, M. *Your Body in Mind*. London: Souvenir Press, 1981.

Carruthers, M. and Murray, A. *F/40—Fitness on Forty Minutes a Week*. London: Futura, 1976.

Craig, M. *Miss Craig's 21 Day Shape-up Program for Men and Women*. New York: Random House, 1970.

Cooper, K. H. *The New Aerobics*. New York: Bantam, 1979.

Cooper, K. H., and Cooper, M. *Aerobics for Women*. New York: Bantam, 1976.

Fixx, J. F. *The Complete Book of Running*, rev. ed. London: Chatto & Windus, 1979.

Gallwey, W. T. *The Inner Game of Tennis*. London: Jonathan Cape, 1975.

Glasser, W. *Positive Addiction*. New York: Harper & Row, 1976.

Hessel, S. *The Articulate Body*. New York: St. Martin's Press, 1978.

Higdon, H. "Can Running Cure Mental Illness?" *Runners World*, 1978, pp. 36–43.

——. "Running and the Mind," *Runners World*, 1978, pp. 36–48.

Jones, F. P. *Body Awareness in Action*. New York: Shocken Books, 1977.

Leonard, G. *The Ultimate Athlete*. New York: Avon Books, 1977.

Mensendeick. B. M. *Look Better, Feel Better*. London: Souvenir Press, 1976.

Mirkin, G. and Hoffman, M. *The Sportsmedicine Book*. Boston: Little, Brown & Co., 1978.

Morehouse, L. E., and Gross, L. *Total Fitness in 30 Minutes a Week*. London: Hart-Davis, MacGibbon, 1976.

Murphy, M. *Beyond Jogging*. Milbrae, Cal.: Celestial Arts, 1976.

Murphy, M., and White, R. *The Psychic Side of Sports*. Reading, Mass.: Addison-Wesley, 1978.

Noble, E. *Essential Exercises for the Childbearing Year*. London: John Murray, 1978.

Runners World. *The Complete Runner*. New York: Avon Books, 1978.

Spino, M., and Warren, J. *Mike Spino's Mind-Body Running Program*. New York: Bantam, 1979.

Stillness

Akishige, Y., ed. *Psychological Studies on Zen*. Tokyo: Zen Institute of Komazawa University, 1970.

Benson, H. *The Relaxation Response*. New York: Morrow, 1975.

Benson, H., Rosner, B. A., and Marzetta, B. R. "Decreased Systolic Blood Pressure in Hypertensive Subjects Who Practice Meditation," *Journal of Clinical Investigation*, Vol. 52 (1973).

Bloomfield, H. H., Caim, W., and Jaffe, R. *TM: Discovering Inner Energy and Overcoming Stress*. New York: Delacorte Press, 1975.

Brown, B. B. *Stress and the Art of Biofeedback*. New York: Harper & Row, 1977.

Friedman, M., Rosenman, R. H. *Type a Behavior and Your Heart*. New York: Knopf, 1974.

Govinda, L. A. *Creative Meditation and Multi-dimensional Consciousness*. Wheaton, Ill.: Theosophical Publishing House, 1976.

Hewitt, J. *Meditation*. London: Hodder & Stoughton, 1978.

Hittleman, R. *Richard Hittleman's 30 Day Yoga Plan*. London: Corgi, 1978.

Iyengar, B.K.S. *Light on Pranayama*. London: George Allen & Unwin, 1981.

Jacobson, E. *You Must Relax*. New York: McGraw-Hill, 1962.

——. *Progressive Relaxation*. Chicago: University of Chicago Press, 1938.

Keers, W., Lewensztain, J., and Malavika, K. *Yoga Art of Relaxation*. London: Watkins, 1979.

LeShan, L. *How to Meditate*. New York: Bantam, 1974.

Luthe, W. *Autogenic Training*. New York: Grune & Stratton, 1965.

——. *Creativity Mobilization Techniques*. New York: Grune & Stratton, 1976.

Madders, J. *Stress and Relaxation*. London: Martin Dunitz, 1979.

Martin, I.C.A. *The Art and Practice of Relaxation*. London: Hodder & Stoughton, 1977.

Mason, L. J. *Guide to Stress Reduction*. Culver City, Cal.: Peace Press, 1980.

Naranjo, C., and Ornstein, R. E. *On the Psychology of Meditation*. New York: Viking, 1971.

Oswald, I. *Sleep*. London: Penguin Books, 1970.

Pelletier, K. R. *Mind As Healer, Mind As Slayer*. New York: Delacorte Press/Seymour Lawrence, 1977.

Schwartz, A. K., and Aaron, N. S. *Somniquest*. London: Wildwood House, 1980.

Selye, H. *Stress Without Distress*. New York: Dutton, 1974.

————. *The Stress of Life*. New York: McGraw-Hill, 1976.

Smith, M. *Kicking the Fear Habit*. London: Bantam, 1978.

Trungpa, C. *Meditation in Action*. Berkeley, Cal.: Shambhala, 1969.

————. *Cutting Through Spiritual Materialism*. Berkeley, Cal.: Shambhala, 1973.

Book Two: Maintenance

The Body

Aron-Brunetiere, R. *Beauty and Medicine*. London: Jonathan Cape, 1978.

Ayalah, D., and Weinstock, I. *Breasts*. London: Hutchinson, 1979.

Birkinshaw, E. *Think Slim—Be Slim*. Santa Barbara, Cal.: Woodbridge Press, 1976.

Bricklin, M. *Lose Weight Naturally*. Emmaus, Pa.: Rodale Press, 1979.

Bruno, F. J. *Think Yourself Thin*. New York: Barnes & Noble, 1972.

Burton, R. *The Language of Smell*. London: Routledge & Kegan Paul, 1976.

Castleton, V. *The Handbook of Herbal Beauty*. Emmaus, Pa.: Rodale Press, 1975.

Downing, G. *The Massage Book*. New York: Random House/Bookworks, 1973.

Gerrard, D. *One Bowl*. New York: Random House/Bookworks, 1974.

Horrocks, L. *Natural Beauty*. London: Angus & Robertson, 1980.

Kloss, J. *Back To Eden*. Riverside, Cal.: Lifeline Books, 1973.

Kneipp, S. *My Water Cure*. Wellingborough, England: Thorsons, 1979.

Lautie, R., and Passebecq, A. *Aromatheraphy*. Wellingborough, England: Thorsons, 1979.

Ledermann, E. K. *Good Health Through Natural Therapy*. London: Kogan Page, 1976.

Little, K. *Kitty Little's Book of Herbal Beauty*. London: Jill Norman, 1980.

Maury, M. *The Secret of Life and Youth*. London: Macdonald, 1964.

Milan, A. R. *Breast Self-examination*. New York: Liberty/Workman, 1980.

Orbach, S. *Fat Is a Feminist Issue*. London: Paddington Press, 1978.

Poesnecker, G. E. *The Clymer Clinic—It's Only Natural*. Quakertown, Pa.: Adventures Ltd. Publication, 1975.

Powell, E. *Health from Earth, Air and Water*. Rustington, England: Health Science Press, 1970.

Reejhsinghani, A. *Be Your Own Beautician*. New Delhi: Orient Paperbacks, 1976.

Simnett, S. *Slimmers in Extremis*. Twickenham, England: Simnett Publications, 1981.

Stern, F. M., Hoch, R. S., and Carper, J. *Mind Trips to Help You Lose Weight*. Chicago: Playboy Press, 1976.

Stuart, R. B. *Act Thin, Stay Thin*. London: Granada, 1978.

Thomson, A., and Smith, E. *Healing Herbs*. London: BBC Publications, 1978.

Tisserand, R. *The Art of Aromatherapy*. London: C. W. Daniel, 1977.

Valnet, J. *Aromathérapie*. Paris: Librairie Maloine, 1974.

The Face

Abbot, D. *New Life for Old*. London: Frederick Muller, 1981.

Aron-Brunetiere, R. *Beauty and Medicine*. London: Jonathan Cape, 1978.

Bahr, R., Gerras, C., and Bingham, J. *The Natural Way to a Healthy Skin*. Emmaus, Pa.: Rodale Press, 1972.

Clark, L. *Face Improvement Through Exercise and Nutrition*. New Canaan, Conn.: Keats Publishing, 1973.

——. *Secrets of Health and Beauty*. New York: Pyramid, 1974.

——. *Rejuvenation*. Old Greenwich, Conn.: Devin-Adair, 1979.

Clements, H. *Skin Troubles*. Wellingborough, England: Thorsons, 1973.

Douglas, J. S. *Making Your Own Cosmetics*. London: Pelham Books, 1979.

Franklin, O. *H3*. London: Arthur Barker, 1964.

Halsell, G. *Los Viejos—Secrets of Long Life*. Emmaus, Pa.: Rodale Press, 1976.

Hayflick, L. "The Biology of Aging," *Natural History*, August–September 1977, pp. 22–25.

——. "On the Facts of Life: How Old Would You Be If You Didn't Know How Old You Were?" *Executive Health*, Vol. 14 (1978).

Kane, J. *How to Use Your Hands to Save Your Face*. New York: Avon Books, 1969.

Kartzman, J., and Gordon, P. *No More Dying: The Conquest of Aging and Extension of Human Life*. New York: Dell, 1977.

Kugler, H. J. *Slowing Down the Aging Process*. New York: Pyramid, 1974.

——. *Doctor Kugler's Seven Keys to a Longer Life*. New York: Fawcett Crest, 1978.

Lamb, L. *Get Ready for Immortality*. London: Hamish Hamilton, 1974.

Lamb, M. J. *Biology of Ageing*. Glasgow: Blackie, 1977.

Liggett, J. *The Human Face*. London: Constable, 1974.

Lindsay, R. *The Pursuit of Youth*. New York: Pinnacle Books, 1976.

Lubowe, I. *The Modern Guide to Skin Care and Beauty*. London: George Allen & Unwin, 1973.

Maxwell-Hudson, C. *Your Health and Beauty Book*. London: Macdonald & Janes, 1979.

——. *The Natural Beauty Book*. London: Macdonald & Janes, 1976.

Messegue, M. *Of Men and Plants*. London: Weidenfeld & Nicolson, 1972.

——. *Maurice Messegue's Way to Natural Health and Beauty*. London: George Allen & Unwin, 1976.

——. *Health Secrets of Plants and Herbs*. London: Collins, 1979.

Null, G. *Handbook of Skin and Hair*. New York: Pyramid, 1976.

——. *The Organic Beauty Book*. New York: Dell, 1973.

Rose, J. *Herbs and Things*. New York: Grosset & Dunlap, 1975.

——. *Herbal Body Book*. New York: Grosset & Dunlap, 1976.

Sperber, P. *Treatment of the Aging Skin and Dermal Defects*. Springfield, Ill.: Charles C. Thomas, 1965.

Winter, R. *Ageless Aging*. New York: Crown, 1973.

The Hair

deCourtais, G. *Women's Headdress and Hairstyles*. London: Batsford, 1973.

Galvin, D. *The World of Hair Colour*. London: Macmillan, 1977.

Kaszas, J. *Hair: Care for It and Keep It*. New York: Barnes & Noble, 1974.

Kingsley, P. *The Complete Hair Book*. London: Magnum, 1980.

Leighton, H. *Haircutting for Everyone*. London: Arthur Barker, 1977.

Lubowe, I. *New Hope for Your Hair*. New York: Belmont/Tower, 1970.

Michael, G., and Lindsay, R. *George Michael's Secrets for Beautiful Hair*. Garden City, N.Y.: Doubleday, 1981.

Savagee, J. *The Biodynamics of Hair Growth*. Brandford, England: Health Science Press, 1977.

Thomson, J. C., and Thomson, L. *Healthy Hair*. Wellingborough, England: Thorsons, 1967.

Zizmor, J., and Foreman, J. *Superhair*. New York: Berkley/Putnam, 1978.

The Fun of It All

Clark, F. *Vogue Guide to Make-up*. London: Penguin Books, 1981.

Daly, B. *Daly Beauty*. London: Macdonald, 1980.

Day, I. *Perfumery with Herbs*. London: Darton, Longman and Todd, 1979.

Hunter, C. *Positive Beauty*. London: Hutchinson, 1980.

Kennett, F. *History of Perfume*. London: Harrap, 1975.

Launert, E. *Scent and Scent Bottles*. London: Barrie & Jenkins, 1975.

Price, J., and Booth, P. *Making Faces*. London: Michael Joseph, 1980.

Sagan, F., and Hanoteau, G. *Il est des parfums* . . . Paris: Jean Dullis Editeur, 1973.

Sagarin, E. *The Science and Art of Perfumery*. London: McGraw-Hill, 1945.

Index